Multiple Sclerosis, Part I: Background and Conventional MRI

Guest Editor

MASSIMO FILIPPI, MD

NEUROIMAGING CLINICS OF NORTH AMERICA

www.neuroimaging.theclinics.com

Consulting Editor
SURESH K. MUKHERJI, MD

November 2008 • Volume 18 • Number 4

SAUNDERS an imprint of ELSEVIER, Inc.

W.B. SAUNDERS COMPANY
A Division of Elsevier Inc.

1600 John F. Kennedy Boulevard • Suite 1800 • Philadelphia, Pennsylvania 19103-2899

http://www.theclinics.com

NEUROIMAGING CLINICS OF NORTH AMERICA Volume 18, Number 4
November 2008 ISSN 1052-5149, ISBN 13: 978-1-4160-6321-6, ISBN 10: 1-4160-6321-8

Editor: Donald Mumford

Neuroimaging Clinics of North America (ISSN 1052-5149) is published quarterly by Elsevier Inc., 360 Park Avenue South, New York, NY 10010-1710. Months of issue are February, May, August, and November. Business and editorial offices: 1600 John F. Kennedy Blvd., Suite 1800, Philadelphia, PA 19103-2899. Business and editorial offices: 6277 Sea Harbor Drive, Orlando, FL 32887-4800. Periodicals postage paid at New York, NY, and additional mailing offices. Subscription prices are USD 264 per year for US individuals, USD 407 per year for US institutions, USD 135 per year for US students and residents, USD 305 per year for Canadian individuals, USD 510 per year for Canadian institutions, USD 388 per year for international individuals, USD 510 per year for international institutions and USD 194 per year for Canadian and foreign students and residents. To receive student/resident rate, orders must be accompanied by name of affiliated institution, date of term, and the *signature* of program/residency coordinator on institution letterhead. Orders will be billed at individual rate until proof of status is received. Foreign air speed delivery is included in all *Clinics* subscription prices. All prices are subject to change without notice. POSTMASTER: Send address changes to *Neuroimaging Clinics of North America*, Elsevier Periodicals Customer Service, 11830 Westline Industrial Drive, St. Louis, MO 63146. Customer Service (orders, claims, online, change of address): Elsevier Periodicals Customer Service, 11830 Westline Industrial Drive, St. Louis, MO 63146. Tel: 1-800-654-2452 (U.S. and Canada); 314-453-7041 (outside U.S. and Canada). Fax: 314-453-5170. E-mail: journalscustomerservice-usa@elsevier.com (for print support); journalsonlinesupport-usa@elsevier.com (for online support).

Reprints. For copies of 100 or more of articles in this publication, please contact the Commercial Reprints Department, Elsevier Inc., 360 Park Avenue South, New York, NY 10010-1710. Tel.: 212-633-3812; Fax: 212-462-1935; E-mail: reprints@elsevier.com.

Neuroimaging Clinics of North America is covered by *Excerpta Medical/EMBASE,* the RSNA Index of Imaging Literature, *MEDLINE/PubMed (Index Medicus),* MEDLINE/MEDLARS, SciSearch, Research Alert, and Neuroscience Citation Index.

Printed in the United States of America.

GOAL STATEMENT

The goal of *Neuroimaging Clinics of North America* is to keep practicing radiologists and radiology residents up to date with current clinical practice in radiology by providing timely articles reviewing the state of the art in patient care.

ACCREDITATION

The *Neuroimaging Clinics of North America* is planned and implemented in accordance with the Essential Areas and Policies of the Accreditation Council for Continuing Medical Education (ACCME) through the joint sponsorship of the University of Virginia School of Medicine and Elsevier. The University of Virginia School of Medicine is accredited by the ACCME to provide continuing medical education for physicians.

The University of Virginia School of Medicine designates this educational activity for a maximum of 60 *AMA PRA Category 1 Credits*™. Physicians should only claim credit commensurate with the extent of their participation in the activity.

The American Medical Association has determined that physicians not licensed in the US who participate in this CME activity are eligible for *AMA PRA Category 1 Credits*™.

Credit can be earned by reading the text material, taking the CME examination online at http://www.theclinics.com/home/cme, and completing the evaluation. After taking the test, you will be required to review any and all incorrect answers. Following completion of the test and evaluation, your credit will be awarded and you may print your certificate.

FACULTY DISCLOSURE/CONFLICT OF INTEREST

The University of Virginia School of Medicine, as an ACCME accredited provider, endorses and strives to comply with the Accreditation Council for Continuing Medical Education (ACCME) Standards of Commercial Support, Commonwealth of Virginia statutes, University of Virginia policies and procedures, and associated federal and private regulations and guidelines on the need for disclosure and monitoring of proprietary and financial interests that may affect the scientific integrity and balance of content delivered in continuing medical education activities under our auspices.

The University of Virginia School of Medicine requires that all CME activities accredited through this institution be developed independently and be scientifically rigorous, balanced and objective in the presentation/discussion of its content, theories and practices.

All authors/editors participating in an accredited CME activity are expected to disclose to the readers relevant financial relationships with commercial entities occurring within the past 12 months (such as grants or research support, employee, consultant, stock holder, member of speakers bureau, etc.). The University of Virginia School of Medicine will employ appropriate mechanisms to resolve potential conflicts of interest to maintain the standards of fair and balanced education to the reader. Questions about specific strategies can be directed to the Office of Continuing Medical Education, University of Virginia School of Medicine, Charlottesville, Virginia.

The faculty and staff of the University of Virginia Office of Continuing Medical Education have no financial affiliations to disclose.

The authors/editors listed below have identified no professional/financial affiliations for themselves or their spouse/partner:
Marco Battaglini, MSc; Christian Confavreux, MD; Nicola De Stefano, MD; Todd Eagar, PhD; Antonio Giorgio, MD; Nitin Karandikar, MD, PhD; Donald Mumford (Acquiring Editor); Stephen M. Smith, DPhil; and Sandra Vukusic, MD, PhD.

The authors listed below have identified the following professional/financial affiliations for themselves or their spouse/partner:
Robert A. Bermel, MD serves on the Speakers Bureau for Biogen-Idec and Teva Neurosciences.
Jeffrey A. Cohen, MD is a consultant for Biogen Idec, Eisai, Eli Lilly, and Genentech and is an industry funded research/investigator for Biogen Idec.
Massimo Filippi, MD (Guest Editor) is an industry funded research/investigator, is a consultant, and serves on the Speakers Bureau for TEVA Pharmaceutical Industries, Merck-Serono, Bayer-Schering, and Biogen Dompé.
Elizabeth Fisher, PhD is a consultant for Biogen Idec, Millennium Pharmaceuticals, and Wyeth, and is an industry funded research/investigator and serves on the Speakers Bureau for Biogen Idec.
Elliot M. Frohman, MD, PhD is a consultant and serves on the Advisory Board for Biogen Idec and TEVA and serves on the Advisory Board for Bayer.
Mark A. Horsfield, PhD is a consultant for Teva Pharmaceutical Industries, owns stock in Xinapse Systems Limited, and is an industry funded research/investigator for Schering AG.
B.K. Kleinschmidt-DeMasters, MD serves on the Speakers Bureau and is a consultant for Teva Neuroscience.
Hans Lassmann, MD serves on the Advisory Committee for Bayer and the Speakers Bureau for Novartis, Biogen/Idec, and Serono.
David K.B. Li, MD is the Director of a UBC MS/MRI Research Group contracted with Angiotech, Bayer, Berlex-Schering, Bio-MS, Centocor, Daiichi Sankyo, Hoffmann-LaRoche, Merck-Serono, Schering-Plough, Teva Neurosciences, Sanofi-Aventis, Transition Therapeutics.
Joseph C. McGowan, PhD, PE is employed by Exponent and is a consultant for Teva Neurosciences.
Nancy Monson, PhD serves on the Advisory Committee for Genentech.
Suresh K. Mukherji, MD (Consulting Editor) is a consultant for Bracco, Bayer, Philips, and Xoran Technologies.
Jack H. Simon, MD, PhD is a speaker for Serono and has received researching funding and is a consultant for Genentech.
Olaf Stüve, MD, PhD is a speaker and a consultant for Teva Neuroscience and EMD Serono, and is a consultant for Novartis, and Genentech.
Anthony Traboulsee, MD serves on the Speakers Bureau for EMD Serono and Teva Neurosciences.

Disclosure of Discussion of Non-FDA Approved Uses for Pharmaceutical and/or Medical Devices.

The University of Virginia School of Medicine, as an ACCME provider, requires that all faculty presenters identify and disclose any off-label uses for pharmaceutical and medical device products. The University of Virginia School of Medicine recommends that each physician fully review all the available data on new products or procedures prior to clinical use.

TO ENROLL

To enroll in the Neuroimaging Clinics of North America Continuing Medical Education program, call customer service at 1-800-654-2452 or sign up online at *http://www.theclinics.com/home/cme*. The CME program is available to subscribers for an additional annual fee of USD 175.

Neuroimaging Clinics of North America

THE CLINICS ARE NOW AVAILABLE ONLINE!

Access your subscription at:
www.theclinics.com

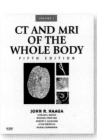 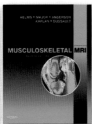 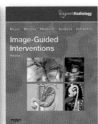 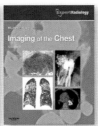 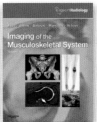
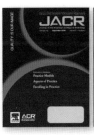 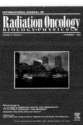 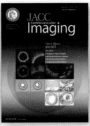 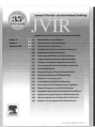 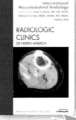 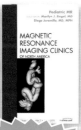
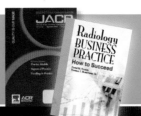

Contributors

CONSULTING EDITOR

SURESH K. MUKHERJI, MD
Professor and Chief of Neuroradiology and
Head and Neck Radiology; Professor of
Radiology, Otolaryngology Head Neck Surgery
and Radiation Oncology, University of
Michigan Health System, Ann Arbor, Michigan

GUEST EDITOR

MASSIMO FILIPPI, MD
Director, Neuroimaging Research Unit,
Department of Neurology, San Raffaele
Scientific Institute and University, Milan, Italy

AUTHORS

MARCO BATTAGLINI, MSc
Neurology and Neurometabolic Unit,
Department of Neurological and Behavioural
Sciences, University of Siena, Siena, Italy

ROBERT A. BERMEL, MD
Mellen Center for Multiple Sclerosis Treatment
and Research, Neurological Institute,
Cleveland Clinic Foundation, Cleveland, Ohio

JEFFREY A. COHEN, MD
Mellen Center for Multiple Sclerosis Treatment
and Research, Neurological Institute,
Cleveland Clinic Foundation, Cleveland, Ohio

CHRISTIAN CONFAVREUX, MD
Professor of Neurology; Head of Department,
Service de Neurologie A, Hôpital Neurologique
Pierre Wertheimer, Lyon-Bron cedex, France

NICOLA DE STEFANO, MD
Neurology and Neurometabolic Unit,
Department of Neurological and Behavioural
Sciences, University of Siena, Siena, Italy

TODD EAGAR, PhD
Assistant Professor, Departments of Neurology
and Immunology, University of Texas
Southwestern Medical Center at Dallas, Dallas,
Texas

ELIZABETH FISHER, PhD
Biomedical Engineering, Lerner Research
Institute, Cleveland Clinic Foundation,
Cleveland, Ohio

ELLIOT M. FROHMAN, MD, PhD
Professor of Neurology and Ophthalmology;
Director, MS Program; Irene Wadel and Robert
Atha Distinguished Chair of Neurology,
Departments of Neurology and Ophthalmology,
University of Texas Southwestern Medical
Center at Dallas, Dallas, Texas

ANTONIO GIORGIO, MD
Neurology and Neurometabolic Unit,
Department of Neurological and Behavioural
Sciences, University of Siena, Siena, Italy;
Oxford University Centre for Functional MRI of
the Brain (FMRIB), Department of Clinical
Neurology, University of Oxford, Oxford,
United Kingdom

MARK A. HORSFIELD, PhD
Medical Physics Section, Department of
Cardiovascular Sciences, University of
Leicester, Leicester Royal Infirmary, Leicester,
United Kingdom

NITIN KARANDIKAR, MD, PhD
Associate Professor, Departments
of Neurology, Immunology, and Pathology,
University of Texas Southwestern Medical
Center at Dallas, Dallas, Texas

B.K. KLEINSCHMIDT-DEMASTERS, MD
Professor, Departments of Pathology,
Neurology and Neurosurgery, University
of Colorado Health Sciences Center, Denver,
Colorado

HANS LASSMANN, MD
Professor, Center for Brain Research,
Medical University of Vienna, Spitalgasse,
Austria

DAVID K.B. LI, MD
Professor of Radiology, Department
of Radiology, University of British Columbia,
Vancouver, British Columbia, Canada

JOSEPH C. McGOWAN, PhD, PE
Visiting Research Associate Professor,
Drexel University, School of Biomedical
Engineering; Exponent, Inc., Philadelphia,
Pennsylvania

NANCY MONSON, PhD
Assistant Professor, Departments of Neurology
and Immunology, University of Texas
Southwestern Medical Center at Dallas, Dallas,
Texas

JACK H. SIMON, MD, PhD
Chief, Imaging, Portland VA Medical
Center; Professor, Departments of
Radiology and Neurology, Oregon Health
and Sciences University, Portland,
Oregon

STEPHEN M. SMITH, DPhil
Oxford University Centre for Functional MRI
of the Brain (FMRIB), Department of Clinical
Neurology, University of Oxford, Oxford,
United Kingdom

OLAF STUVE, MD, PhD
Assistant Professor, Departments of Neurology
and Immunology, University of Texas
Southwestern Medical Center at Dallas, Dallas,
Texas

ANTHONY TRABOULSEE, MD
Assistant Professor of Medicine, Department
of Medicine, Division of Neurology, University
of British Columbia, Vancouver, British
Columbia, Canada

SANDRA VUKUSIC, MD, PhD
Service de Neurologie A, Hôpital Neurologique
Pierre Wertheimer, Lyon-Bron cedex, France

Contents

Multiple sclerosis (MS) pathology is originally defined by the presence of focal white matter lesions, characterized by inflammation, primary demyelination, and reactive glial scaring. More recently, however, it became clear that focal white matter plaques in MS comprise of a broad spectrum of different lesion types, reflecting different stages of activity and different degrees of neurodegeneration or repair. In addition, the MS brain is affected by global changes in the normal-appearing white matter and gray matter. All types of changes in the MS brain and spinal cord occur on the background of inflammation; the type of inflammation, however, differs between different stages and forms of the disease.

Multiple sclerosis is widely recognized as the most commonly identified cause of progressive neurologic disability in young adults throughout the developed world. The disorder is clinically suspected when patients experience either acute attacks of neurologic compromise or instead are afflicted by a steadily progressive deterioration in functional capabilities. The pathophysiology of acute exacerbations is thought to be related to the development of inflammation and its consequences, within strategic and often discrete central nervous system tract systems. Although a myriad of hypotheses have been formulated to explain the underpinnings of the mechanisms that contribute to both the predilection and triggering of the multiphasic inflammatory events that personify multiple sclerosis, much remains to be done to understand fully the specific set and sequence of events that produce the disease and its cardinal features.

A comprehensive knowledge of the natural course and prognosis of multiple sclerosis is of utmost importance for a physician to make it affordable in simple descriptive terms to a patient when personal and medical decisions are to be taken. It is still topical because the currently acknowledged disease-modifying agents only marginally alter the overall prognosis of the disease. It provides reference for evaluating the efficacy of a therapeutic intervention in clinical trials; clues for public health services, health insurance companies, and pharmaceutical industry in their respective activities; and insights into the pathophysiology and the treatment of multiple sclerosis. Precise, consistent, and reliable data from appropriate cohorts have become available and knowledge is fairly comprehensive.

Magnetic resonance (MR) imaging has become the dominant clinical imaging modality with widespread, primarily noninvasive, applicability throughout the body and across many disease processes. The flexibility of MR imaging enables the development of purpose-built optimized applications. Concurrent developments in digital image processing, microprocessor power, storage, and computer-aided design have spurred and enabled further growth in capability. Although MR imaging may be viewed as "mature" in some respects, the field is rich with new proposals and applications that hold great promise for future research health care uses. This article delineates the basic principles of MR imaging and illuminates specific applications.

Computerized image analysis is becoming more routine in multiple sclerosis research. This article reviews the common types of task that are performed when producing quantitative measures of disease status, progression, or response to treatment. These tasks encompass uniformity (bias) correction, registration, segmentation, image algebra and fitting, diffusion tensor imaging and tractography, perfusion assessment, and three-dimensional visualization. The aim of these steps is to output reproducible, quantitative assessments of MR imaging scans that can be performed on data generated by the many different scanning sites that may be involved in multicenter studies.

Conventional MR imaging refers to techniques that are readily available and widely used in the diagnosis and monitoring of individuals with multiple sclerosis (MS). MR imaging is helpful in establishing an early diagnosis of MS after a single clinical event consistent with demyelination. A standardized imaging protocol is invaluable for diagnosis and monitoring disease evolution and response to treatment over time. The characteristic lesions of MS are varied and not always evident at the earliest stages of the disease. Furthermore, MR imaging is highly sensitive for detecting these lesions but remains pathologically nonspecific. Careful communication among clinicians and radiologists will optimize the interpretation of important abnormalities on MR imaging.

The use of MR imaging–derived methods to provide sensitive and reproducible assessments of brain volume (eg, to estimate atrophy) has increased the interest in this measure as a reliable indicator of disease progression in many neurologic disorders, including multiple sclerosis (MS). After an overview of the most commonly used methods for assessing brain atrophy state and changes in MS, this article discusses the clinical relevance of the most recent developments and reflects on its interpretation in a complex disease such as MS. Some caveats of these measurements are considered and possible future approaches discussed for improving the potential of this measure in assessing and monitoring pathologic evolution and treatment efficacy in this disease.

MR imaging is an integral part of multiple sclerosis (MS) clinical trials. It provides the primary efficacy outcome of preliminary proof-of-concept studies and important corroborating data as secondary and exploratory outcomes in pivotal trials. At all stages of drug development, MR imaging provides important information on the kinetics and magnitude of treatment effect and insight into potential mechanisms of action. Attention to issues in scan acquisition, quantitative image processing, and statistical analysis is critical to generate high-quality data. Although it is unlikely that one single outcome measure can capture all aspects of the MS disease process, there is potential for MR imaging outcomes to evaluate inflammatory and degenerative components within clinical trials.

The classic multiple sclerosis variants including Devic's neuromyelitis optica (NMO), Balo's concentric Sclerosis, Schilder's disease, and Marburg MS are both interesting and instructive from a disease pathophysiology perspective. Although rare, the variants are important as they often arise in the differential diagnosis for severe, acute demyelinating disease, including MS and acute disseminated encephalomyelitis. In the case of NMO, an originally unsuspected and entirely new pathophysiology based on water channels has been described, only after the recent original description of the more specific diagnostic test for NMO based on serum immunoglobulin.

Foreword

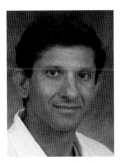

Suresh K. Mukherji, MD
Consulting Editor

We are very honored to have Dr. Massimo Filippi as our guest editor for this issue of *Neuroimaging Clinics of North America*. Dr. Fillipi is a recognized expert in multiple sclerosis (MS), and his numerous contributions are known throughout the world. He is Director of the Neuroimaging Research Unit in the Department of Neurology at the San Raffaele Scientific Institute and University in Milan, Italy. He also has academic affiliations at Temple University and the University of Belgrade.

Dr. Filippi's contribution to *Neuroimaging Clinics of North America* is unique and comprised of two separate issues. This two-part series is a dedicated translational treatise covering all aspects of MS. This work provides a comprehensive and state-of-the-art review of the technical, molecular, methodological, imaging, and clinical issues related to MS. Part I is entitled "Background and Conventional MRI." The first issue reviews the pathology, epidemiology, immunology, and clinical manifestations of MS. The information herein is necessary for understanding this complex disease and forms the foundation for subsequent chapters on the imaging findings.

The comprehensive and translational nature of this contribution will be beneficial to all individuals involved in ongoing research and the care of patients with MS. All of us in the scientific community sincerely thank Dr. Filippi, not only for this contribution to *Neuroimaging Clinics of North America*, but for his continuing efforts that permit us to better understand this complex disease. It is our hope that this issue will assist those dedicated individuals who have devoted their career to treating and potentially eradicating this disorder.

Suresh K. Mukherji, MD
Neuroradiology and Head and Neck Radiology
Radiology, Otolaryngology Head Neck Surgery
and Radiation Oncology
University of Michigan Health System
1500 E. Medical Center Drive
Ann Arbor, MI 48109-0030, USA

E-mail address:
mukherji@med.umich.edu (S.K. Mukherji)

Neuroimag Clin N Am 18 (2008) xiii
doi:10.1016/j.nic.2008.09.006
1052-5149/08/$ – see front matter

Preface

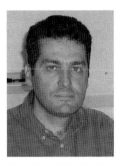

Massimo Filippi, MD
Guest Editor

Multiple sclerosis (MS), the major non-traumatic cause of permanent disability in young adults, is a heterogeneous condition that hits the central nervous system (CNS) haphazardly and repeatedly over time. The multifaceted nature of the disease is manifested pathologically and clinically. Indeed, various pathological features, ranging from edema to permanent loss of myelin and axons, have been demonstrated in focal macroscopic lesions and in the normal–appearing white matter (NAWM), where astrogliosis, microglial activation, increased permeability of the blood-brain barrier, demyelination, and axonal loss have all been shown to occur. In the gray matter (GM), less inflammatory changes are seen, but numerous lesions can be identified ex vivo, which may be associated to irreversible tissue injury. Clinically, MS heterogeneity is made evident not only by the existence of different disease phenotypes characterized by variable combinations of relapse-occurrence and disability accumulation, but also by differences in age of onset, gender prevalence, and rate of progression.

During the past two to three decades, due to its exquisite sensitivity towards MS-related damage, magnetic resonance imaging (MRI) has become an established tool not only to diagnose MS, but also to monitor its course—either natural or modified by treatment. The conventional MRI measures typically applied to monitor MS patients include assessment of T2-visible and gadolinium-enhancing lesions, which demonstrate the spatial and temporal dissemination of the disease earlier than on clinical ground alone. In patients with established MS, these MRI metrics are five to ten times more sensitive for detecting disease activity than the assessment of clinical relapses.

Additional conventional MRI metrics include the quantification of T1-hypointense lesions and brain atrophy, which are thought to reflect the more destructive aspects of MS pathology.

Overall, MRI is a useful diagnostic tool because it provides objective and reliable measures, allowing an accurate estimate of disease burden, and because it contributes significantly to exclude other WM affections that mimic MS clinically. Despite this, conventional MRI is only partially helpful in disentangling the heterogeneous features of MS pathology, both in focal lesions and in the normal–appearing tissues of the brain and spinal cord. This is perhaps the main reason why conventional MRI metrics are only weakly associated to patients' clinical status. As a consequence, a large effort has been devoted to the development and application of modern, quantitative MR techniques able to overcome such limitation, with the ultimate goal of improving our understanding of MS pathophysiology and the mechanisms responsible for the accumulation of irreversible disability.

This issue of *Neuroimaging Clinics of North America* (the first of two) aims at providing a complete and up-to-date overview of technical, methodological, and clinical issues related to the application of MRI in MS. In this issue, the main aspects of the disease (pathology, epidemiology, immunology, and clinical manifestations) are reviewed to provide the necessary background for the subsequent contributions in the second issue, all devoted to MRI aspects.

The first article herein describes the pathological features of MS lesions, as well as of the brain and spinal cord tissue outside focal WM plaques. The

Neuroimag Clin N Am 18 (2008) xv–xvi
doi:10.1016/j.nic.2008.09.001

neuroimaging.theclinics.com

pathological aspects of MS variants, including neuromyelitis optica and Balo's concentric sclerosis are also illustrated. The subsequent article discusses the major disease clinical phenotypes and their immunological patterns followed by a review of the epidemiology of the disease. The MRI articles follow, introduced by a technical background on the basic principles of MR physics, hardware components, and characteristics of the pulse sequences more commonly used to assess MS patients. A description of the tasks that are needed for an adequate postprocessing of MR images (ie, uniformity correction, registration, and segmentation) in order to obtain reliable quantitative measures is the topic of the next review. In this article, strategies for postprocessing nonconventional MRI techniques—such as magnetization transfer, diffusion tensor, and perfusion MRI—are also briefly illustrated. The last articles of this issue describe how conventional MRI is used to monitor disease evolution. A specific focus is devoted to the discussion of the clinical relevance of the assessment of brain atrophy, with an overview of the methods most commonly used for such an assessment, as well as a critical consideration of their possible caveats. Strategies for improving the potential of this measure in monitoring evolution and treatment efficacy in MS are also proposed. Given the growing use of MR-derived metrics as primary or secondary measures of outcome in clinical trials, an in-depth review of this important field of MRI application in MS is offered by assessing the role of standard MRI measures of disease activity (ie, gadolinium-enhancing lesions and new or enlarging T2 lesions)

and severity (T2 lesion volume, T1-hypointense lesions, brain atrophy). The potentialities, as exploratory trial end points, of measures derived from modern MR-based techniques, which have been applied in a few seminal studies, is considered as well. In addition, scan acquisition, quantitative image postprocessing, and statistical analysis (which are critical to generate high-quality trial data) are discussed critically. The final article presents the clinical and MRI features of the major variants of MS (neuromyelitis optica, Balo's concentric sclerosis, acute MS [Marburg type], Schilder's disease, and acute disseminated encephalomyelitis). The second issue of this two-part topic will review the most promising MRI approaches to the study of MS that have recently emerged or that are under development/refinement and which are likely to enter the clinical arena in the near future.

The hope is that the material presented here will be of help to clinicians and researchers in all cases when MRI might be successfully applied to the study of MS. This is, indeed, an ever-growing and exciting field of research in which much has been accomplished in the past few years, but there is still a long journey ahead of us.

Massimo Filippi, MD
Neuroimaging Research Unit
Department of Neurology
San Raffaele Scientific Institute and University
Via Olgettina, 60-20132, Milan, Italy

E-mail address:
filippi.massimo@hsr.it (M. Filippi)

The Pathologic Substrate of Magnetic Resonance Alterations in Multiple Sclerosis

Hans Lassmann, MD

KEYWORDS

- Multiple sclerosis • Pathology • Demyelination
- Remyelination • Neurodegeneration

Multiple sclerosis (MS) is defined as an inflammatory demyelinating disease of the central nervous system (CNS). Its pathologic hallmark is the presence of focal demyelinated plaques with reactive glial scaring in the white matter of the brain and spinal cord. Seminal studies, performed in the late nineteenth and early twentieth centuries have defined the key pathologic features of the disease.[1–4] The studies showed that demyelinated lesions develop around small veins and venules and occur on the background of an inflammatory reaction, mainly composed of lymphocytes and macrophages. Primary demyelination, as defined by selective destruction of myelin with preservation of axons, is the dominant structural alterations within MS plaques;[1] the process of demyelination is accompanied by reactive astrocytic scar formation. Axons are preserved within the lesions in relation to the complete myelin destruction, but this preservation is not absolute. In fact, axonal injury and loss are seen in all MS lesions; the degree, however, is highly variable.[3,5] In addition to these destructive aspects in MS lesions, there are also attempts of remyelination and repair. Signs of remyelination, defined by the appearance of newly formed thin myelin sheaths with widened nodes of Ravier can be seen quite frequently even in newly formed lesions.[3] In addition, shadow plaques, defined by a global appearance of thin myelin sheaths throughout the whole lesion,[6] suggest that whole MS lesions can be repaired by remyelination.

For more than one hundred years, this plaque-centered view was regarded sufficient to explain the pathology of MS. It allowed clinicians to distinguish MS from other inflammatory diseases of the CNS. The perspective, at least in part, explained the clinical deficits of the patients and it was generally believed that preventing the formation of new demyelinating lesions in the CNS should stop the disease process. During recent decades, however, this view was fundamentally challenged by clinical studies on the natural course of the disease[7,8] and on the response to disease modifying treatments.[9] Most importantly, recent observations, obtained in cross-sectional and longitudinal studies, on the development of brain changes seen by magnetic resonance (MR) imaging, suggest, that MS pathology is much more complicated than it was assumed before.[10–15] These observations, which were unpredicted by previous disease concepts, stimulated extensive research efforts to redefine MS pathology, in particular focusing on alterations, affecting the brain and spinal cord outside classical white matter plaques. From these investigations, it became clear that the CNS of MS patients is affected not only by white matter plaques but also by global changes in the gray matter and the normal-appearing white matter (NAWM). Furthermore, longitudinal MR imaging studies revealed dynamic changes within the classical MS plaques, for which the pathologic substrate had still to be elucidated.[16,17]

FOCAL WHITE MATTER LESIONS

Focal MS lesions can be present in any location of the CNS. However, since they arise around veins

Center for Brain Research, Medical University of Vienna, Spitalgasse 4, A-1090 Wien, Austria
E-mail address: hans.lassmann@meduniwien.ac.at

Neuroimag Clin N Am 18 (2008) 563–576
doi:10.1016/j.nic.2008.06.005

and venules,[2,4] areas of the CNS with high venular density are more frequently affected than others. Such predilection sites are the periventricular and the subcortical white matter of the forebrain, the optic nerves and chiasm, the cerebellar peduncles and the lateral columns of the spinal cord.[18]

MS plaques are sharply demarcated focal white matter lesions, characterized by primary demyelination, a variable extent of axonal injury and reactive astrocytic scar formation. Several different types of lesions can be distinguished.[19] Active lesions contain numerous inflammatory infiltrates, which are mainly composed of T- and B-lymphocytes, some plasma cells, and activated macrophages or microglia cells. Remnants of the myelin sheaths or of destroyed axons are contained within the lysosomes of macrophages; the molecular composition of the degradation products can be used to define stages of demyelinating activity within a given lesion.[20] In inactive lesions, inflammation is sparse. The cell density in the inactive lesions is low, due to the profound loss of oligodendrocytes. Demyelinated fibers are embedded in a glial scar, formed by densely packed fibrillary astrocytic cell processes. In remyelinated lesions or lesion areas, myelin sheaths are surrounded by unusually thin myelin sheaths, which frequently show widened nodes of Ranvier.[21] The cell density in remyelinated lesions, in general, is high and the number of oligodendrocytes may even exceed that seen in the surrounding NAWM. Fully remyelinated plaques are sharply demarcated areas with reduced myelin density, due to the homogeneously thin myelin sheaths throughout the plaque. Such lesions are called "shadow plaques."[6,21,22]

MR imaging, even when restricted to the analysis of conventional T2-weighted images, is very sensitive in regard to detecting focal white matter lesions. Indeed, early studies, correlating T2 images with pathology showed good agreement in the detection of white matter plaques. However, when postmortem MR imaging was performed and T2 lesion areas were specifically sampled for pathologic analysis, the situation became more complicated.[23,24] In the study by Barkhof and colleagues,[24] 161 T2 lesion areas were sampled. From those, 78% revealed focal white matter lesions. Based on the T2 signal, it was, however, not possible to distinguish demyelinated from partially or fully remyelinated lesions. Furthermore, 22% of the lesion areas which were identified by MR imaging showed no pathologic substrate and, in particular, no demyelination.

There are several possible explanations for this unexpected finding. First, it is possible that remyelination in MS lesions may become so complete that a reduction of myelin density due to the thinly remyelinated fibers is no longer visible. Currently, neuropathology does not offer a technique to unequivocally prove or disprove this scenario. Alternatively, these abnormal T2 areas shown in MR imaging may reflect a subtle pathology, which currently escapes neuropathological detection. One such subtle pathology may be focal areas of edema. A similar problem with the correlation between MR imaging and pathologic findings is also seen in leukoarayosis.

AXONAL INJURY AND WIDENING OF THE EXTRACELLULAR SPACE

Axonal destruction within the plaques is an important feature of MS pathology because axonal destruction appears to be the major substrate for permanent functional deficit.[25] The extent of axonal destruction is variable between different lesions within a given patient and between different patients; the variation ranges from 20% to more than 80%. Most pronounced acute axonal injury occurs during the active stage of the lesion.[26–28] In active lesions, an average reduction of axonal density by 30% may be seen, which is in part due to true axonal destruction, but also in part to inflammation and edema, which is pronounced during this stage. A partial normalization of axonal density values is generally seen, when lesions mature, due to the clearance of edema. Therefore, the average axonal loss in lesions in the late active stage is only between 10% and 20%. Similar values for axonal density are also seen in remyelinated shadow plaques. Within permanently demyelinated lesions, which are present in the late chronic stage of the disease, axonal loss is much more dramatic. In such lesions, axonal density is reduced on average by 60% to 70%.[25,29] These data indicate that, in MS lesions, two different patterns of axonal injury occur. Massive and synchronous axonal injuries occur during the active stage of the lesions, while there is a further accumulation of axonal loss in demyelinated plaques at late stages.[27] Whether this chronic loss of axons is due to repeated demyelination of remyelinated lesion areas or to a slow and continuous injury of chronically demyelinated axons is not yet clear. It should, however, be emphasized that active axonal injury in the acute stages, as well as in the late chronic stage, is invariably associated with inflammation and microglia activation.[26,27]

Demyelination and axonal loss within MS lesions are associated with a widening of the extracellular space, which in extremely destructive lesions may be reflected in cystic tissue necrosis. This widening of the extracellular space seems to have a correlate in the reduced density within lesions in T1-weigted scans.[30] In fact, quantitative MR imaging and pathology reveal that the extent of T1 signal reduction in part correlates with the degree of axonal loss in the lesions.[31] It has, however, to be emphasized that tissue loss and widening of the extracellular space is due to axonal and myelin loss as well as to edema. All three factors, therefore, may influence dynamic changes of T1 signal intensity during lesion evolution.

REMYELINATION

Although evidence for remyelination in MS lesions has been provided in the earliest neuropathological accounts of this disease,[3] it was believed for a long time, that repair of myelin is sparse or absent in white matter lesions of the CNS. However, systematic ultrastructural studies provided unequivocal evidence for myelin repair within the lesions.[21,32,33] Furthermore, these studies showed that remyelinated lesions may become affected by new demyelinating attacks.[34] Remyelination is seen in parts of the lesions or it may lead to complete restoration of myelin within the entire plaque. Recruitment of new oligodendrocytes

and formation of new thin myelin sheaths are frequent findings in most MS lesions in early stages of lesional activity.[35–37] This early stage of remyelination occurs on the background of massive macrophage infiltration within the lesions. Based on these findings, it was suggested that remyelination is extensive in the early stage of MS,[38] where classical active lesions are frequently seen, but that remyelination fails in the later progressive stage of the disease.

A systematic analysis of stable remyelination, which was seen in the form of shadow plaques or plaque areas, revealed a different picture.[39] Extensive remyelination is seen in a subset of patients, although other patients show very little myelin repair; (**Fig. 1**). In fact, MS patients can be separated into two distinct groups. In one group, extensive remyelination was seen in most lesions, with the exception of those that were still in the process of active demyelination. In others, remyelination was sparse and was restricted to small areas at the plaque margins. Contrary to previous views, the most extensive remyelination was seen in patients who were dying at very old ages and with long-standing disease.[39,40] These data indicate that remyelination is initiated in the early stages of lesion formation in many cases, but

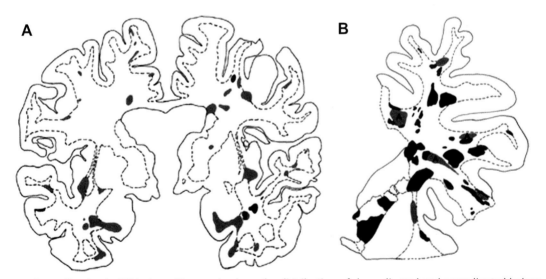

Fig. 1. Remyelination in MS lesions. The graphs show the distribution of demyelinated and remyelinated lesions in the brain of two MS patients. The demyelinated lesions are shown in red and the remyelinated lesions in blue. (*A*) Double hemispheric section of a brain from a patient with secondary progressive MS (with disease duration of 20 years). Most of the lesions are completely demyelinated (red). There are only few and small lesions, which are remyelinated "shadow plaques" (blue). (*B*) Hemispheric section of a patient with relapsing-remitting MS (with a disease duration of 13 years). The majority of the lesions are remyelinated "shadow plaques" (blue). The remaining demyelinated lesions (red) are in the active stage of demyelination. (*From* Patrikios P, Stadelmann C, Kutzelnigg A, et al. Remyelination is extensive in a subset of multiple sclerosis patients. Brain 2006;129:3165–72; with permission.)

this newly formed myelin may be instable and subject to subsequent demyelination. Only when the inflammatory disease process becomes inactive, remyelination may become stable and permanent. However, remyelination is extensive in some patients, but fails in others. The reason for these interindividual differences is so far unknown.

Although there is no specific MR imaging sequence that distinguishes remyelinated from demyelinated areas in MS brains, indirect information about remyelination can be obtained by assessing dynamic changes in T1-weighted scans[30] or in voxel-based analysis of magnetization transfer ratio (MTR) changes.[41] Using this technology, it was shown recently that, within a given patient, the dynamic changes within multiple lesions are strikingly similar and, in a subset of patients, lesions changed from hypointense to isointense on T1-weighted scans.[42] These data are consistent with neuropathological findings that suggest pronounced remyelination in a subpopulation of MS patients.

BLOOD BRAIN BARRIER DAMAGE AND INFLAMMATION

Assessing blood–brain barrier (BBB) damage in MS lesions through the leakage of gadolinium (Gd) became a very useful tool to determine the activity of the disease process in clinical diagnosis and therapeutic trials.[43–45] There is good agreement between studies showing that Gd-enhancement is a characteristic feature of newly forming lesions in the brain and spinal cord. Brain biopsies in early MS lesions have shown that Gd-enhancement is associated with inflammation.[46,47] Based on these observations, a common dogmatic view has been established that equates Gd-enhancement with inflammation in the MS brain. This view, however, is incorrect and misleading.

Neuropathological studies have provided ample evidence that the BBB is disturbed in MS not only in active lesions, but also in inactive plaques and in the NAWM.[48–52] There is, however, a difference in the degree of BBB disturbance, it being most pronounced in classical active plaques. Thus, the selective Gd-leakage in active MS lesions is due to the low sensitivity of this technique to detect changes in BBB alterations (**Fig. 2**).

Even more complicated is the relation between BBB disturbance and inflammation (**Fig. 3**).[53] In classical active MS plaques, massive BBB disturbance is seen and this is generally associated with intravascular and perivascular inflammatory infiltrates. However, in the vicinity of active lesions, numerous vessels are seen that show profound leakage of serum protein and evidence for leaky endothelial cells in the absence of inflammatory infiltrates. It is likely that, in such vessels, BBB function is disturbed by soluble inflammatory mediators that are liberated from inflammatory cells in the adjacent lesions. Despite this dissociation between inflammation and BBB damage in individual vessels, these data are still consistent with MR imaging observations, linking active lesions with Gd-enhancement.

The situation, however, is different in the late (progressive) stage of the disease where Gd-enhancing lesions are rare or absent.[15,44,54] However, there is pronounced inflammation within the brain tissue in such patients, which is reflected

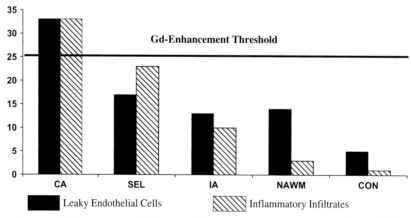

Fig. 2. Inflammation and BBB damage in MS lesions. This graph shows average numbers of inflammatory infiltrates and leaky cerebral endothelial cells, visualized by the expression of dysferlin[51] in different types of MS lesions. *Abbreviations*: CA, classical active lesions; SEL, slowly expanding active lesions; IA, inactive lesions; NAWM, normal-appearing white matter of MS patients; CON, white matter of control patients. The line indicates the hypothetical threshold for Gd-enhancement to be seen on MR imaging scans.

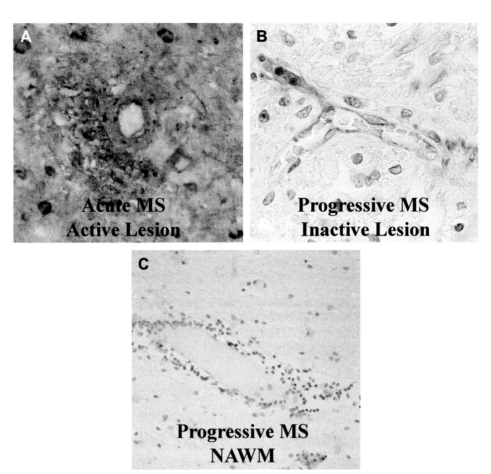

Fig. 3. BBB damage in relation to inflammation in MS lesions. (*A*) Classical active MS lesion; endothelial cells highly express dysferlin as a marker for leaky vessels (blue endothelial cells). In addition, there is massive leakage of fibrin (red) into the tissue. Double labeling immunocytochemistry for dysferlin and fibrin. (*B*) Slowly expanding lesion in primary progressive MS; dysferlin staining shows a vessel with leaky endothelial cells (brown) with only very sparse inflammation. (*C*) Normal-appearing white matter in primary progressive MS. A vessel shows profound perivascular inflammation (blue cells) without leaky endothelial cells (absence of brown staining in endothelial cells).

by perivascular inflammatory cuffs as well as by diffuse infiltration of the tissue by lymphocytes and macrophages.[53,55] Mild disturbance of the BBB, which seems to be below the detection limit of Gd-enhancement, is seen in some of the inflamed or not inflamed vessels at this stage. In addition, many vessels with profound perivascular inflammatory infiltrates are seen that do not show any evidence for increased permeability (see **Fig. 3**). At this stage of the disease, inflammation also accumulates in the meninges and perivascular spaces in the form of lymph follicle–like structures.[56] Thus, in the progressive stage of MS, inflammation becomes trapped or compartmentalized behind a closed or repaired BBB. Lack of Gd-enhancement in the progressive stage of MS does not mean that there is an absence of

inflammation. This is important to consider when discussing MS-based neurodegeneration in relation to inflammation.

BBB DAMAGE AND ACTIVE DEMYELINATION

Active white matter lesions, which are defined by Gd-enhancement, are frequent in the early stages of MS, but they are rather rare in the progressive stage. In the progressive stage, up to three enhancing lesions have been described per scan and time point in the entire brain[45,54]. In contrast, in pathology, active demyelination is described in more than 50% of all lesions in patients with primary or secondary progressive MS.[57,58] Thus, there is a major discrepancy between the active lesions seen on MR imaging scans in progressive

MS and those lesions identified within comparable brains by pathology.

This discrepancy may be partly explained by the fact that pathology allows researchers to distinguish between different types of active MS lesions (**Fig. 4**).[55] Classical active lesions are characterized by pronounced inflammation and extensive BBB damage. They are infiltrated by macrophages throughout the lesion and, depending upon the time after onset of demyelination, these macrophages contain myelin degradation products in different stages of digestion.[20] Such lesions apparently represent those seen on MR imaging scans with homogeneous Gd-enhancement. Other classical, active plaques have a peripheral rim of ongoing myelin destruction that, similarly to other classical active plaques, show dense inflammatory infiltrates and a broad rim of activated macrophages. The center of these lesions is also densely packed with macrophages, but these cells contain late (sudanophilic) remnants of myelin degradation such as cholesterol and free fatty acids. Such lesions, in general, show ring enhancement and a small hypointense rim in T2-weighted images, delineating the zone of dense macrophage infiltration.[46] Classical active lesions, as described here, are mainly found in patients with acute and early relapsing disease, but they are rare in patients with progressive MS.

The other type of actively demyelinating lesions is the slowly expanding pre-existing plaque.[55] Such lesions have an inactive center, which is surrounded at the plaque margin by a rim of densely packed activated microglia cells and a low to moderate number of macrophages (see **Fig. 4**). Only few of the macrophages and activated microglia cells contain early myelin degradation products, suggesting a very slow, active expansion of the lesions. Inflammation and BBB damage in such lesions is generally mild.[53] It is thus unlikely that such lesions show Gd-enhancement at least when standard doses of contrast material are used. Slowly expanding lesions are already present in the brains from patients with relapsing-remitting MS, but they become the dominant active lesions in patients with progressive MS.[55] Thus, in practical terms, the absence of Gd-enhancement on MR imaging scans does not

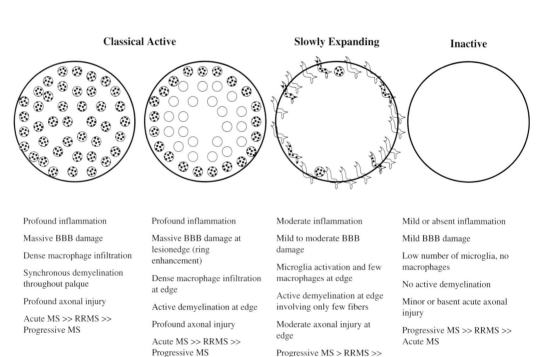

Classical Active		Slowly Expanding	Inactive
Profound inflammation	Profound inflammation	Moderate inflammation	Mild or absent inflammation
Massive BBB damage	Massive BBB damage at lesionedge (ring enhancement)	Mild to moderate BBB damage	Mild BBB damage
Dense macrophage infiltration			Low number of microglia, no macrophages
Synchronous demyelination throughout palque	Dense macrophage infiltration at edge	Microglia activation and few macrophages at edge	No active demyelination
Profound axonal injury	Active demyelination at edge	Active demyelination at edge involving only few fibers	Minor or basent acute axonal injury
Acute MS >> RRMS >> Progressive MS	Profound axonal injury	Moderate axonal injury at edge	Progressive MS >> RRMS >> Acute MS
	Acute MS >> RRMS >> Progressive MS	Progressive MS > RRMS >> Acute MS	

Fig. 4. Different types of focal white matter lesions in MS. This graph summarizes the key alterations within classical active slowly expanding, and inactive MS lesions. Small open circles: macrophages with late myelin degradation products; small dotted circles: macrophages with early myelin degradation products; open bipolar cells: microglia cells; dotted bipolar cells: microglia with early myelin degradation products. Classical active lesions have a profound infiltration of macrophages either throughout the whole extent or at the margins, all containing early myelin degradation products. Slowly expanding lesions show a rim of activated microglia cells at the margin, and some microglia cells and few macrophages contain early myelin degradation products. Inactive lesions have a sharp border without activated microglia or macrophages.

necessarily mean that the corresponding lesions are inactive in terms of inflammation, ongoing demyelination, or tissue injury.

FOCAL WHITE MATTER CHANGES PRECEDING THE APPEARANCE OF A DEMYELINATING LESION

For a long time, it was assumed that focal disturbance of the BBB, as seen on Gd-enhanced MR imaging scans, is the initial event in the formation of a new white matter lesion of MS.[43,44,60] However, subsequent studies, performing serial MR imaging investigations separated by small time intervals, showed that, at least in some lesions, subtle changes in the white matter can be seen in areas, which days to weeks later develop into classical Gd-enhancing active lesions. These changes consisted of reduction of the MTR signal[16] and a mild to moderate reduction of N-acetyl aspartate.[17] These observations suggested that subtle changes within the tissue may precede inflammation in MS plaques.

In an attempt to define the pathologic substrate of such lesions, De Groot and colleagues[23] analyzed the neuropathology of white matter areas that were abnormal on T2-weighted MR imaging scans. They identified a specific lesion type, described as (p)reactive lesions, which was characterized by mild inflammation, edema, and microglia activation, in patients with progressive MS. The incidence of such lesions within the brains, however, was more than 25% of all lesions analyzed, and was thus much higher than expected for initial stages of active plaques in patients with late progressive disease. No attempts were made to differentiate in these (p)reactive lesions areas from remyelination or secondary (Wallerian) tract degeneration.

A different approach was taken by Barnett and Prineas.[61] They described the pathology in the brain stem of an individual MS patient, who died within a few days after the onset of a new attack of the disease. The authors found, besides classical active lesions, areas of microglia activation and oligodendrocyte apoptosis surrounding the established demyelinating plaque. Inflammation in these areas of oligodendrocyte death was sparse and restricted to the perivascular space. The authors also found similar lesion areas in other patients with active disease. From these data, it was concluded that the earliest stages of the formation of MS lesions may be driven by microglia activation and may be independent from lymphocytic inflammatory infiltrates.

A more recent study addressed this question by analyzing the global pathology of the brain in patients dying in the course of fulminating MS, using an approach that was similar to that described by Barnet and Prineas, but using large hemispheric or double hemispheric brain sections.[62] In such patients, multiple active lesions develop in a very short time window of a few weeks to months and, therefore, the chance to find initial tissue alterations, preceding the formation of new classical plaques, is high. The authors found areas of tissue alteration either in close vicinity to active plaques or even topographically unrelated to existing plaques that fulfilled the criteria for initial lesions predicted by MR imaging studies. In these areas, there was a mild perivascular inflammatory reaction associated with mild edema and BBB damage, which is likely to be below the threshold of detection by Gd-enhancement. Precipitation of fibrin adjacent to the surface of microglia was associated with profound expression of inducible nitric oxide synthase and myeloperoxidase. In addition, there was a moderate acute axonal injury, seen by the accumulation of amyloid precursor protein within the axoplasm. Such pre-lesional tissue alterations were only found in a subset of MS patients, in whom demyelinated plaques follow a hypoxia-like tissue injury (pattern III),[63] but not in patients with other patterns of demyelination. In patients following pattern II (antibody and complement associated demyelination), inflammation, demyelination, and tissue injury occurs in parallel. Thus, in such lesions, inflammation and massive BBB damage is the earliest event in lesion development.

DIFFUSE CHANGES IN THE NORMAL-APPEARING WHITE MATTER

Diffuse signal abnormalities on MR imaging scans, global reduction of N-acetyl aspartate, or other quantitative MR indices are seen in the NAWM, in particular from patients with progressive MS. The extent of these changes in the NAWM can only partly be explained as a secondary consequence of axonal destruction in focal white matter lesions.[13,54,64–66] Only a few studies have concentrated on the neuropathology of tissue damage in the NAWM.

One explanation for the appearance of tissue damage in the NAWM is axonal and neuronal loss in demyelinated lesions in the white matter or the cortex, which will lead to secondary (Wallerian) degeneration of respective fiber tracts. As described above, axonal loss in focal white matter lesions is profound, affecting, in late chronic lesions, on average 60% to 70% of the total axonal population. In addition, loss of neurons has been seen in the cortex of MS patients.[67,68] Wallerian tract degeneration has been assessed with neuropathological techniques in several studies. As an example, focal white matter lesions in the brain hemispheres give rise to tract degeneration in the corpus callosum.[69] Similar tract degeneration is also frequently seen in the spinal cord.[70,71] However, a meticulous analysis of plaque load in the spinal cord in relation to spinal cord atrophy suggests that additional factors other than axonal loss within lesions may account for loss of axons in the NAWM.[72,73]

There are a few reports describing diffuse white matter changes in MS brains that may develop independently from focal white matter lesions. They consist of some perivascular inflammatory infiltrates, small perivenous demyelinating lesions, and diffuse astroglia and microglia activation.[74,75] Small microglia nodules can also be seen in the periplaques white matter.[59] A more systematic study, comparing NAWM between early and late stages of MS, revealed diffuse reduction of myelin density, chronic perivascular and parenchymal infiltration of the tissue with T-lymphocytes, and profound microglia activation, which was most pronounced in patients with primary and secondary progressive MS. This diffuse inflammation was associated with widespread axonal injury in the absence of primary demyelination.[55] The extent of inflammation and tissue injury in the NAWM did not correlate with the size or location of focal inflammatory demyelinating lesions, suggesting that diffuse white matter damage may develop at least in part independently of focal plaques. As in most focal lesions seen in the progressive stage of MS, these diffuse changes were accompanied only by mild blood brain damage, although they invariably were associated with persistent inflammation in the brain. These data suggest that in the later stages of MS and, in particular, in progressive MS, white matter becomes affected in a global sense and this diffuse white matter damage may be driven by a compartmentalized inflammatory reaction within the brain compartment.

CORTICAL AND GRAY MATTER PATHOLOGY

MS is commonly regarded as a disease affecting the white matter exclusively. It has, however, been noted already in early studies that gray matter, and in particular the cerebral cortex, is affected by demyelination.[18,76,77] Although cortical demyelination can so far hardly be seen directly on MR imaging, cortical atrophy and subtle changes in cortical MTR have been reported in MS patients, in particular in the progressive stage of the disease.[14,78] The current view in neuropathology is that the cerebral cortex is affected in MS patients

in two different ways: cortical demyelination and diffuse neuronal loss with cortical atrophy.

Cortical Demyelination

The global extent of cortical demyelination in MS became clear only recently, when sensitive techniques were introduced to visualize the thin cortical myelinated fibers.[67] Using these techniques, three different types of cortical demyelinated lesions were identified. The first are cortico-subcortical lesions, due to white matter lesions, which expand into the cortical tissue. The second are small intracortical, perivascular lesions. The third type, which is most abundant in MS and is mainly found in patients with progressive disease, are subpial lesions.[67,79,80] These lesions are oriented toward inflammatory infiltrates located in the leptomeninges.[55] They appear as band-like subpial zones of demyelination, affecting the outer layers of the cortex and may span over large distances involving several adjacent gyri and sulci (**Fig. 5**). Subpial cortical lesions are not evenly distributed throughout the entire cortex but affect certain cortical areas more frequently than others.[55,81] They are mainly found in cortical sulci and – even more prominently – in deep invaginations of the outer surface of the brain. Thus, they are seen most frequently in the insular cortex, the cingulated gyrus, and in the deep cortical invaginations in the frontobasal, temporobasal and occipital lobes. Other predilection sites for cortical demyelination are the cerebellum[82] and the hippocampus.[83] Although cortical lesions can be present already in the early stages of acute and relapsing MS, the extent of cortical demyelination increases with disease duration, being highest in patients with primary or secondary progressive MS. In such patients, cortical demyelination may affect up to 80% of the cortical ribbon in the forebrain and up to 95% in the cerebellum.[55,82] Subpial demyelination appears to be highly specific for MS. It is not seen in other inflammatory–demyelinating diseases, such as adrenoleukodystrophy or progressive multifocal leukoencephalopathy (PML). In PML, only some intracortical and cortico-subcortical demyelination is seen, which is associated with virus antigen expression in the respective areas; subpial demyelination is absent.[84]

Cortical lesions differ from white matter plaques in several fundamental aspects. Lymphocytic inflammation is sparse or absent within the cortical parenchyma,[85] but profound T- and B-cell infiltrates are invariably present in the meninges, adjacent to active cortical lesions. Particularly aggressive cortical lesional activity is seen in patients

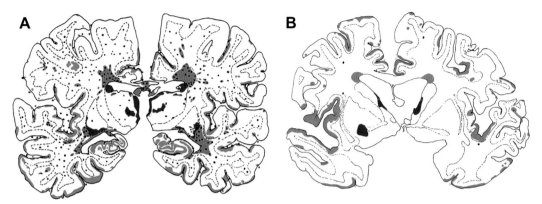

Fig. 5. Demyelinated lesions in MS brains. White matter lesions are shown in green; cortical lesions appear in red; and lesions in the deep gray matter are shown in blue. Cortical lesions are mainly found in invaginations of the cortical surface (sulci, insular cortex, cingulated cortex). In some patients profound cortical demyelination is seen with only a very few and small white matter lesions. (*A*) Secondary progressive MS; (*B*) Primary progressive MS. (*From* Kutzelnigg A, Lucchinetti CF, Stadelmann C, et al. Cortical demyelination and diffuse white matter injury in multiple sclerosis. Brain 2005;128:2705–12; with permission.)

with lymph follicle–like inflammatory infiltrates in the meninges.[86] Active cortical demyelination is associated with activated microglia cells. BBB damage and edema is sparse or absent in cortical lesions, even when they are actively demyelinating.[87] Thus, Gd-enhancement is not seen in such lesions with one exception: in cortico-subcortical lesions, BBB damage in the white matter parts of the lesions may lead to protein extravasation and edema, which may penetrate also into the adjacent cortical areas.

There is good agreement that neuronal density is reduced in cortical lesions but is also reduced in the adjacent normal appearing cortex.[68,82,88] In active cortical lesions, some neuronal apoptosis and some dystrophic axons are seen.[67] Data on synaptic loss in cortical plaques are discordant. Some studies found profound loss, although in others no loss was seen.[68,82,88] Remyelination is frequently encountered in cortical MS lesions and appears to be more pronounced as in white matter lesions.[89]

Direct comparison with neuropathology revealed that at this time only some of the cortico-subcortical and intracortical, but none of the other cortical, lesions can be seen on MR images.[90,91] This is even the case when brain slices are imaged with an 8T magnet with very long data acquisition time.[92] Whether the loss of myelin sheaths in the cortex of MS patients is clinically relevant is, at present, not clear.

Cortical Atrophy

There is clear evidence from MR imaging studies that cortical volume decreases with time in MS patients. The pathologic substrate of the cortical

atrophy is, however, so far not well understood. In a detailed quantitative study, Wegner and colleagues[68] found a general reduction of cortical thickness by 10% in demyelinated as well as the normal-appearing cortex. In addition, neuronal and glial cell loss was seen in the amount of 10% and 36% in demyelinated, but not in the normal cortex. A similar amount of neuronal loss was seen in demyelinated cortex in other studies.[82,88] These studies suggest that neuronal loss in the cortex is in part due to inflammatory tissue damage, but, in addition, they also suggest that it might be a secondary consequence of axonal transection in the white matter. Indeed, when cortex is analyzed in the vicinity of destructive subcortical white matter lesions, neuronal alteration reminiscent for retrograde degeneration can be seen. These diffuse cortical changes in MS have to be separated from MS-unrelated cortical damage. In aging MS patients, cortical alterations of Alzheimer's disease are seen in a similar frequency as the one seen in a cohort of normal aging individuals.[93]

SPECIFIC ASPECTS OF MS VARIANTS
Neuromyelitis Optica (Devic's Disease)

A specific subtype of MS-like inflammatory-demyelinating diseases is neuromyelitis optica (NMO).[94,95] Originally described as a monophasic disease, it recently became clear that the disease process in NMO can also affect other brain regions and chronic relapsing disease courses are frequent. Characteristic features of this disease are longitudinally extensive lesions in the spinal cord, expanding over several cord segments.[96] In contrast to classical MS,[97] NMO lesions in the spinal cord target the central portions, including the gray matter columns, more frequently that the subpial white matter. Involvement of optic nerves and chiasm is typical and bilateral optic nerve affection is frequent. In a small subset of patients, additional lesions are seen at predilection sites for MS lesions, such as the forebrain white matter or the brain stem. Another typical predilection site for NMO lesions are the circumventricular organs.[98]

In recent years, an auto-antibody response has been described that appears to be specific for patients with NMO.[99] The antibodies are directed against the astrocytic water channel aquaporin 4[100] and the above described predilection sites for lesions in NMO patients are sites with high expression of this antigen.[101] The pathology of NMO lesions suggests that the antibody response against astrocytic aquaporin 4 plays a major role in their pathogenesis.[102] In early lesional stages, astrocyte processes at the glia limitans are dressed with immunoglobulins and activated complement, and astrocytes are specifically lost and destroyed in later stages of lesional development.[98] Demyelination and axonal loss is seen at later stages and may represent a secondary consequence of immune-mediated astrocytic destruction. These tissue alterations occur on the background of an inflammatory reaction, consisting of T-lymphocytes, a few B-cells, activated macrophages, and microglia cells. In contrast to classical MS lesions, granulocytes represent a major component of the inflammatory infiltrates.[102] Chronic established lesions are characterized by massive tissue destruction, resulting in tissue loss and cyst formation.

It is currently not clear whether NMO is part of the disease spectrum of MS or represents a distinct disease entity.[94] It is unlikely that aquaporin 4 antibodies alone are able to induce lesions in the CNS of NMO patients because the intact BBB does not allow circulating antibodies to reach the brain or spinal cord in concentrations sufficient to induce disease and lesions. Thus, a T-cell mediated inflammatory response, similar to that seen in classical MS, may be necessary to initiate the lesions.

Balo's Concentric Sclerosis

The lesions in Balo's concentric sclerosis are characterized by alternating rims of myelinated and demyelinated tissue.[103] At low magnification, such lesions show a concentric patterning resembling that seen in a transected onion. Classical Balo's disease is only seen when very large lesions with a diameter of several centimetres are present. However, some concentric banding is a typical feature of more classical MS lesions, following a pattern of demyelination with hypoxia-like tissue injury (pattern III).[61,63,104] Within the concentric layers of preserved myelin, stress proteins and molecules involved in tissue preconditioning are highly expressed. This finding suggests that the concentric pattern of lesions is induced by the balance between neuroprotection and neurodegeneration in rapidly expanding large brain lesions.[104] Concentric demyelination can be seen in all areas of the brain and spinal cord. Thus, Balo's concentric sclerosis is not a distinct disease entity but is a variant of MS with rapidly progressive formation of exceptionally large lesions in the CNS.

SUMMARY

Neuropathology is generally regarded as the gold standard for defining MS lesions in diagnosis and research. However, the neuropathologist's view of MS was for a long time restricted to focal white matter lesions, the classical MS plaques. Detailed cross-sectional and longitudinal MR imaging studies in MS patients, however, have identified aspects of MS pathology that could not be explained by the plaque-centered view of the disease and that have stimulated intense research efforts aimed at redefining the pathology of the disease. Although focal plaques of primary demyelination are still the pathologic hallmark of MS, it became clear in recent years that the brains of affected MS patients are damaged in a much more global sense. It is likely that diffuse changes in the NAWM and the pathology in the cortex or deep gray matter nuclei are similarly important for explaining the complex clinical deficits in the patients – in particular in the progressive stages of the disease.

REFERENCES

1. Babinski J. Recherches sur ĺanatomie pathologique de la sclerose en plaque et etude comparative des diverses varietes de la scleroses de la moelle. Archives de Physiologie (Paris) 1885;5–6:186–207.
2. Charcot JM. Lecons sur les maladies du systeme nerveux faites a la Salpetriere. 4e edition. Paris: Tome 1; 1880.
3. Marburg O. Die sogenannte "akute multiple sklerose". Jahrbücher für Psychiatrie und Neurologie 1906;27:211–312.
4. Rindfleisch E. Histologisches Detail zur grauen Degeneration von Gehirn und Rückenmark. Arch Pathol. Virchows Archiv 1863;26:474–83.
5. Doinikow B. Über De- und Regenerationserscheinungen an Achsenzylindern bei der multiplen

Sklerose. Zeitschrift für die gesamte Neurologie und Psychiatrie 1915;27:151–78.

6. Schlesinger H. Zur Frage der akuten multiplen Sklerose und der encephalomyelitis disseminata im Kindesalter. Arbeiten aus dem Neurologischen Institu (Wien) 1909;17:410–32.

7. Confavreux C, Vukusic S, Adeleine P. Early clinical predictors and progression of irreversible disability in multiple sclerosis: an amnesic process. Brain 2003;126:770–82.

8. Confavreux C, Vukusic S, Moreau T, et al. Relapses and progression of disability in multiple sclerosis. N Engl J Med 2000;343:1430–8.

9. Coles AJ, Cox A, Le Page E, et al. The window of therapeutic opportunity in multiple sclerosis. Evidence from monoclonal antibody therapy. J Neurol 2006;253:98–108.

10. Fu L, Matthews PM, De-Stefano N, et al. Imaging axonal damage of normal-appearing white matter in multiple sclerosis. Brain 1998;121:103–13.

11. Leary SM, Davie CA, Parker GJ, et al. 1H magnetic resonance spectroscopy of normal appearing white matter in primary progressive multiple sclerosis. J Neurol 1999;246:1023–6.

12. De-Stefano N, Narayanan S, Francis SJ, et al. Diffuse axonal and tissue injury in patients with multiple sclerosis with low cerebral lesion load and no disability. Arch Neurol 2002;59:1565–71.

13. Rocca MA, Iannucci G, Rovaris M, et al. Occult tissue damage in patients with primary progressive multiple sclerosis is independent of T2-visible lesions—a diffusion tensor MR study. J Neurol 2003;250:456–60.

14. Dehmeshki J, Chard DT, Leary SM, et al. The normal appearing grey matter in primary progressive multiple sclerosis: a magnetization transfer imaging study. J Neurol 2003;250:67–74.

15. He J, Inglese M, Li BS, et al. Relapsing remitting multiple sclerosis; metabolic abnormality in nonenhancing lesions and normal-appearing white matter at MR imaging; initial experience. Radiology 2005;234:211–7.

16. Filippi M, Rocca MA, Martino G, et al. Magnetization transfer changes in the normal appearing white matter precede the appearance of enhancing lesions in patients with multiple sclerosis. Ann Neurol 1998;43:809–14.

17. Narayanan PA, Doyle TJ, Lai D, et al. Serial proton magnetic resonance spectroscopic imaging, contrast-enhanced magnetic resonance imaging, and quantitative lesion volumetry in multiple sclerosis. Ann Neurol 1998;43:56–71.

18. Lumsden CE. The neuropathology of multiple sclerosis. In: Vinken PI, Bruyn GW, editors. "Handbook of clinical neurology", vol 9. New York: Elsevier; 1970. p. 217–309.

19. Lassmann H, Raine CS, Antel J, et al. Immunopathology of multiple sclerosis: report on an international meeting held at the Institute of Neurology of the University of Vienna. J Neuroimmunol 1998; 86:213–7.

20. Brück W, Porada P, Poser S, et al. Monocyte/macrophage differentiation in early multiple sclerosis lesions. Ann Neurol. 1995;38:788–96.

21. Prineas JW. The neuropathology of multiple sclerosis. In: Koetsier JC, editor. "Handbook of clinical neurology", vol 47. New York: Elsevier; 1985. p. 337–95.

22. Lassmann H. Comparative neuropathology of chronic experimental allergic encephalomyelitis and multiple sclerosis. Springer Schriftenr. Neurol 1983;25:1–135.

23. De Groot CJ, Bergers E, Kamphorst W, et al. Postmortem MRI-guided sampling of multiple sclerosis brain lesions: increased yield of active demyelinating and (p)reactive lesions. Brain 2001;124:1635–45.

24. Barkhof F, Brück W, De-Groot CJ, et al. Remyelinated lesions in multiple sclerosis: magnetic resonance image appearance. Arch Neurol 2003;60: 1073–81.

25. Bjartmar C, Kidd G, Mork S, et al. Neurological disability correlates with spinal cord axonal loss and reduced N-acetyl aspartate in chronic multiple sclerosis patients. Ann Neurol. 2000;48:893–901.

26. Ferguson B, Matyszak MK, Esiri MM, et al. Axonal damage in acute multiple sclerosis lesions. Brain 1997;120:393–9.

27. Kornek B, Storch M, Weissert R, et al. Multiple sclerosis and chronic autoimmune encephalomyelitis: a comparative quantitative study of axonal injury in active, inactive and remyelinated lesions. Am J Pathol 2000;157:267–76.

28. Trapp BD, Peterson J, Ransohoff RM, et al. Axonal transection in the lesions of multiple sclerosis. N Engl J Med. 1998;338:278–85.

29. Mews I, Bergmann M, Bunkowski S, et al. Oligodendrocyte and axon pathology in clinically silent multiple sclerosis lesions. Mult Scler 1998;4:55–62.

30. Bitsch A, Kuhlmann T, Stadelmann C, et al. A longitudinal MRI study of histopathologically defined hypointense multiple sclerosis lesions. Ann Neurol 2001;49:793–6.

31. Van Waesberghe JH, Kamphorst W, De-Groot CJ, et al. Axonal loss in multiple sclerosis lesions: magnetic resonance imaging insights into substrates of disability. Ann Neurol 1999;46:747–54.

32. Prineas JW, Connell F. Remyelination in multiple sclerosis. Ann Neurol 1979;5:22–31.

33. Prineas JW, Kwon EE, Cho ES, et al. Continual breakdown and regeneration of myelin in progressive multiple sclerosis plaques. Ann N Y Acad Sci 1984;436:11–32.

34. Prineas JW, Barnard RO, Revesz T, et al. Multiple sclerosis. Pathology of recurrent lesions. Brain 1993;116:681–93.

35. Lucchinetti C, Brück W, Parisi J, et al. A quantitative analysis of oligodendrocytes in multiple sclerosis lesions. A study of 117 cases. Brain 1999;122:2279–95.

36. Prineas JW, Kwon EE, Goldenberg PZ, et al. Multiple sclerosis. Oligodendrocyte proliferation and differentiation in fresh lesions. Lab Invest 1989;61:489–503.

37. Raine CS, Scheinberg L, Waltz JM. Multiple sclerosis: Oligodendrocyte survival and proliferation in an active established lesion. Lab Invest 1981;45:534–46.

38. Prineas JW, Barnard RO, Kwon EE, et al. Multiple sclerosis: remyelination of nascent lesions. Ann Neurol 1993;33:137–51.

39. Patrikios P, Stadelmann C, Kutzelnigg A, et al. Remyelination is extensive in a subset of multiple sclerosis patients. Brain 2006;129:3165–72.

40. Patani R, Balaratnam M, Vora A, et al. Remyelination can be extensive in multiple sclerosis despite a long disease course. Neuropathol Appl Neurobiol 2007;33:277–87.

41. Chen JT, Kuhlmann T, Jansen GH, et al. Canadian MS/BMT Stdy Group. Voxel-based analysis of the evolution of magnetization transfer ratio to quantify remyelination and demyelination with histopathological validation in a multiple sclerosis lesion. Neuroimage 2007;36:1152–8.

42. Minneboo A, Uitdenhaag BM, Ader HJ, et al. Patterns of enhancing lesion evolution in multiple sclerosis are uniform within patients. Neurology 2005;65:56–61.

43. Miller DH, Rudge P, Johnson G, et al. Serial gadolinium enhanced magnetic resonance imaging in multiple sclerosis. Brain 1988;111:927–39.

44. Grossman RI, Braffman BH, Brorson JR, et al. Multiple sclerosis: serial study of gadolinium enhanced MR imaging. Radiology 1988;169:117–22.

45. Kappos L, Moeri D, Radue EW, et al. For the gadolinium MRI meta-analysis group. Predictive value of gadolinium-enhancement magnetic resonance imaging for relapse rate and changes in disability or impairment in multiple sclerosis: a meta-analysis. Lancet 1999;353:964–9.

46. Brück W, Bitsch A, Kolenda H, et al. Inflammatory central nervous system demyelination: correlation of magnetic resonance imaging findings with lesion pathology. Ann Neurol 1997;42:783–93.

47. Katz D, Taubenberger JK, Cannella B, et al. Correlation between magnetic resonance imaging findings and lesion development in chronic, active multiple sclerosis. Ann Neurol 1993;34:661–9.

48. Broman T. Blood brain barrier damage in multiple sclerosis. Supra-vital test observations. Acta Neurol Scand 1964;10:21–4.

49. Kwon EE, Prineas JW. Blood brain barrier abnormalities in longstanding multiple sclerosis lesions. An immunohistochemical study. J Neuropathol Exp Neurol 1994;53:625–36.

50. Claudio L, Raine CS, Brosnan CF. Evidence for persistent blood-brain barrier abnormalities in chronic-progressive multiple sclerosis. Acta Neuropathol 1995;90:228–38.

51. Vos CM, Geurts JJ, Montagne L, et al. Blood brain barrier alterations in both focal and diffuse abnormalities on postmortem MRI in multiple sclerosis. Neurobiol Dis 2005;20:953–60.

52. Kirk J, Plumb J, Mirakhur M, et al. Tight junctional abnormality in multiple sclerosis white matter affects all calibers of vessel and is associated with blood-brain barrier leakage and active demyelination. J Pathol 2003;201:319–27.

53. Hochmeister S, Grundtner R, Bauer J, et al. Dysferlin is a new marker for leaky brain blood vessels in multiple sclerosis. J Neuropathol Exp Neurol 2006;65:855–65.

54. Ingle GT, Sastre-Garriga J, Miller DH, et al. Is inflammation important in early PPMS? A longitudinal MRI study. J Neurol Neurosurg Psychiatr 2008;76:1255–8.

55. Kutzelnigg A, Lucchinetti CF, Stadelmann C, et al. Cortical demyelination and diffuse white matter injury in multiple sclerosis. Brain 2005;128:2705–12.

56. Serafini B, Rosicarelli B, Magliozzi R, et al. Detection of ectopic B-cell follicles with germinal centers in the meninges of patients with secondary progressive multiple sclerosis. Brain Pathol 2004;14:164–74.

57. Breij EC, Brink BP, Veerhuis R, et al. Homogeneity of active demyelinating lesions in established multiple sclerosis. Ann Neurol 2008;63:16–25.

58. Newcombe J, Hawkins CP, Henderson CL, et al. Histopathology of multiple sclerosis lesions detected by magnetic resonance imaging in unfixed post-mortem central nervous system tissue. Brain 1991;114:1013–23.

59. Prineas JW, Kwon EE, Cho ES, et al. Immunopathology of secondary-progressive multiple sclerosis. Ann Neurol 2001;50:646–57.

60. Cotton F, Weiner HL, Jolesz FA, et al. MRI contrast uptake in new lesions in relapsing-remitting MS followed at weekly intervals. Neurology 2003;60:640–6.

61. Barnett MH, Prineas JW. Relapsing and remitting multiple sclerosis: pathology of the newly forming lesion. Ann Neurol 2004;55:458–68.

62. Marik C, Felts P, Bauer J, et al. Lesion genesis in a subset of patients with multiple sclerosis: a role for innate immunity? Brain 2007;130:2800–15.

63. Lucchinetti C, Brück W, Parisi J, et al. Heterogeneity of multiple sclerosis lesions: implications for the pathogenesis of demyelination. Ann Neurol 2000; 47:707–17.

64. De-Stefano N, Narayanan S, Matthews PM, et al. In vivo evidence for axonal dysfunction remote from focal cerebral demyelination of the type seen in multiple sclerosis. Brain 1999;122:1933–9.

65. Rovaris M, Bozzali M, Santuccio G, et al. In vivo assessment of the brain and cervical cord pathology of patients with primary progressive multiple sclerosis. Brain 2001;124:2540–9.

66. Pelletier D, Nelson SJ, Oh J, et al. MRI lesion volume heterogeneity in primary progressive MS in relation with axonal damage and brain atrophy. J Neurol Neurosurg Psychiatr 2003;74:950–2.

67. Peterson JW, Bo L, Mork S, et al. Transsected neurites, apoptotic neurons and reduced inflammation in cortical multiple sclerosis lesions. Ann Neurol. 2001;50:389–400.

68. Wegner C, Esiri MM, Chance SA, et al. Neocortical neuronal, synaptic and glial loss in multiple sclerosis. Neurology 2006;67:960–7.

69. Evangelou N, Konz D, Esiri MM, et al. Regional axonal loss in the corpus callosum correlates with cerebral white matter lesion volume and distribution in multiple sclerosis. Brain 2000;123:1845–9.

70. Ganter P, Prince C, Esiri MM. Spinal cord axonal loss in multiple sclerosis: a post-mortem study. Neuropathol Appl Neurobiol 1999;25:459–67.

71. Lovas G, Szilagyi N, Majtenyi K, et al. Axonal changes in chronic demyelinated cervical spinal cord plaques. Brain 2000;123:308–17.

72. Evangelou N, DeLuca GC, Owens T, et al. Pathological study of spinal cord atrophy in multiple sclerosis suggests limited role of focal lesions. Brain 2005;128:29–34.

73. De Luca GC, Williams K, Evangelou N, et al. The contribution of demyelination to axonal loss in multiple sclerosis. Brain 2006;129:1507–16.

74. Allen IV, McKeown SR. A histological, histochemical and biochemical study of the macroscopically normal white matter in multiple sclerosis. J Neurol Sci. 1979;41:81–91.

75. Allen IV, McQuid S, Miradkhur M, et al. Pathological abnormalities in the normal-appearing white matter in multiple sclerosis. Neurol Sci 2001;22: 141–4.

76. Brownell B, Hughes JT. The distribution of plaques in the cerebrum in multiple scleosis. J Neurol Neurosurg Psychiatr. 1962;25:315–20.

77. Gilmore CP, Bo L, Owens T, et al. Spinal cord grey matter demyelination in multiple sclerosis: a novel pattern of residual plaque morphology. Brain Pathol 2006;16:202–8.

78. Khaleeli Z, Cercignani M, Audoin B, et al. Localized grea matter damage in early primary progressive multiple sclerosis contributes to disability. Neuroimage 2007;37:253–61.

79. Bo L, Vedeler CA, Nyland HI, et al. Subpial demyelination in the cerebral cortex of multiple sclerosis patients. J Neuropathol Exp Neurol 2003;62: 723–32.

80. Kidd T, Barkhof F, McConnell R, et al. Cortical lesions in multiple sclerosis. Brain 1999;122:17–26.

81. Kutzelnigg A, Lassmann H. Cortical demyelination in multiple sclerosis: a substrate for cognitive deficits? J Neurol Sci 2006;245:123–6.

82. Kutzelnigg A, Faber-Rod JC, Bauer J, et al. Widespread demyelination in the cerebellar cortex in multiple sclerosis. Brain Pathol 2007;17:38–44.

83. Geurts JJ, Bo L, Roosendaal SD, et al. Extensive hippocampal demyelination in multiple sclerosis. J Neuropathol Exp Neurol 2007;66:819–27.

84. Moll NM, Rietsch AM, Ransohoff AJ, et al. Cortical demyelination in PML and MS: similarities and differences. Neurology 2007;70:336–43.

85. Bo L, Vedeler CA, Nyland H, et al. Intracortical multiple sclerosis lesions are not associated with increased lymphocyte infiltration. Mult Scler 2003;9:323–31.

86. Magliozzi R, Howell O, Vora A, et al. Meningeal B-cell follicles in secondary progressive multiple sclerosis associate with early onset of disease and severe cortical pathology. Brain 2007;130:1089–104.

87. Van Horssen J, Brink BP, de Vries HE, et al. The blood brain barrier in cortical multiple sclerosis lesions. J Neuropathol Exp Neurol 2007;66:321–8.

88. Vercellino M, Plano F, Votta B, et al. Grey matter pathology in multiple sclerosis. J Neuropathol Exp Neurol 2005;64:1101–7.

89. Albert M, Antel J, Brück W, et al. Extensive cortical remyelination in patients with chronic multiple sclerosis. Brain Pathol 2007;17:129–38.

90. Geurts JJ, Bo L, Pouwels PJ, et al. Cortical lesions in multiple sclerosis: combined postmortem MR imaging and histopathology. ANJR Am J Neuroradiol 2005;26:572–7.

91. Geurts JJ, Blezer EL, Vrenken H, et al. Does highfield MR imaging improve cortical lesion detection in multiple sclerosis? J Neurol 2008;255:183–91.

92. Kangariu A, Bourekas EC, Ray-Chaudhury A, et al. Cerebral cortical lesions detected by MR imaging at 8 Tesla. Amer J Neuroradiol 2007;28:262–6.

93. Dal Bianco A, Bradl M, Frischer J, et al. Multiple sclerosis and Alzheimer's disease. Ann Neurol 2008;63:174–83.

94. Wingerchuck DM, Lennon VA, Pittock SJ, et al. Revised diagnostic criteria for neuromyelitis optica. Neurology 2006;66:1485–9.

95. Devic E. Myelite subaigue compliquee de nevrite optique. Bull Med 1984;8:1033.

96. Weinshenker BG, Wingerchuk DM, Vukusic S, et al. Neuromyelitis optica IgG predicts relapse after longitudinally extensive transverse myelitis. Ann Neurol 2006;59:566–9.

97. Fog T. Topographic distribution of plaques in the spinal cord in multiple sclerosis. Arch Neurol Psychiat 1950;63:382–414.

98. Roemer SF, Parisi JE, Lennon VA, et al. Distinct pattern of aquaporin-4 expression in neuromyelitis optica lesions. Brain 2007;130:1194–205.

99. Lennon VA, Wingerchuk DN, Kryzer TJ, et al. A serum autoantibody marker of neuromyelitis optica: distinction from multiple sclerosis. Lancet 2004; 364:2106–12.

100. Lennon VA, Kryzer TJ, Pittock SJ, et al. IgG marker of optic-spinal multiple sclerosis binds to the aquaporin-4 water channel. J Exp Med 2005;202:473–7.

101. Pittock SJ, Weinshenker BG, Lucchinetti CF, et al. Neuromyelitis optica brain lesions localized at sites of high aquaporin-4 expression. Arch Neurol 2006; 63:964–8.

102. Lucchinetti CF, Mandler R, McGavern D, et al. A role for humoral mechanisms in he pathogenesis of Devic's neuromyelitis optica. Brain 2002;125: 1450–61.

103. Balo J. Encephalitis periaxialis concentrica. Arch Neurol 1928;19:242–64.

104. Stadelmann C, Ludwin S, Tabira T, et al. Tissue preconditioning may explain concentric lesions in Balo's type of multiple sclerosis. Brain 2005;128:979–87.

Immunologic Mechanisms of Multiple Sclerosis

Elliot M. Frohman, MD, PhD[a,b,]*, Todd Eagar, PhD[a,c],
Nancy Monson, PhD[a,c], Olaf Stuve, MD, PhD[a,c],
Nitin Karandikar, MD, PhD[a,c,d]

KEYWORDS

- Multiple sclerosis
- Optical coherence tomography • Pupillometry
- Retinal nerve fiber layer • Macular volume

Multiple sclerosis (MS) is widely recognized as the most commonly identified cause of progressive neurologic disability in young adults throughout the developed world. The disorder is clinically suspected when patients experience either acute attacks of neurologic compromise or instead are afflicted by a steadily progressive deterioration in functional capabilities. In the former circumstance, attacks or so-called "exacerbations" can literally produce any neurologic symptom (Table 1) with a persistence of at least 24 hours (but often lasting much longer) followed by a period of partial and in some cases nearly complete recovery. The pathophysiology of acute exacerbations (as part of relapsing remitting MS [RRMS]) is thought to be related to the development of inflammation and its consequences, within strategic (often referred to as "eloquent") and often discrete central nervous system (CNS) tract systems.[1] Although a myriad of hypotheses have been formulated to explain the underpinnings of the mechanisms that contribute to both the predilection and triggering of the multiphasic inflammatory events that personify MS, much remains to be done to understand fully the specific set and sequence of events that produce the disease and its cardinal features.

In contrast to the RRMS phase of the disease, many patients are afflicted with either a wholly progressive and insidiously changing course of disability from the inception without any evidence of acute attacks (primary progressive MS), or RRMS patients later transition into this phase of the disease (secondary progressive MS) after years of having intermittently active inflammatory events (clinically characterized by exacerbations and radiographically by new MR imaging lesions).[2] Despite vigorous debate, most who actively manage MS patients understand that the accrual of permanent physical and intellectual disability can be a derivative of the exacerbating (most patients do not fully recover from their attacks), progressive, and even subclinical aspects of the disease.[3]

Historically, MS is not a newly recognized disorder. Perhaps the first individual identified with a disease course thought to be indistinguishable from MS was St. Ludwina of Schiedam, a Dutch girl who lived in the fourteenth century, and who at the age of 16 fell in an ice skating accident, which was subsequently followed by a relapse-remitting course of neurologic attacks and remissions.[4] She later became permanently disabled and died before her sixtieth birthday. The work of

[a] Department of Neurology, University of Texas Southwestern Medical Center at Dallas, 5323 Harry Hines Boulevard, Dallas, TX 75235, USA
[b] Department of Ophthalmology, University of Texas Southwestern Medical Center at Dallas, 5323 Harry Hines Boulevard, Dallas, Texas 75390, USA
[c] Department of Immunology, University of Texas Southwestern Medical Center at Dallas, 5323 Harry Hines Boulevard, Dallas, Texas 75390, USA
[d] Department of Pathology, University of Texas Southwestern Medical Center at Dallas, 5323 Harry Hines Boulevard, Dallas, Texas 75390, USA
* Corresponding author.
E-mail address: elliot.frohman@utsouthwestern.edu (E.M. Frohman).

Neuroimag Clin N Am 18 (2008) 577–588
doi:10.1016/j.nic.2008.06.009

Table 1
Clinical manifestations of multiple sclerosis

Exacerbations	Symptoms	Progression Features	Interventions
Optic neuritis	Blurred vision Eye pain Color loss Field defects	Acuity loss Visual field loss Reduced reading	Maximize refraction Magnification

Myelitis	Numbness
	Pain
	Dysesthesias
	Pressure sensations
	Weakness
	Ataxia (sensory)
	Gait dysfunction
	Neurogenic bladder
	Neurogenic bowel
	Sexual dysfunction
	Spasticity
		Sensory disturbances
		Chronic pain syndromes
		Weakness
		Exercise intolerance
		Poor gait mechanics
		Foot drop
		Falling
		Bladder retention
		Chronic constipation
		Anorgasmia
		Erectile dysfunction
		Tonic and phasic
		  spasticity
		Impact on activities of
		  daily living
		Reduced driving safety
			Membrane stabilizers
			Exercise training
			Physiotherapy
			Stretching
			Orthotic devices
			Assist devices
			Anticholinergics
			Alpha antagonists
			Fiber, fluid, stimulants
			Vibrator stimulation
			Proerectile agents
			Baclofen,
			  benzodiazepine

Ocular, motor,
  vestibular
	Double vision
	Oscillopsia
	Vertigo
	Nausea, vomiting
	Disorientation
	Gait dysfunction
		Double vision
		Eye strain ($\pm$ headaches)
		Poor reading
		Difficulty driving
		Falling
			Patching, prismatic
			  correction
			Magnification
			Driving assessments
			Assist devices

Paroxysms	Seizures Focal dystonias Tonic spasms Dysarthria Ataxia Speech arrest Transient aphasias	Tend to be transient	Membrane stabilizers

Uhthoff's	Virtually any physical or
	  cognitive deficit in
	  multiple sclerosis can
	  be stereotypically and
	  reversibly intensified
	  or exacerbation with
	  infection, heat,
	  prolonged exercise, or
	  stress.
		This phenomenon
		becomes more
		prominent as the
		disease advances.
		Uhthoff's
		phenomenon
		represents one of the
		most vexing and
		disabling aspects of
		multiple sclerosis and
		is highly limiting to
		many patients. It
		signifies reversible
		conduction block
		secondary to
		demyelination.
			Cooling devices
			Avoid temperature
			  extremes
			4-aminopyridine
			Titrate exercise
			Stress reduction
			Treat infection
			Antipyretics when
			  febrile

(continued on next page)

Table 1
(continued)

Exacerbations	Symptoms	Progression Features	Interventions
Cognitive	Slow processing speed Poor multitasking Reduced memory Rarely aphasic syndrome	Reduced work performance Altered activities of living Medication errors Driving accidents Altered communication	Neuropsychologic tests Mental activities Avoid Uhthoff's stimuli Acetylcholinesterase inhibitor Memantine Psychostimulant use Modafinil Treat B_{12} deficiency Treat hypothyroidism Treat depression Treat anemia
Fatigue	Literally affects all aspect of an multiple sclerosis patient's life. Often related to sleep disturbance, mood dysregulation, Uhthoff's phenomenon, altered properties of physical functions (eg, faulty gait mechanics, spasticity, and so forth).	Reduced activities Poor work performance Cognitive compromise Depression Demoralization Altered thinking Reduced walking	Treat depression Evaluate sleep Physiotherapy Exercise training Rest periods Cooling strategies Pychostimulants Modafinil Acetyl-L-carnitine D-Ribose 4-Aminopyridine Amantadine Atomoxetine

Charcot[5] in the nineteenth century was seminal in that he and his group at the Salpetiere in Paris exhaustively chronicalized the longitudinal changes in the disease course and its impact on clinical disability over the life of patients with MS. Further, his group systematically performed neuropathologic studies on the brain and spinal cord on these same patients after death, and thereby established the two cardinal tenets of neurologic practice: where is the lesion that is responsible for the resulting clinical signs and symptoms, and what is the nature or etiology of this lesion? Although Charcot did not discover MS clinically or pathologically, he and his collaborators did institute the framework on which much progress has been made in the understanding of the relationship between the development of tissue injury in the CNS and its relevance to clinical disability.

The first MS diagnostic criteria was known as "Charcot's triad" and consisted of scanning speech, intention tremor, and nystagmus. Further, his early work emphasized the central tenet of MS diagnosis, that of being a disorder that is multiphasic in producing clinical attacks occurring at different times in a patient's life, and affecting distinctly different CNS injury targets (hence the adage "multiple events in space and time"). Since

the time of Charcot, clinicians have witnessed an expanded and more precise series of diagnostic criteria that have refined the ability to confirm the diagnosis with greater sensitivity and specificity.[6-9] Perhaps what has changed most profoundly in the last few decades has been the recognition that the presentation of a clinically isolated demyelinating syndrome, the first recognizable clinical event, is most typically associated with clear and unmistakable dissemination of ineloquent brain or spinal cord lesions.[10] This suggests that most of those evaluated with a clinically isolated demyelinating syndrome already have MS (once the mimics have been excluded) as their working diagnosis. This observation underscores the difficulty in trying to identify the true onset of the disease process, making proclamations about early diagnosis and treatment intervention erroneous in most circumstances. There have now been three published early treatment clinical trials that demonstrate benefit to those patients randomized to active disease-modifying therapy with interferon at the time of their clinically isolated demyelinating syndrome, when compared with those receiving placebos.[11-13] This suggests that the rubric of MS only being declared at a time when a patient has experienced multiple attacks or exacerbations in "space and time" is outdated and likely of detriment to patients. Instead, it now seems appropriate to use the "working diagnosis" of MS when patients present with a single (or more than one) event, not explained by an alternative etiology, and when there is evidence of disease dissemination anatomically as defined by MR imaging criteria. There is little debate today that MS is radiographically substantially more active (perhaps as much as 5–10 times) than what is anticipated observing clinically over time. This confirms that the disease process in MS is much more active than previously appreciated and likely constitutively. An important point of emphasis here is that this level of heightened activity observed by MR imaging is done so with conventional technical applications. With the advent of nonconventional MR imaging techniques, such as with diffusion tensor, magnetization transfer, and spectroscopic applications, it seems that nearly the entire central neuraxis of MS is affected by the disease process (see other sections in this issue for further discussion). Perhaps MS is not truly characterized by "multiple" areas of sclerosis, but rather the true representation of the disease and its associated histopathologic profile is one of a "diffuse" sclerosis.

The inflammatory hypothesis as an underlying and unifying principle for understanding how the course and tempo of tissue injury proceeds in MS is not a contemporary advance. Instead, it was known for quite some time that a distinguishing feature of this disease has been related to the conspicuous and exuberant presence of mononuclear cell infiltrates that seem to congregate around postcapillary venules within the brain and spinal cord. The initial and most rigorous observation of this classic pathologic profile was published by Rindfleisch[14] in 1863. Using rudimentary microscopic techniques, he was able to identify perivenular inflammation in tissues derived from patients with MS. This observation has been corroborated innumerable times, and has been the basis and pretext for widespread research on the mechanisms of mononuclear cell trafficking from the circulation into the various tissue compartments of the body.

Although is it fully appreciated that the interaction of specific families of adhesion molecules facilitates the redistribution of lymphocytes and macrophages from the circulation to the blood vessel endothelium for physical tethering and stabilization, and ultimately transmigration into the CNS, in general there is a paucity of endothelial expression of these molecules in normal subjects. Alternately, in MS patients, there is an unmistakable up-regulation in the expression of cell adhesion molecules on cerebrovascular endothelium

that can serve as a scaffolding for the migration of circulating mononuclear cells into the brain and spinal cord.[15] On their entry, these cells can then participate in a complex orchestration of injury cascades that seem to culminate in inflammation; demyelination; remyelination; axonal dysfunction or degeneration; oligodendrocyte apoptosis; and ultimately neurodegeneration and gliosis (the sclerosis component of MS).

WHAT IS THE EVIDENCE FOR INFLAMMATORY MECHANISMS UNDERLYING TISSUE INJURY IN MULTIPLE SCLEROSIS?

Although those who have worked in this field recognize and appreciate the contributions made by modeling inflammation and cellular trafficking mechanisms in animal models of MS, it is abundantly evident that these models do not fully parody the full complexity of molecular processes that are being elucidated in human inflammatory demyelinating disease. As such, this section avoids any discussion whatsoever as it relates to the use of animal experimentation as it may be related to MS pathophysiology, immunology, or immunogenetics. Instead, it is now patently clear that much has actually been learned from the direct investigation of the MS disease process in those afflicted with the condition.

MS is similar to a number of other immune-mediated disorders in that there seems to be fundamental derangements in a series of regulator mechanisms that allow the proceedings of the immune system normally to be telescoped on the identification and neutralization of foreign invaders (eg, virus, bacteria, fungi, parasites). Unfortunately, in MS there is also a corresponding capability inherent within the immune system that allows for the inappropriate recognition of self-epitopes fomenting a series of inflammatory reactions that lead to tissue injury. The ability precisely to distinguish between self-antigens and foreign antigens is related to these regulatory mechanisms that collectively might be referred to as "tolerance." A breach in tolerance has been considered as a central hypothesis within the landscape of autoimmune disorders. In a sense, the behavior of the immune system is likely akin to that of the system when confronted with a transplanted organ (a kidney, heart, and so forth). As such, MS may be highly related to processes that are germane to transplant rejection. It is not surprising that a number of therapeutic strategies applied to MS and related diseases involve treatments that are mainstays of transplant medicine.

An important disclaimer in any discussion related to the underlying principles of how inflammation is integrated into the grand schema of MS pathophysiology, is that the primary genetic and environmental factors that predispose to and trigger the disease process remain enigmatic. Despite this, much has been learned about the phenomenology that ensues after the inception of the disease process. For instance, it has been demonstrated that MS patients do have T cells that are actively primed against myelin antigens (albeit not exclusively).[16,17] Relevant to this observation has been that the presence of these cellular clones is strongly correlated with clinical disease activity and resultant disability.[18] An interesting feature of these differentiated and potentially pathogenic (at least partially) lymphocytes is that they exhibit features that render them more resistant to programmed cell death (ie, apoptosis), implicating a failure of an adaptive process that serves to screen and edit the evolution and expansion of autoaggressive responses. Studies using anti-CD4 strategies may have failed on the basis of this disease-related inherent resistance.[19,20]

The indiscriminate depletion of T cells may not be a viable treatment strategy for patients with MS for a variety of reasons. A subpopulation of CD4$^+$ T helper cells was recently characterized as regulatory T (Treg) cells. The biologic function of these cells seems to be the maintenance of immune homeostasis[1,2,21,22] The transcription factor forkhead box p3 (FOXp3) seems to be a key regulator of Treg function[1,2,21,22] It was recently demonstrated that FOXp3 transcription and protein levels are decreased in patients with MS[6,23]

Pathologic investigations of human MS brain tissue have revealed various histopathologic substrates, with some degree of heterogeneity.[15,24–26] The parenchymal CNS infiltrate has been shown to consist of B and T cells along with macrophages. Although both CD4 and CD8 T cells are redistributed from the peripheral circulation into the perivenular space and CNS parenchyma, importantly, CD8 T cells seem to be enriched and clonally expanded in MS[27] indicating that they must play an important local role. The antigenic specificity of these cells and their role (pathogenic versus immune regulatory), however, is still unclear. Importantly, CNS-specific autoreactive CD8 T-cell responses are classically noted in RRMS.[28] In contrast, a deficiency of CD4 and CD8 T-cell regulatory functions may underlie the proinflammatory state in MS.[29] For instance, therapy with glatiramer acetate results in the restoration of this regulatory capacity of CD8 T cells, which may serve as an important anti-inflammatory mechanism associated with mitigation of the disease both clinically and radiographically.[29,30]

In addition to the role posited for T-cell dysregulation in MS, a number of lines of evidence have implicated humoral mechanisms as a central element of MS disease pathogenesis. In 1942, Kabat and colleagues[31] reported that cerebrospinal fluid derived from MS patients contained evidence of antibody synthesis (the oligoclonal band) that seemed to be compartment driven (corresponding synthesis was not observed in the peripheral blood). These early studies have been corroborated and expanded (including refined recommendations for using isoelectric focusing techniques to optimize sensitivity) such that it is now recognized that most MS patients have cerebrospinal fluid findings of oligoclonal bands and that their presence at the time of clinically isolated demyelinating syndrome strongly predicts conversion to clinically definite MS.[32] It is important to underscore, however, that a vast array of inflammatory and infectious etiologies can also result in the production of cerebrospinal fluid oligoclonal bands.

Humoral immune responses involve a complex series of molecular changes within B cells that ultimately result in the production of antibodies. On stimulation of B cells there is an initial process of somatic hypermutation within immunoglobulin genes to commence the process of epitope recognition and binding to the business end of antibodies. With time and repeated stimulation (as with booster immunizations) affinity maturation is promoted. Initial development of early IgM antibodies is later transitioned to a class switch to long-term IgG classed antibodies.

A humoral mechanism of potential relevance (albeit not yet proved in MS) to the mechanisms of inflammation in MS is molecular mimicry. An active infection normally generates B cell–derived antibodies targeted against infectious epitopes, which can be structurally (sequence or spatial domain) homologous to self tissue epitopes thereby establishing the possibility of cross-reactivity and the development of autoaggressive immune responses. There is some evidence for this process in patients infected with human T-lymphotropic virus 1 who develop an associated myelopathy (also known as "tropical spastic pareparesis").[33] It is important to recognize that the human immune system has an inherent capability to generate autoaggressive responses but that a series of adaptive regulatory control mechanisms averts most of these. For instance, the evolution of B cell–derived self-targeted antibodies can provoke replacement of the immunoglobulin light chains with newly arranged molecular variations.[34] This process has been referred to as "receptor revision" or "editing" and has been documented in B cells derived from the cerebrospinal fluid of MS patients.[35] Nevertheless, a failure in the competency of these editing mechanisms may underlie some aspects of humorally mediated tissue injury in MS. The role of B-cell regulation in the pathogenesis and perpetuation of MS has been further appreciated by a recent study that showed that a selective monoclonal antibody against a B-cell developmental protein, CD20, was able significantly to reduce both clinical and MR imaging measures of disease activity in a small cohort of RRMS patients.[36]

EPITOPE SPREADING

Another process that seems to be relevant to the pathophysiology of MS involves the diversification of the antigenic specificity of immune responses over the course of the disease.[37] Such changes influence both cellular and humor limbs of the immune response and represent an important adaptive strategy for ensuring the recognition and neutralization of infectious agents.[38] If, however, such reactions are targeted against self-antigens, then the steady amplification and diversity of these molecular interactions can similarly enhance the fidelity and hard-wiring of such responses thereby establishing the basis for a maladaptive low threshold, and nearly constitutive (given the pervasive presence of self-antigens and their exposure to antigen-presenting cells, T and B cells) disease activity in MS patients.

LYMPHOCYTE NOMENCLATURE AND PHENOTYPE

General principles and corresponding generalizations that stem from them can often represent the nidus of great misunderstanding, oversimplification, and strongly held erroneous concepts about how highly complex processes can be codified and reduced to a few concrete models of interaction. When it comes to understanding immune regulation in health or illness, nothing is further from reality. The immune system rivals any of the great creations of the universe. It is endowed with the ability to learn, memorize, refine memory, distort memory, lie about its memory, lose its memory, and can be dynamically influenced for a lifetime. With all of this, the immune system has "legs," it moves and provides surveillance diffusely and compartmentally to the entire physical milieu. With these points in mind, it is preposterous to assume that one can honestly segregate immune responses into functional stratifications of proinflammatory or anti-inflammatory patterns of behavior. And yet, this is exactly what has been achieved (with some important limitations) over the last 50 years. The most salient

and recognizable framework for characterizing the behavior of T cells has been the rubric of TH_1 and TH_2 phenotypes, which are classically partitioned into inflammatory and regulatory behavioral patterns, respectively. Although the ultimate function and behavior of these cells is modifiable, their classification is based largely on the cytokines they produce when assayed.[39] For instance, TH_1 cells are typically associated with the preferential release of proinflammatory cytokines, such as interferon-γ and tumor necrosis factor-β, and may be educated in an interleukin (IL)-12–rich environment. IL-12 and tumor necrosis factor-β are thought to be associated with MS-related disease activity.[40–42] Analysis of peripheral blood mononuclear cells derived from MS patients shows augmented expression of IL-12 when compared with cells derived from control subjects,[43] supporting the notion of a "TH_1" bias. In contrast, TH2 cells elaborate IL-4, IL-5, IL-6, and IL-13[44] and are thought of as anti-inflammatory or protective in this context. TH_{17} cells that produce IL-17, under the influence of IL-23 or IL-6 and transforming growth factor-β, are gaining a great deal of prominence as pathogenic cells in MS and other diseases.[45] At the same time, different types of CD4 regulatory cells, such as FOXP3+ CD4CD25+ classic Tregs, the IL-10–producing Tr1 cells, and the transforming growth factor-β–producing "TH_3" cells also seem to be involved in down-regulation of inflammation. The relationships between many of these populations is only beginning to be unveiled and it may be possible that there is more plasticity in these populations than previously imagined, including the secretion of effector and regulatory cytokines by the same cells.

Important lessons have been learned concerning the differential regulation of immune system cytokines and chemokines, some of which are particularly relevant to the clinical course of the disease. For instance, interferons are well recognized to have anti-inflammatory, antiviral, and antiproliferative immune effects. An early MS treatment trial used interferon-γ to treat a RRMS population of patients and was shown to provoke new exacerbations.[46] This cytokine is known to increase the expression of the major histocompatibility complex type II antigen, which is required for the process of antigen presentation and the subsequent development of cellular and humoral immune responses.[47] Treatment with a different interferon-β seems to help in reducing clinical MS disease activity, the mechanisms of which are unclear. Other drugs, such as glatiramer acetate and statins, seem to promote a TH_1 to TH_2 shift but the relationship between this shift and the clinical effects remains poorly understood.[48,49]

The more recently characterized TH_{17} cells,[9] which produce IL-17 and IL-22, may also play a critical role in MS pathogenesis.[50] Research in this regard is ongoing, and the effect of currently used pharmaceuticals on these cells is incompletely understood at this time.

MANAGING CELLULAR TRAFFICKING IN MULTIPLE SCLEROSIS

One of the most important research advances in modern biology has been the elucidation of cellular adhesion pathways. Cellular trafficking (eg, immune system surveillance) across the various tissue compartments of the body is contingent on the use of specific molecular motifs that serve the purpose of physically stabilizing cells to prepare them for transmigration into organ parenchyma. With respect to MS, it is now recognized that an expanded number of cells enter the brain and spinal cord, at least partially enabled by the heightened expression of adhesion molecules on the endothelial surface of postcapillary venules. Selectins are adhesion molecules on endothelium that interact with cell surface mucin motifs on mononuclear cells. This interaction facilitates slowing and rolling of these cells on the vessel surface. Subsequently, cell surface integrins (eg, very late antigen-4) receptors on lymphocytes and macrophages interact with endothelially expressed members of the immunoglobulin supergene family proteins (they structurally resemble antibodies and serve to mediate adhesion), such as vascular cell adhesion molecule 1. This interaction facilitates physical and firm stabilization. Once these cells are anchored to the endothelium, they then use matrix metalloproteinases, which serve to digest fibronectin and basement membrane collagen to create a channel of passage for the migration of lymphocytes into the brain and spinal cord. On their entry, these cells then have the ability to mediate damage through a variety of injury cascades involving cytokines, chemokines, free radicals, superoxides, antibody and complement-dependent reactions, and changes in ion channels and excitatory amino acid mechanisms.[15] The development of a selective adhesion molecule inhibitor against very late antigen-4 (natalizumab) has resulted in the most effective therapy yet available for MS and powerfully corroborates the contention that basic understanding of the mechanisms of the disease process (including inflammation) is germane to advancing treatment for the disease (**Fig. 1**).[51]

One of the most interesting aspects of MS pathobiology has been the expanded view of MS as a disorder that targets both white and gray matter; produces inflammation and neurodegeneration; and involves both adaptive (eg, remyelination, transition of oligodendrocyte precursors to adult myelinating cells) and maladaptive changes (eg, gliosis) in response to injury. An emerging hypothesis to help explain the transition from inflammation to neurodegeneration has focused on the role of excitotoxicity as a basis for irreversible damage to key neural tissue elements, such as the axon.[52] Following active demyelination, there is altered axonal conduction mechanisms caused by loss of salutatory properties that are afforded by normal myelin internodes punctuated by nodes of Ranvier (the location of sodium channels). Demyelinated axonal segments can then incorporate new sodium channels into the membrane to reconstitute normal conduction physiology. Exaggerated amounts of sodium are then admitted to the intraxonal segments, however, thereby driving molecular strategies to reduce sodium. One strategy involves reversal of the sodium-calcium exchanger, the increased activity of which results in excessive calcium entry, activation of calcium-dependent proteases, culminating in axonal damage and potentially even transaction.[53,54] Further, nitric oxide is increased in MS lesions and this noxious agent can serve to provoke mitochondrial energy failure, and thereby contribute to axonal injury.[55] These observations have prompted the suggestion that sodium channel blockers may serve as a potentially mitigating influence on the progressive aspects of the disease process.[56,57]

CENTRAL NERVOUS SYSTEM NEUROPROTECTION AND REGENERATION

An expanded appreciation now exists for a number of novel injury and potential repair processes within the CNS. A number of neurodevelopmental sequences are activated during the embryologic period that may shed light on potential mechanisms with implications for neuroprotection and potentially even neurorestoration. At the end of development, a receptor signaling system serves to arrest further growth and sprouting of neuritis to ensure their proper distribution and anatomic position. One system is the NOGO receptor apparatus and it has been further characterized to be influenced by a number of molecular agonists, such as NOGO, myelin-associated glycoprotein, oligodendrocyte myelin glycoprotein, and leucine-rich repeat and Ig domain-containing NOGO receptor-interacting protein (LINGO).[58] Arresting the inhibition of the NOGO receptor could potentially be harnessed as a method for potentially promoting regrowth of axons in MS patients. The protein LINGO-1 is a repressor protein that inhibits the

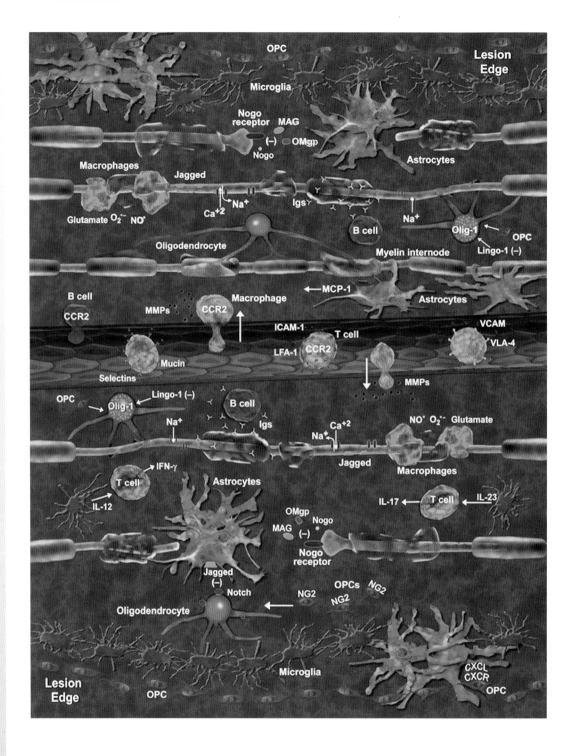

terminal differentiation of oligodendrocyte progen-
itors. A reservoir of these cells persists after development, and may represent storage of a recovery
capability if the inhibitory influence of this protein
can be removed. An inhibitor of LINGO-1 has
been developed and has been proposed to be
used in MS clinical trials in the near future for the
purpose of myelin repair. A number of other pathway interactions (eg, NOTCH and Jagged) also
seem poised to instruct how CNS tissue changes
in MS proceed during injury and what can be
done to encourage molecular events that promote
recovery.

GENETIC AND ENVIRONMENTAL FACTORS

For quite some time it has been realized that MS is
a disorder with both genetic and environmental ru-
diments.[1] Despite this, clinicians continue to
search vigorously for new clues on how such factors interact with each other either to protect
against MS, or heighten the predilection for developing this autoimmune disorder. It has been
learned that the disease is more common in
women and whites; is more ominously progressive
in African Americans; is more common in family
members than in the general population; and that
a restricted set of immune response genes may

Fig. 1. The inflammatory penumbra of the MS plaque. This figure illustrates a myriad of mechanisms that potentially underlie a number of injury cascades that ultimately culminate in the histopathologic substrate of the MS
plaque. The center portion of the figure shows a postcapillary venule in longitudinal section with mononuclear
cells trafficking across the endothelial tight junctions. Mononuclear cells are redistributed from the axial stream
of circulation to the endothelial surface through a series of adhesions interactions involving selectins (that mediate slowing and rolling by interaction with mucin) and the integrin family of cell surface receptors (eg, very late
antigen [VLA-4] and lymphocyte functional associated antigen [LFA-1]) that interact with endothelially expressed
members of the immunoglobulin supergene family of proteins (eg, vascular cell adhesion molecule [VCAM] and
intercellular adhesion molecule [ICAM]). These cells use matrix metalloproteinases (MMPs) to digest basement
membrane type IV collagen and fibronectin to establish a pathway for diapedesis (and a consequent breach in
the integrity of the blood-brain barrier, radiographically evident by gadolinium enhancement). Once these cells
gain entry into the CNS in large numbers, a number of diverse injury processes can become established including
antibody-mediated demyelination; macrophage-associated release of free radicals and superoxides; and the exaggerated release of excitatory amino acids, such as glutamate (acting by the NMDA receptor). Further, demyelination leads to a compromise of axonal conduction, resulting in the incorporation of new sodium channels on
the axonal surface to restore electrical transmission of frequency-coded messages. This can lead to excessive in-
flux of sodium, which prompts reversal of the sodium-calcium exchanger. The eventual accumulation of intra-ax-
onal calcium can lead to the activation of calcium-dependent proteases; release of excitatory amino acids; and
the eventual demise and destruction of the axon (transaction with consequent dying back and wallerian degeneration). In addition to the evident injury cascades illustrated, a number of potential mechanisms may influence
neuroprotection and thereby salvage the inflammatory penumbra. For instance, chemokines and their corresponding receptor interactions may facilitate redistribution of oligodendrocyte progenitor cells (OPCs) from
the lesion edge into the plaque proper, where reconstruction of tissue architecture may be achieved. Chemokine
receptors (CCR) that are important for the processing of cellular trafficking into the CNS are shown distributed on
entering mononuclear cells. The chemokine CCR2 (shown on the surface of entering macrophages, T and B cells)
interacts with monocyte chemoattractant protein (MCP-1), which is elaborated by glial cells, such as astrocytes.
Also important for inflammation is the association of CCR5 with RANTES (not shown). On inflammatory demyelination, a series of repair processes can be initiated, potentially resulting in reconstitution of functioning axons
and olidgodendroglia. At the plaque edge (top and bottom of the figure) microglia are aligned at the perimeter,
intermixed with astrocytes. OPCs with cell surface expression of NG2 (which inhibits oligodendrocyte function)
are developmentally converted into oligodendrocytes with notch expression. Notch interacts with Jagged molecules expressed on astrocytes and axons to prevent myelin production. Withdrawal of this developmental arrest
may be a cardinal step toward the process of remyelination. In the lower right portion of the figure, a chemokine
ligand (CXCL) positive astrocyte interacts with a chemokine receptor (CXCR) positive OPC. Other OPCs are converted into oligodendrocytes where a developmental gene product Olig-1 is shuttled from the nucleus into
the cytoplasm, signaling an activated (potentially myelinating) state of these cells. A recently characterized negative modulator of oligodendrocyte myelination is LINGO-1 (a developmental repressor protein), which can be
manipulated to promote myelin repair in experimental animal models. At sites where axons have been transected, astrocytes accumulate, which represents a potential obstacle for establishing recontinuity of axonal
ends. Astrocytic proliferation at these zones constitutes a major component of the gliotic scar, which character-
izes sclerosis. At the transected ends of axons the NOGO receptor is designated, which when activated by NOGO,
oligodendrocyte myelin glycoprotein (OMgp), or myelin-associated glycoprotein (MAG), prevents the process of
axonal growth and repair. Therapies in the future may focus on NOGO receptor blockade to promote axonal
growth.

modify the risk of MS, particularly in those who are exposed to some cofactor triggering event (perhaps a viral infection). For some time clinicians have known about the association of MS and the histocompatibility leukocyte antigen gene, HLA-DRB*1501. The presence of this gene haplotype is associated with higher risk of MS and with a tumor necrosis factor promoter polymorphism that seems to modulate the expression of TH_1 cytokines.[59] Large-scale robotic sequence techniques have analyzed messenger RNA derived from MS plaques and have shown the abundant presence of alpha-beta crystallin and inducible heat shock protein and osteopontin.[60–62] Osteopontin seems to be capable of influencing the polarization of immune responses toward a phenotype associated with release of interferon-γ and IL-12 (proinflammatory).[60,62] Further, increased levels of osteopontin have been seen in the plasma derived from MS patients during relapses and may represent a potential surrogate of activity.[63]

Most recently, genetic studies have revealed that two additional gene polymorphisms, IL-2 receptor and IL-7, might participate in the susceptibility to MS.[64]

THE FUTURE: WHERE IS IT?

Enormous progress has been achieved in the capability to diagnose and treat both the disease process itself and its resultant symptoms. Despite these important capabilities, clinicians continue to impact only modestly the most important element of the disease process: progression. A deeper interrogation of the mechanisms that ignite the earliest and perpetuate the latest and constitutive processes in MS will likely reveal cascades of injury that are fundamental to injury and whose modification is equally crucial for arresting tissue injury and its resultant impact on physical and intellectual life in patients.

REFERENCES

1. Noseworthy JH, Lucchinetti C, Rodriguez M, et al. Medical progress: multiple sclerosis. N Engl J Med 2000;343:938–52.
2. Frohman EM. Multiple sclerosis. Med Clin N Am 2003;87:867–97.
3. Lublin FD, Baier M, Cutter G. Effect of relapses on development of residual deficit in multiple sclerosis. Neurology 2003;61(11):1528–32.
4. Maeder R. Does the history of multiple sclerosis go back as far as the 14th century? Acta Neurol Scand 1979;60:189–92.
5. Charcot JM. Histologie de la sclerose en plaques. Gaz Hop Civils Milit (Paris) 1868;41:554–8.
6. Schumacher FA, Beeve GW, Kibler RF, et al. Problems of experimental trials of therapy in multiple sclerosis. Ann NY Acad Sci 1965;122:552–68.
7. Poser CM, Paty DW, Scheinberg L, et al. New diagnostic criteria for multiple sclerosis: guidelines for research protocols. Ann Neurol 1983;13:227–31.
8. McDonald WI, Compson A, Edan G, et al. Recommended diagnostic criteria for multiple sclerosis: guidelines from the international panel on the diagnosis of multiple sclerosis. Ann Neurol 2001;50:121–7.
9. Polman CH, Reingold SC, Edan G, et al. Diagnostic criteria for multiple sclerosis: 2005 revisions to the McDonald Criteria. Ann Neurol 2005;58(6):840–6 [review].
10. Frohman EM, Goodin D, Calabresi P, et al. The utility of MRI in suspected MS. The Therapeutics and Technology Assessment Committee of the American Academy of Neurology. Neurology 2003;61:602–11.
11. Comi G, Filippi M, Barkhof F, et al. Effect of early interferon treatment on conversion to definite multiple sclerosis: a randomized study. Lancet 2001;357:1576–82.
12. Jacobs LD, Beck RW, Simon JH, et al. Intramuscular interferon beta-1a therapy initiated during a first demyelinating event in multiple sclerosis. N Engl J Med 2000;343:898–904.
13. Kappos L, Freedman MS, Polman CH, et al. BENEFIT Study Group. Effect of early versus delayed interferon beta-1b treatment on disability after a first clinical event suggestive of multiple sclerosis: a 3-year follow-up analysis of the BENEFIT study. Lancet 2007;370(9585):389–97.
14. Rindfleisch E. Histologische detail zu der grauen degeneration von gehirn and ruckenmark. Virchow Arch Path Anat Physiol 1863;26:474–83.
15. Frohman EM, Raine C, Racke MK. Multiple sclerosis: the plaque and its pathogenesis. N Engl J Med 2006;354:942–55.
16. Lovett-Racke AE, Trotter JL, Lauber J, et al. Decreased dependence of myelin basic protein-reactive T cells on CD28 mediated costimulation in multiple sclerosis patients: a marker of activated memory T cells. J Clin Invest 1998;101:725–30.
17. Scholz C, Patton KT, Anderson DE, et al. Expansion of autoreactive T cells in multiple sclerosis is independent of exogenous B7 costimulation. J Immunol 1998;160:1532–8.
18. Moldavan IR, Rudick RA, Cotleur AC, et al. Interferon gamma responses to myelin peptides in multiple sclerosis correlate with a new clinical measure of disease progression. J Neuroimmunol 2003;141:132–40.
19. van Oosten BW, Lai M, Hodgkinson S, et al. Treatment of multiple sclerosis with monoclonal anti-CD4 antibody cM-T412: results of a randomized, double-blind, placebo-controlled, MRI-monitored phase II trial. Neurology 1997;49:351–7.

20. Rep MH, van Oosten BW, Roos MT, et al. Treatment with depleting CD4 monoclonal antibody results in a preferential loss of circulating naïve T cells but does not affect IFN gamma secreting TH1 cells in humans. J Clin Invest 1997;99:2225–31.
21. Hori S, Nomura T, Sakaguchi S. Control of regulatory T cell development by the transcription factor Foxp3. Science 2003;299:1057–61.
22. Sakaguchi S, Powrie F. Emerging challenges in regulatory T cell function and biology. Science 2007; 317:627–9.
23. Huan J, Culbertson N, Spencer L, et al. Decreased FOXP3 levels in multiple sclerosis patients. J Neurosci Res 2005;81:45–52.
24. Trapp B, Peterson J, Ransohoff RM, et al. Axonal transection in the lesions of multiple sclerosis. N Engl J Med 1998;338:278–85.
25. Lucchinetti CF, Brueck W, Rodriquez M, et al. Distinct patterns of multiple sclerosis pathology indicates heterogeneity in pathogenesis. Brain Pathol 1996;6:259–74.
26. Lucchinetti CF, Brueck W, Rodruquez M, et al. Multiple sclerosis: lessons from neuropathology. Semin Neurol 1998;18:337–49.
27. Babbe H, Roers A, Waisman A, et al. Clonal expansions of CD8+ T cells dominate the T cell infiltrate in active multiple sclerosis lesions as shown by micromanipulation and single cell polymerase chain reaction. J Exp Med 2000;192:393–404.
28. Crawford MP, Yan SX, Ortega S, et al. High prevalence of autoreactive neuroantigen-specific CD8+ T cells in multiple sclerosis revealed by novel flow cytometric assay. Blood 2004;103: 4222–31.
29. Karandikar NJ, Crawford MP, Yan X, et al. Glatiramer acetate (Copaxone) therapy induces CD8+ T cell responses in patients with multiple sclerosis. J Clin Invest 2002;109:641–9.
30. Johnson KP, Brooks MD, Cohen JA, et al. Copolymer 1 reduces relapse rate and improves disability in relapsing-remitting multiple sclerosis: results of a phase III multicenter, double-blind, placebo-controlled trial. Neurology 1995;45:1268–76.
31. Kabat EA, Moore DH, Landow H. An electrophoretic study of the protein components in cerebrospinal fluid and their relationship to the serum proteins. J Clin Invest 1942;21(5):571–7.
32. Villar LM, García-Barragán N, Sádaba MC, et al. Accuracy of CSF and MRI criteria for dissemination in space in the diagnosis of multiple sclerosis. J Neurol Sci 2008;266(1–2):34–7.
33. Levin MC, Lee SM, Kalume F, et al. Autoimmunity due to molecular mimicry as a cause of neurological disease. Nat Med 2002;8:509–13.
34. Nemazee D, Hogquist KA. Antigen receptor selection by editing or downregulation of V(D)J recombination. Curr Opin Immunol 2003;15:182–9.
35. Owens G, Ritchie A, Burgoon M, et al. Single cell repertoire analysis demonstrates clonal expansion is prominent feature of the B cell response in multiple sclerosis spinal fluid. J Immunol 2003;171: 2725–33.
36. Hauser SL, Waubant E, Arnold D, et al. B cell depletion with rituximab in relapsing-remitting multiple sclerosis. N Engl J Med 2008;358:676–88.
37. Lehmann PV, Forsthuber T, Miller A, et al. Spreading of T-cell autoimmunity to cryptic determinants of an autoantigen. Nature 1992;358:155–7.
38. Tian J, Gregori S, Adorini L, et al. The frequency of high avidity T cells determines the hierarchy of determinant spreading. J Immunol 2001;166:7144–50.
39. O'Garra A. Cytokines induce the development of functionally heterogeneous T helper cell subsets. Immunity 1998;8:275–83.
40. Balashov KE, Smith DR, Khoury SJ, et al. Increased IL-12 production in progressive multiple sclerosis: induction by activated CD4+ T cells via CD40 ligand. Proc Natl Acad Sci U S A 1997;94: 599–603.
41. Sharief MK, Hentges R. Association between tumor necrosis factor-alpha and disease progression in patients with multiple sclerosis. N Engl J Med 1991;325:467–72.
42. Mosmann TR, Cherwinski H, Bond MW, et al. Two types of murine helper T cell clone. I. Definition according to profiles of lymphokine activities and secreted proteins. J Immunol 1986;136:2348–57.
43. Comabella M, Balashov K, Issazadeh S, et al. Elevated interleukin-12 in progressive multiple sclerosis correlates with disease activity and is normalized by pulse cyclophosphamide therapy. J Clin Invest 1998;102:671–8.
44. Seder RA, Paul WE. Acquisition of lymphokine-producing phenotype by CD4+ T cells. Annu Rev Immunol 1994;12:635–73.
45. Langrish CL, Chen Y, Blumanschein WM, et al. IL-23 drives a pathogenic T cell population that induces autoimmune inflammation. J Exp Med 2005;201: 233–40.
46. Panitch HS, Hirsch RL, Haley AS, et al. Exacerbations of multiple sclerosis in patients treated with gamma interferon. Lancet 1987;1:893–5.
47. Steimle V, Siegrist CA, Mottet A, et al. Regulation of MHC class II expression by interferon-gamma mediated by the transactivator gene CIITA. Science 1994;265:106–9.
48. Duda PW, Schmied MC, Cook SL, et al. Glatiramer acetate (Copaxone) induces degenerate, Th2-polarized immune responses in patients with multiple sclerosis. J Clin Invest 2000;105:967–76.
49. Youssef S, Stuve O, Patarroyo JC, et al. The HMG-CoA reductase inhibitor, atorvastatin, promotes a Th2 bias and reverses paralysis in central nervous system autoimmune disease. Nature 2002;420:78–84.

50. Harrington LE, Hatton RD, Mangan PR, et al. Interleukin 17–producing CD4+ effector T cells develop via a lineage distinct from the T helper type 1 and 2 lineages. Nat Immunol 2005;6:1123–32.

51. Polman CH, O'Connor PW, Havrdova E, et al. AFFIRM Investigators. A randomized, placebo-controlled trial of natalizumab for relapsing multiple sclerosis. N Engl J Med 2006;354:899–910.

52. Ransom BR, Waxman SG, Davis PK. Anoxic injury of CNS white matter: protective effect of ketamine. Neurology 1990;40:1399–404.

53. Stys PK, Waxman SG, Ransom BR. Ionic mechanisms of anoxic injury in mammalian CNS white matter: role of Na_-Ca2_ exchanger. J Neurosci 1992;12:430–9.

54. Craner MJ, Newcombe J, Black JA, et al. Molecular changes in neurons in MS: altered axonal expression of Nav1.2 and Nav1.6 sodium channels and Na_/C2_ exchanger in the human CNS. Proc Natl Acad Sci U S A 2004;101:8168–73.

55. Smith KJ, Kapoor R, Hall SM, et al. Electrically active axons degenerate when exposed to nitric oxide. Ann Neurol 2001;49:470–6.

56. Kapoor R, Davies M, Blaker PA, et al. Blockers of sodium and calcium entry protect axons from nitric oxide mediated degeneration. Ann Neurol 2003;53: 174–80.

57. Waxman SG. NO and the axonal death cascade. Ann Neurol 2003;53:150–4.

58. Domeniconi M, Cao Z, Spencer T, et al. Myelin-associated glycoprotein interacts with the Nogo66 receptor to inhibit neurite outgrowth. Neuron 2002;35: 283–90.

59. Garcia-Merino A, Alper CA, Usuku K, et al. Tumor necrosis factor microsatellite haplotypes in relation to extended haplotypes, susceptibility to diseases associated with the major histocompatibility complex, and TNF secretion. Hum Immunol 1996;50: 11–21.

60. Chabas D, Baranzini S, Mitchell D, et al. The influence of the pro-inflammatory cytokine, osteopontin, on autoimmune demyelinating disease. Science 2001;294:1731–5.

61. Lock C, Hermans G, Pedotti R, et al. Gene microarray analysis of multiple sclerosis lesions yields new targets validated in autoimmune encephalomyelitis. Nat Med 2002;8:500–8.

62. Steinman L, Zamvil S. Transcriptional analysis of targets in multiple sclerosis. Nat Rev Immunol 2003;3: 483–93.

63. Vogt M, Lopatinskaya L, Smits M, et al. Elevated osteopontin levels are associated with disease activity in relapsing-remitting MS patients. Ann Neurol 2003; 53:819–22.

64. International Multiple Sclerosis Genetics Consortium, Hafler DA, Compston A, et al. Risk alleles for multiple sclerosis identified by a genomewide study. N Engl J Med 2007;357(9):851–62.

The Clinical Epidemiology of Multiple Sclerosis

Christian Confavreux, MD*, Sandra Vukusic, MD, PhD

KEYWORDS
- Multiple sclerosis • Natural history
- Course • Prognosis • Epidemiology

A comprehensive knowledge of the natural course and prognosis of multiple sclerosis (MS) is of utmost importance for a physician to make it affordable in simple descriptive terms to a patient when personal and medical decisions are to be taken. It is still topical because the currently acknowledged disease-modifying agents (DMAs) only marginally alter the overall prognosis of the disease. It provides reference for evaluating the efficacy of a therapeutic intervention in clinical trials; clues for public health services, health insurance companies, and the pharmaceutical industry in their respective activities; and insights into the pathophysiology and treatment of MS. Since the pioneering works of McAlpine,[1,2] many authors have tackled the description of the overall course and prognosis of MS.[3] Thanks to them, precise, consistent, and reliable data from appropriate cohorts have become available and knowledge is fairly comprehensive at least at the level of groups of patients.

METHODOLOGIC CONSIDERATIONS

For a comprehensive analysis of the natural history of MS, several methodologic criteria must be fulfilled.[3–5] This includes considerations on population sampling, clinical assessments, and techniques of data analysis.

Population Sampling

The population of patients with MS under study must be representative of the disease. Ideally, all the cases of the disease present in a well-defined geographic area must have been ascertained and included in the cohort, which is population-based. Such a complete ascertainment is always a difficult challenge in MS, notably in hospital- or clinic-based studies. Benign cases, which do exist, are not so prone to come to neurologic attention. This is even more evident with the well-known patients incidentally found to have the disease at autopsy[6–10] or at neuroimaging examinations.[11,12] This bias leads to an overestimation of the disease severity.[13,14]

Another key point is diagnostic accuracy. No specific diagnostic test is available for MS. The criteria of Poser and colleagues[15] and McDonald and colleagues[16] provide useful safeguards for a secure diagnosis. It must be kept in mind, however, that they are not MS-specific.

A minimum sample size is also needed for the sake of statistical power in such a clinically variable disease as MS. It is difficult to state where the lower limit stands, however, but presumably it is in a range of some hundreds. In principle, the higher the better but this may be at the expense of accuracy, homogeneity, and frequency of assessments. An interesting solution is to pool data from different sources, which is best achieved when they have been collected following the same standards on the same databasing system, such as the EDMUS system.[17,18]

Last but not least, a cohort of patients can be considered as appropriate for the study of the natural history provided that DMAs have not been administered to these patients. This is no longer the case in MS since the mid-1990s with the approval

Service de Neurologie A, Centre de Coordination EDMUS et INSERM U842, Hôpital Neurologique Pierre Wertheimer, 59 Boulevard Pinel, 69677 Lyon-Bron cedex, France
* Corresponding author.
E-mail address: christian.confavreux@chu-lyon.fr (C. Confavreux).

Neuroimag Clin N Am 18 (2008) 589–622
doi:10.1016/j.nic.2008.09.002

and wide prescription of β-interferon, glatiramer acetate, and more recently mitoxantrone and natalizumab. The number of natural history MS cohorts is definitively limited.

Assessments

Ideally, the follow-up must be from the very onset of the disease until death for all included patients. It must be made prospectively, and at regular and as close as possible intervals, because ascertainment of relapses in MS is positively correlated to the frequency of neurologic assessments.[19–21] It is also important to work on robust, easily assessable variables, even in retrospect. Assessments must be made homogeneously. This means that the same acknowledged language, definitions, and scales are to be used for all the patients throughout the study. Standardization and computerization of the data with the adoption of a database system facilitate a uniform description throughout the disease.[17,22–25] Training sessions of examiners allow one to reduce interexaminer variability. All these tools are to be recommended. Unfortunately, for many easily understandable reasons in a disease with such a long duration, these goals are essentially unattainable for the standard follow-up of large cohorts of patients in the long-term.

Data Analysis

Analyses would be straightforward if it were possible to deal with the complete data of the overall sample population until the death of each included individual. Assuming the sample population to be representative of the disease, the results would reflect the truth at least for the area and time under study. Unfortunately, especially in a chronic disease with such a long duration, the researcher is expected to provide results well in advance and has to deal with incomplete data and to provide estimates.

For a population of patients studied at the time of closure of the study with respect to a given end point (or outcome or dependent-variable) as, for instance, a given level of irreversible disability or the onset of progression, any individual fits one of three categories: (1) the end point has already been reached, (2) the individual is still under scrutiny but has not reached the end point, or (3) the patient has been lost to follow-up since a given date at which the end point had not been reached (**Fig. 1**). The last two categories make up the group of censored patients.[3]

In elementary statistical analyses of the past, only the patients who had reached the end point

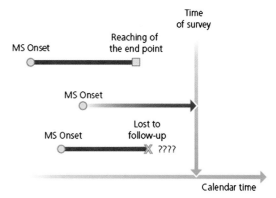

Fig. 1. Schematic representation of the distribution of patients in a cohort at the time of survey, according to their status with respect to reaching the end point under scrutiny. Top line, patients who have reached the end point before the closing of the survey; middle line, patients who have not reached the end point at the time of closure; bottom line, patients who had not reached the end point at the time they were lost to follow-up. (*From* Confavreux C, Compston A. The natural history of multiple sclerosis. In: Compston A, editor. McAlpine's multiple sclerosis. 4th edition. London: Churchill Livingstone Elsevier; 2006. p. 183–272; with permission.)

when the survey closes were taken into account. Patients who had not yet reached this end point by the time of closure, but would do so later, were not included. This approach invariably led to underestimation of the true time interval from the starting point to the end point. Nowadays, more sophisticated survival analyses, such as those produced by the Kaplan-Meier technique, are preferred because the patients who have already reached the end point but also the patients censored at the time of closure of the study are taken into account in the probabilistic estimates of time intervals.[26,27] As compared with the former statistical analyses restricted to observed data, survival analyses provide longer estimates that are closer to reality. These estimates, however, are not necessarily accurate. Noticeably, the proportion of censored patients has a clear influence on these statistics. This can be well illustrated in MS when studying the time to reach disease-related milestones, such as onset of progression or irreversible levels of disability: the higher the proportion of censored patients, the longer the estimated time intervals.[3] For instance, as shown in **Fig. 2** for the Lyon cohort, when the proportion of censored patients was experimentally decreased from 75% to 25%, the median time to reach a score of Disability Status Scale (DSS) 4 decreased from 25.1 to 5.1 years.[28]

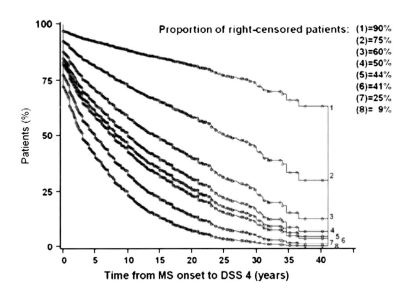

Fig. 2. Kaplan-Meier survival curves for the time from the onset of MS to the assignment of an irreversible score of 4 on the Kurtzke Disability Status Scale (DSS), depending on the proportion of right-censored patients, among the 1844 patients in the Lyon, France, MS cohort. (*From* Confavreux C, Ritleng C, Debouverie M, et al. Defining the natural history of multiple sclerosis: the need for complete data and rigorous definitions. Answer to Tremlett et al. Mult Scler 2008;14:1144–7; with permission.)

MATERIAL AVAILABLE FOR STUDIES ON THE NATURAL HISTORY OF MULTIPLE SCLEROSIS

Schematically, there are two different kinds of material for such a purpose. Both of them have strengths and weaknesses that, in many respects, are complementary. Geographically well-defined long-term natural history cohorts can be considered as representative of MS and provide robust information regarding long-term outcomes. Data related to the initial period of the disease are generally not optimal, however, because in many cases they have been assessed only in retrospect. More generally, for the reasons discussed previously, precision and reliability of the data are heterogeneous from one patient to the other, but also for a given patient during the course of the disease. By contrast, prospective short-term studies, either observational or within the scope of placebo arms of therapeutic trials, can provide precise and robust information regarding the course and prognosis of the disease during the study period. The latter, by design, however, is limited to several months or years. Such studies cannot provide robust results regarding the periods coming before and after the study period and, more generally, the long-term course and prognosis of the disease. Furthermore, the representativeness of the cohort is often limited, as inversely correlated to the tightness of the inclusion criteria.

For the description of the long-term natural history of MS, observational long-term studies are clearly the most valuable, especially those with a systematic longitudinal follow-up and special attention to the assessment of major outcome criteria, being it relapse occurrence, onset of

progression, or time to reach selected landmarks of irreversible disability. In this respect, three cohorts combine the qualities of a relevant information source on the natural history of MS as for the large size and disease representativeness of the selected population; the prospective long-term longitudinal follow up with numerous, comprehensive, standardized clinical assessments at rather close intervals; the absence of significant DMAs; and the appropriate statistical analyses, notably survival techniques: (1) Lyon, France;[29–34] (2) Gothenburg, Sweden;[35–37] and (3) London, Ontario.[38–45]

THE CLINICAL LANDMARKS OF MULTIPLE SCLEROSIS

There are two approaches to describe the natural history of MS. One is qualitative, based on the interplay between relapses and progression, leading to a delineation of the course of the disease. The other one is quantitative, referring to the accumulation of neurologic disability, allowing for assessing the prognosis. Both can serve also in therapeutic trials.

Course-Related Dependent Variables

It has long been recognized that the course of MS may be considered as the expression of two clinical phenomena, relapses and progression,[2,46,47] which correspond to distinct physiopathologic processes within the central nervous system (CNS). The clinical interplay between relapses and progression leads to the consideration of two phases in the disease and three main types of evolution.

Relapses, which may also be called "exacerbations," "attacks," or "bouts," are the clinical counterpart of acute focal inflammation of the CNS.[48] More precisely, they correspond to the occurrence of a new focal acute inflammatory lesion or the reactivation of an older one. They are defined as the occurrence, the recurrence, or the worsening of symptoms of neurologic dysfunction marked by a subacute onset over a few hours or days before plateauing and usually ending with a remission, either partial or complete. They last more than 24 hours but, for some authors, 48 hours is the minimum required duration. Symptoms occurring within a month are considered as part of the same relapse.[15–17,49] Fatigue alone is not considered as a relapse. Similarly, transient fever or exercise-related worsening of symptoms is not considered as a relapse. Indeed, they reflect only transient impairment of the nervous conduction within pre-existing lesions in relation to transient physicochemical changes associated with increase in body temperature or physical exercise (Uhthoff's phenomenon). By contrast, paroxysmal neurologic symptoms occurring in isolation but repeatedly in a given patient for more than 24 hours might qualify for a relapse.

Progression is defined as the steady worsening of symptoms and signs over 6 months at least[15,17,49] or even 12 months according to other authors.[16,50] As soon as progression has started, it goes on continuously throughout the disease, although occasional plateaus and temporary minor improvements may be observed.[51] Most likely, the progression is the clinical manifestation of the chronic, progressive, diffuse degeneration of the CNS, which is the other hallmark of MS, besides the acute, multifocal, recurrent inflammatory process. The date of onset of progression is assessed in retrospect, once the required 6- or 12-month duration of continuous neurologic worsening has been confirmed. There is always some uncertainty regarding this parameter.

The occurrence of relapses and progression leads to the consideration of two distinct phases in the course of MS. The relapsing-remitting (RR) phase is characterized by relapses alternating with periods of clinical inactivity. Neurologic sequelae may be caused by relapses but remain stable (ie, they do not worsen) between relapses. The progressive phase is characterized by the clinical progression defined previously. Relapses may be superimposed onto progression, either at its onset or during its course, or both, as observed in around 40% of the cases.[31,34]

Since Charcot,[46] it has been acknowledged that the disease can enter a steadily progressive stage after successive relapses and remissions, or follow this steadily progressive course right from clinical onset. Concretely, a given patient may present only one of the two phases or both, with in the second case an orderly sequence of the RR phase coming first and followed by a conversion to the progressive phase. To standardize the terminology used in the description of the pattern and course of MS and to improve a mutual understanding of clinicians and researchers, an international survey of clinicians involved in MS has been performed and a consensus has been reached to classify the disease course in four different categories (**Fig. 3**):[51]

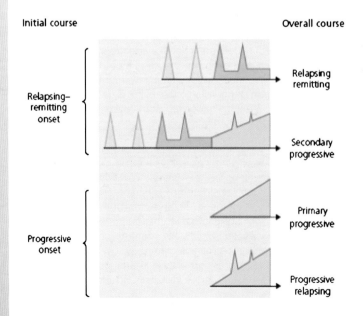

Initial course

Overall course

Relapsing–remitting onset

Relapsing remitting

Secondary progressive

Progressive onset

Primary progressive

Progressive relapsing

Fig. 3. Classification of the course of MS. (*Adapted from* Lublin FD, Reingold SC, for the National Multiple Sclerosis Society (USA) Advisory Committee on Clinical Trials of New Agents in Multiple Sclerosis. Defining the clinical course of multiple sclerosis: results of an international survey. Neurology 1996;46:907–11; with permission.)

1. Relapsing-remitting MS: clearly defined relapses with full recovery or with sequelae and residual deficit on recovery; periods between disease relapses characterized by a lack of disease progression.
2. Secondary progressive MS: initial relapsing-remitting disease course followed by progression with or without occasional relapses, minor remissions, and plateaus.
3. Primary progressive MS: disease progression from onset with occasional plateaus and temporary minor improvements allowed.
4. Progressive-relapsing MS: progressive disease from onset, with clear acute relapses, with or without full recovery; periods between relapses characterized by continuing progression.

It must be noted that in this classification the presence or absence of superimposed relapses were both allowed in secondary progressive (SP) MS cases, whereas primary progressive (PP) cases with superimposed relapses were split from PP cases without (progressive-relapsing [PR] MS versus PPMS).

Prognosis-Related Dependent Variables

The second dimension in the history of MS is quantitative with the appearance of disability, which may be transitory, partially reversible, or definitely irreversible. A way of describing the natural outcome of MS is to assess the time course of disability accumulation. This leads one to address the issue of scoring in MS. The scale, which has been used in most of the works devoted to the description of the natural history of MS, is the DSS[52,53] and its detailed version, the Expanded Disability Status Scale (EDSS).[54] Such a scale, however, has acknowledged shortcomings and limitations.[55–57] It has repeatedly been shown to have only moderate interrater reliability.[18,55,58–63] It must also be realized that the EDSS scale is ordinal and categorical but neither quantitative nor continuous. The assumption that disability, as measured by the EDSS scale, naturally continues to progress at a similar rate all over the course of the disease is clearly contradicted by empiric observations.[38,41,64,65] Despite this impressive list of limitations and criticisms, the EDSS scale has gained unrivalled familiarity and most popularity in the community of clinicians involved in MS. Only a small number of the many other scales suggested for MS are used, particularly in clinical trials, such as the MS functional composite, which is more sensitive and multidimensional than its elder.[56,57] To date, however, no scale fulfills the requirements of the international MS community.[55,63,66]

For the specific purpose of epidemiologic studies requiring long-term follow-up of numerous patients, such as natural history studies of MS, it has proved valuable to focus on robust landmarks of disability that could be easily identified through successive neurologic assessments and through retrospective interview of the patient whenever necessary. For the study of the 1844 patients of the Lyon cohort, selected landmarks of disability were DSS 4, limited walking ability but able to walk more than 500 m without assistance and without resting; DSS 6, ability to walk only with unilateral support and no more than 100 m without resting; and DSS 7, ability to walk no more than 10 m without using a wall or furniture for support. Other series have also addressed other landmarks usually defined as follows: DSS 3, moderate dysfunction (monoparesis, mild hemiparesis, and so forth; and DSS 8, restricted to bed, but with effective use of arms).

Long-term natural history studies also focus on the accumulation of irreversible disability. In the Lyon studies, disability was defined as irreversible when a given score persisted at least 6 months, excluding transient worsening of disability related to relapses. By definition, when a given score of irreversible disability had been assigned to a patient, all the scores of disability that could be subsequently assessed during the follow-up of this same patient were either equal to or higher than the initial score.[31,67]

THE ONSET OF MULTIPLE SCLEROSIS

The demographic and disease-related characteristics of the onset of MS are currently well-delineated thanks to the numerous series devoted to this issue.[3] A female predominance is apparent in all representative studies. The usual ratio is two females for one male. The highest proportion for females has been found at 71% and the lowest at 51%.

Age at Onset of Multiple Sclerosis

There is a consensus for peak onset around 30 years of age. In most representative series, the distribution of patients by age at onset of the disease is essentially bell-shaped, with onset before the age of 20 years in around 10%, from ages 20 to 40 years in 70%, and after the age of 40 years in 20% of the cases. Onset after 55 years of age is rare and should question the diagnosis of MS. Females often seem to have a slightly younger mean age at onset than males. Furthermore, the female/male ratio is usually found to decrease as age at onset increases.

Initial Symptoms

There is no alternative, for many patients, to have their initial symptomatology assessed other than in retrospect, with an interval of months or years between the clinical onset of the disease and the first clinical evaluation. In such circumstances, it is difficult, if not erroneous, to try to go into discrete details for the description and the classification of the initial symptoms and signs. Furthermore, many wordings, although in large use, are poorly defined and may prove misleading. This is the case, for instance, for such terminologies as "motor symptoms," "cerebellar," "pyramidal," "monosymptomatic," "polysymptomatic," "monoregional," and "polyregional." It is wise to classify initial symptoms conservatively in broad categories.[17,31] That said, there is some consensus among the different long-term natural history series in the literature with respect to the distribution of initial symptoms in MS:[3] an incidence of around 15% for isolated optic neuritis, 10% for isolated brainstem dysfunction, 50% for isolated dysfunction of long tracts, and 25% for various combinations of these symptoms are reasonable estimates.

The influence of gender on the initial symptomatology of MS has usually been found to be either nil or marginal. By contrast, an obvious influence of the age at onset of the disease has consistently been found, with a higher percentage of optic neuritis and diplopia in the patients with an earlier onset and of motor disturbances in the patients with a later onset.[38,68–71]

Initial Course

It has become commonplace to call "clinically isolated syndrome" any initial neurologic episode suggestive of MS, provided its onset is acute or subacute; its course is RR; its symptomatology can be attributed to a dysfunction of optic nerves, brainstem, or spinal cord; and appropriate paraclinical investigations have been performed to discard any alternative diagnosis to that of suspected MS.[72–76] It is clear, however, that this denomination is used in different ways according to different authors, from purely monosymptomatic presentations attributable to a single lesion in the CNS, to any RR initial episode. Classical wordings seem still preferable, such as "first neurologic episode" or "inaugural demyelinating episode."

Some differences emerge among the literature as to the actual relative proportions between the two types of initial course of the disease. Indeed, the frequency of cases with progression from onset relatively to cases with an RR onset has been found to range from 5%[65] to 37%.[64] These

extreme figures are likely to be related to recruitment differences. They can also result from classification bias, as has been shown in the London, Ontario, cohort.[38,39] When the Canadian authors updated the data on their total cohort of 1099 patients in 1996, they had to reassign a significant number of patients with respect to the overall clinical course of the disease, because these patients were able to recall a remote first relapse only after several previous visits. From the currently available literature, the initial course of MS can be reasonably estimated to be RR in 85% of the cases and progressive in 15%.[30–32,36,37,42–44]

Since Müller's work,[68,69] it has been repeatedly found that men are more exposed than women to a progressive onset of MS, and that symptoms related to dysfunction of long tracts are relatively more frequent, whereas optic nerve and brainstem symptoms are relatively less frequent in progressive-onset cases compared with RR-onset cases.[2,30,77,78] The strongest correlation between the initial course of the disease and clinical variables assessable at the onset of MS is related to age: the proportion of progressive-onset cases rises steadily with age.[2,29,38,68,69,79–82]

THE OVERALL COURSE OF MULTIPLE SCLEROSIS

Most patients with MS experience successive, distinct, neurologic events: relapses for the most part and onset of progression for a number of them. The focus here is on the events' timing during the course of the disease.[70]

Recovery from the First Neurologic Episode

The key predictive factor of remission is the duration of the ongoing neurologic episode before admission to the hospital: the longer this duration, the lower the probability of improvement.[83,84] The estimates regarding the proportion of cases matching the definition of incomplete recovery following a first acute episode suggestive of MS range from 16% to 30%.[32,37,78]

Development of the Second Neurologic Episode

This topic has recently received renewed attention with the advent of DMAs. Indeed, the development of a second neurologic episode allows one to qualify a case of possible MS for conversion to definite MS provided the second episode involves a new site within the CNS.[15] Following such a conversion, there is additional rationale to offer DMAs.

The first issue is the overall rate of occurrence of the second neurologic episode during the disease. McAlpine and Compston[2] are the first clearly to demonstrate that the highest chance to develop a second neurologic episode comes immediately after the initial episode and that it diminishes progressively thereafter. A remarkably similar distribution was observed in the Lyon series with a median at 1.9 years (**Fig. 4**)[30–32] in agreement with other series.[37,85]

Another source of information comes from the placebo arms of the randomized controlled trials having specifically enrolled patients with a first neurologic episode suggestive of MS. The ONTT trial[86–88] has enrolled only patients suffering from an acute optic neuritis whatever the results of the brain MR imaging. The CHAMPS trial[89,90] enrolled patients with a monofocal episode and two T2 lesions at least on the baseline brain MR image. The episode involved the optic nerve in 50% of the cases, the spinal cord in 28%, or the brainstem-cerebellum in 22%. In the ETOMS trial,[91] patients were enrolled following either a monofocal (61% of the cases) or a multifocal (39%) episode with at least four T2 lesions. Last, for being enrolled in the BENEFIT trial,[92] patients had to present with a monofocal (53% of the cases) or a multifocal (47%) episode, and at least two T2 lesions. The cumulative probability according to Kaplan-Meier estimates of developing a second neurologic episode qualifying for MS at 2 years has been 18% in ONTT, 38% in CHAMPS, 45% in ETOMS, and 45% in BENEFIT. With the exception of the ONTT trial, the median time to the second neurologic episode was close to 2 years, in agreement with what has been observed in the long-term natural history series.

Differences in the recruitment criteria explain the lower likelihood of developing a second neurologic episode within 2 years of follow-up in the ONTT trial. Indeed, enrolment was restricted to a first episode of optic neuritis only for that trial. It is well known that a significant proportion of isolated acute optic neuritis never evolves to MS, notably in cases with normal brain MR imaging.[93] For instance, in a Swedish cohort of 86 patients of isolated unilateral acute optic neuritis followed prospectively for up to 31 years, the cumulative probability of developing a second neurologic episode was 40% at 15 years of disease evolution and this proportion did increase only marginally during the subsequent years of follow-up.[94] A similar conclusion can be drawn from the prospective evaluation of 320 patients suffering from a clinically isolated syndrome in Barcelona.[95] By comparison with cases with brainstem syndromes, spinal cord syndromes, or other localizations, cases with optic neuritis were twice more likely to exhibit a normal baseline MR image and less likely to suffer from a second neurologic episode during the follow-up. It can be argued whether optic neuritis is more benign than other localizations of first neurologic episodes suggestive of MS or, more likely, optic neuritis with normal baseline MR imaging is essentially not MS.

A large multicenter collaborative study of 532 patients with a first neurologic episode suggestive of MS and a mean follow-up of 3.6 years[96] provided a Kaplan-Meier estimate of 7.1 years for the median time to conversion to clinically definite MS (CDMS). This estimate is markedly at odds with the former data analyzed previously and the clinical experience of the neurologist familiar with MS. It must be noted, however, that the outcome in this study was not the occurrence of a second neurologic episode but the conversion to CDMS, which, according to accepted criteria,[15] requires that the new clinical episode affects other parts of the CNS compared with the first clinical episode. Furthermore, this cohort was overrepresented with optic neuritis cases (52%) and included a large proportion (30%) of cases without asymptomatic lesions (mostly patients with no lesions at all) on the baseline brain MR imaging scan. As discussed, a substantial proportion of such patients never convert to MS. Awaiting results from the further follow-up of this cohort, the median time to the second neurologic episode can be reasonably estimated to be 2 years (ie, the proportion of patients suffering from a second neurologic episode is around 50% at 2 years of follow-up).

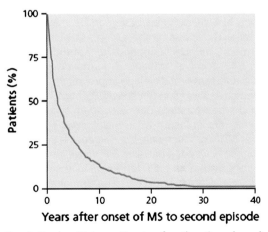

Fig. 4. Kaplan-Meier estimates for the time (years) from onset of MS to the second episode, among the 1562 patients with an exacerbating-remitting initial course in the Lyon, France, MS cohort. (*Adapted from* Confavreux C, Vukusic S, Adeleine P. Early clinical predictors and progression of irreversible disability in multiple sclerosis: an amnesic process. Brain 2003;126:770–82; with permission.)

A second issue concerns the clinical factors that may influence the rate of occurrence of the second neurologic episode in MS. According to the long-term natural history series, there is no such clinical predictive factor, be it gender, age at onset of the disease, monofocality or multifocality of initial symptoms, degree of recovery from the initial episode, and a RR or SP overall course of the disease.[30,37] According to the CHAMPS trial, the 2-year cumulative probability of developing a second episode was similar for optic neuritis, spinal cord syndromes, and brainstem-cerebellar syndromes[90] in agreement with the observations made in Barcelona when optic neuritis cases with abnormal baseline MR imaging only were compared with other inaugural topographic syndromes.[95] This probability was twice higher for multifocal than monofocal presentations in the ETOMS trial,[91] whereas no difference was found in the BENEFIT trial.[92]

The third issue deals with the paraclinical factors that may influence the transition to a second neurologic episode. Results clearly show a strong effect of brain MR imaging abnormalities that may be observed at baseline. The four randomized controlled trials focusing on a first neurologic episode have consistently shown that the higher the number of T2 lesions on the baseline brain MR image, the higher the probability of developing a second episode.[87,91,92,97,98] Presence of enhancing lesions on the baseline MR image seemed the strongest predictor of the development of a second episode in CHAMPS.[98] It was also influential in BENEFIT,[92] but not in ETOMS.[91] Prospective observational studies devoted to patients presenting with a first neurologic episode suggestive of MS have also shown that the presence or the number of multifocal brain MR imaging abnormalities markedly increases the probability of a second neurologic episode within 1 to 3 years,[74,76,95,99–108] but also 5 years,[72] 10 years,[75] and 14 years of follow-up.[109] For instance, in the Queen Square series of 89 patients, conversion to CDMS was observed within 5 years in 65% of the 57 cases with abnormal baseline MR image (defined as one or more lesions compatible with MS) compared with 3% of the 32 cases with normal MR imaging.[72] For the 81 patients still followed at 10 years, the corresponding figures were 83% and 11%.[75] At 14 years, among the 71 patients still under scrutiny, figures were 88% and 19%, respectively.[109] In the previously mentioned cohort of 532 patients with a first neurologic episode suggestive of MS,[96] the Kaplan-Meier estimates at 2 years of survival time for the occurrence of a new clinical episode qualifying for CDMS ranged from about 10% for the group

of patients without asymptomatic lesions (mostly patients with no lesion at all) to about 45% for the group of patients fulfilling the Barkhof-Tintoré dissemination in space criteria (**Fig. 5**). The T2 lesion volume on brain MR imaging at presentation does also play a role: the higher this volume, the higher the risk of developing a second episode.[73,109] Several studies have shown that the presence of gadolinium-enhancing lesions on T1-weighted brain MR imaging is a stronger predictor than the presence of T2 lesions for the probability of developing a second episode.[74,107] An extensive analysis of the T2 and T1 parameters has also demonstrated that the presence of juxtacortical lesions, infratentorial lesions, and periventricular lesions are all independent predictors of the occurrence of a second neurologic episode in the short term.[74] These data have served as a rationale for developing the MR imaging Barkhof criteria qualifying for the dissemination in space, which are used in the current diagnostic classification of MS.[16,110]

Data gathered from repeating early brain MR imaging add significance to the predictions. The presence of new T2 lesions or gadolinium-enhancing lesions on a brain MR image performed 3 months after the baseline MR image[107] or 12 months after the initial episode[108] are both predictors of the occurrence of a second episode. For instance, among 68 patients presenting with a monofocal episode in the British study,[107] development of a second episode at 1 year was observed in 33% of the "baseline MR imaging T2-positive" patients; 52% of the "baseline MR imaging T1-positive" patients; 57% of the "repeatedly T2-positive" patients (defined by the presence of T2 lesions on baseline MR imaging and of new T2 lesions on the second MR image performed 3 months later); and 70% of the "repeatedly T1-positive" patients. Information gathered from the second MR image improves the positive predictive value and the specificity of MR imaging for the development of a second episode. These results are obtained while maintaining sensitivity over 80% for T2 criteria, but decreasing sensitivity from 61% with the baseline MR image only, down to 39% with both brain MR imaging scans for the T1 criteria. These data served as a rationale for using the results of serial early brain MR imaging for satisfying dissemination in time in patients still at the clinical stage of a single neurologic episode.[16]

Typical abnormalities in the baseline cerebrospinal fluid, abnormal results of baseline evoked potentials, and presence of HLA-DR2 antigen are all associated with a shorter time to a second episode. Their predictive value, however, has generally been found to be lower than that of brain MR imaging.[72,101–104,106] Lately, in a study involving

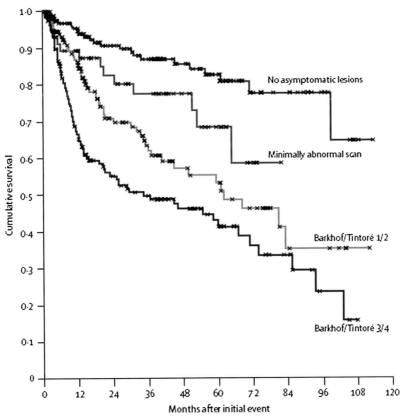

Fig. 5. Kaplan-Meier estimates for the time (years) from the first neurologic episode suggestive of MS to a second neurologic episode qualifying for clinically definite MS according to the Poser and colleagues[15] criteria, among 532 patients with a clinically isolated syndrome. Influence of the number and the spatial distribution of hyperintense lesions observed on proton density T2-weighted sequences on baseline brain MR imaging. Log-rank test, *P* < .001. Minimally abnormal scan = at least one asymptomatic lesion but not fulfilling any of the Barkhof-Tintoré criteria. Barkhof-Tintoré 1/2 and 3/4 refers to the number of fulfilled criteria. (*From* Korteweg T, Tintore M, Uitdehaag B, et al. MRI criteria for dissemination in space in patients with clinically isolated syndromes: a multicentre follow-up study. Lancet Neurol 2006;5:221–27; with permission.)

103 patients with an initial monofocal episode, the presence of antimyelin antibodies in the serum was associated with a dramatically increased risk of developing a second episode, as compared with the seronegative patients.[111] These results have not been confirmed, however, by subsequent studies.[112]

Relapse Frequency

Considerable variations have been reported, from 0.1 to more than one relapse per year. Such a variability is not surprising because of the frequent difficulties encountered by clinicians in defining a relapse and discarding a pseudorelapse. Furthermore, clear-cut differences in the estimates of the relapse frequency emerge when comparing retrospective and prospective assessments, the latter technique leading to higher figures than the former.[19,21] The frequency of assessments is also important; the higher it is, the more sensitive the detection of relapses.[19] That said, in the cross-sectional studies with ensuing retrospective assessment of relapses, the yearly relapse rate is usually found to be lower than 0.5.[2,79,85,113] By contrast, in the studies with longitudinal prospective assessments, the yearly relapse rate is usually found to be higher than 0.5.[19,21,30,114] Results from these prospective studies are fairly consistent with the figure of 2 years found for the median time from onset of MS to the second episode and for the subsequent relapses during the RR phase of the disease (the authors' unpublished data). It may be concluded that 0.5 or slightly more is a reasonable estimate of the yearly relapse rate in a standard, representative RR population of MS patients.

Many authors consider that the relapse rate declines as the disease duration increases.[2,21,35,68,79,85,113] This has been recently challenged by a North American study in which the relapse rate determined prospectively was stable during the 3-year follow-up and was not influenced by overall disease duration.[114] The authors favor this latter conclusion, at least for the RR phase of the disease.[30] Furthermore, as soon as the disease has entered its progressive and chronically disabling stages, relapse detection likely becomes less prioritized and more easily overlooked, resulting in an underascertainment.

Onset of Progression

Despite the methodologic difficulties already discussed, the interexaminer reliability in assessing the onset of progression is good,[18,64] and thanks to the long-term natural history series currently available, knowledge of the onset of progression in MS can be considered evidence-based.

For an overall cohort of patients with MS, including cases with a progressive onset, estimates of the time from onset of MS to onset of progression are quite consistent. With calculations based on observed data only, Müller[68,69] found a median time to progression of 10 years. Using survival techniques, median time to progression turned out to be 11 years in the Lyon series[29,30] and 9 years in the Gothenburg series.[36,37] In the London, Ontario, series, the corresponding figure was only 5.8 years,[38] but it must be remembered here that the proportion of the cases classified as progressive from onset was unusually high in this cohort for reasons previously discussed. In all of these studies, an older age at onset of MS was associated with a shorter time to progression.

The other way of addressing the issue of the onset of progression is to consider specifically the population of cases with an RR onset of MS. This leads one to assess the risk of secondary progression. McAlpine and Compston[2] are to be credited with being the first to demonstrate clearly that "there is a fairly constant rate of change from a remitting to a progressive course, and that there is a gradual rise in the total percentage of progressive cases as the disease advances." A similar distribution has been found with analyses restricted to observed data by Broman and colleagues[35] and with survival analyses in the Lyon series (Fig. 6).[29,30,115] The median time to secondary progression turned out to be 19.1 years among the 1562 patients with an RR onset in the Lyon series,[115] 19 years among the 220 patients in the Gothenburg series,[37] and 18.9 years among the 2484 patients from the British Columbia MS database.[116] These results are consistent with others coming from smaller series.[85,117,118] It may be

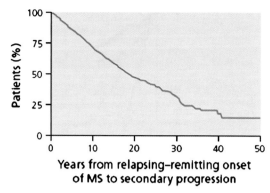

Fig. 6. Kaplan-Meier estimates for the time (years) from the onset of MS to the onset of the secondary progressive phase among the 1562 patients with an exacerbating-remitting initial course in the Lyon, France, MS cohort. (*From* Vukusic S, Confavreux C. Prognostic factors for progression of disability in the secondary progressive phase of multiple sclerosis. J Neurol Sci 2003;206:135–7; with permission.)

concluded that 19 years is a reasonable estimate for the median time to secondary progression following an RR onset in MS and that, each year, 2% to 3% of the patients with a RR form of MS enter secondary progression.

Age at onset of MS is, by far, the strongest predictor of the conversion to secondary progression: the older the age at onset, the shorter the time to onset of progression.[30,36,37,68,69,77,78,115] The influence of other clinical variables on the time to secondary progression is weaker than that of age at onset, or even nil.[3] In general, a shorter time to secondary progression has usually been found to be associated with male gender; spinal cord–related symptoms as compared with optic nerve– or sensory- and, sometimes, brainstem-related symptoms; an incomplete recovery from the initial attack; a shorter time from onset of MS to the second neurologic episode; a higher number of relapses during the first 2 or 5 years of the disease; and a higher disability score or a greater number of the affected functional systems observed 5 years after the onset of MS.[2,30,32,36,37,68,69,77,78,115,118]

THE PROGNOSIS OF MULTIPLE SCLEROSIS

Current knowledge of the overall time course of irreversible disability in MS is well documented. Results obtained at the level of a population of patients with MS lead to the description of a homogeneous picture of the disease. This is dramatically contrasted with the broad heterogeneity that can be observed from one patient to another. A third and a priori surprising characteristic of MS is the steady and stable rate of accumulation of neurologic abnormalities, which can be observed at an individual level.

Overall Accumulation of Irreversible Disability

The Kaplan-Meier estimates for the median time from onset of MS to assignment of DSS 3 has been 7.7 years in the London, Ontario, series[38] and 11 years in the Turkish series.[119] As for DSS 4, it has been estimated at 8.4 years[31,32] and 12.7 years.[118] It is regarding the DSS 6 outcome that the largest amount of data has become available, with fairly consistent results. The median time to DSS 6 has been estimated at 15 years in the London, Ontario, series,[38] 18 years in the Gothenburg study,[36] 18 years in the Turkish study,[119] 20.1 years in Lyon series,[31,32] 14.1 years in the Florence series,[118] and 20 years in the Norwegian series.[85] It has been estimated at 27.9 years in the British Columbian cohort of 2319 patients,[120] but there are several peculiarities in this series that may concur to overestimating the time to reaching disability outcomes.[28,67] Noticeably, however, the smaller series of 201 patients with MS in the Olmsted County, United States, provided results quite close to the Canadian's with median times to reach a DSS score of 3, 6, and 8 at 23, 28, and 52 years, respectively.[121] As for DSS 7, the estimated median time has been 29.9 years in Lyon,[31,32] whereas the 76th percentile time turned out to be 15 years in the Myhr and colleagues study.[85] Lastly, for DSS 8, the median time was 46.4 years in the London, Ontario, series and the 75th percentile time 28 years in Turkish series. **Fig. 7** displays Kaplan-Meier estimates for the times from onset of MS to assignment of irreversible disability scores among the 1844 patients with MS in the Lyon cohort. The median times to DSS 4, DSS 6, and DSS 7 were 8.4 years (95% confidence interval: 7.6–9.2), 20.1

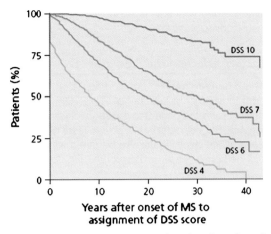

Fig. 7. Kaplan-Meier estimates for the time (years) from the onset of MS to the assignment of an irreversible score of 4, 6, 7, and 10 on the Kurtzke Disability Status Scale (DSS), among the 1844 patients in the Lyon, France, MS cohort. (*From* Confavreux C, Compston A. The natural history of multiple sclerosis. In: Compston A, editor. McAlpine's multiple sclerosis. 4th edition. London: Churchill Livingstone Elsevier; 2006. p. 183–272; with permission.)

years (18.2–22.0), and 29.9 years (25.8–34.1), respectively.

Interindividual Variability Versus Intraindividual Fixity

Contrasting with the wide interindividual variability in the rate of accumulation of irreversible disability, it is rather surprising to observe that, for a given patient, the rate of accumulation of neurologic abnormalities is remarkably steady and stable throughout the course of the disease. This has been independently demonstrated by Fog and Linnemann[19] from 73 patients, and by Patzold and Pocklington[21] from 102 patients (**Fig. 8**). What

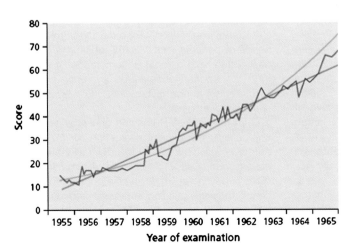

Fig. 8. Serial quantitative neurologic examinations over several years in a patient with MS. The observed clinical sawtoothed curve could, after regression analysis, be transformed into mathematical curves. The best fitting curve was selected from the highest correlation coefficient with the clinical curve. (*Adapted from* Fog T, Linnemann F. The course of multiple sclerosis: in 73 cases with computer designed curves. Acta Neurol Scand Suppl 1970;46:1–175; with permission.)

differs among patients is the individual slope of the neurologic deterioration.

Factors Affecting the Prognosis

The prognosis varying considerably from one patient to another, it is of utmost importance for the clinician and the patient to get some clues for making predictions, notably in the first years of the disease, when decisions are to be taken with regard to personal and professional life but also treatment.

Regarding demographic and clinical variables, the results from the long-term longitudinal studies[30–32,35–40] and from cross-sectional studies[65,68–71,77,79–82,84,85,113,118,119,122–132] provide robust and consistent clues. A shorter time to reach disability landmarks has usually been found associated with the factors listed in **Box 1**.

This list of clinical factors with a predictive value of the outcome in MS seems impressively long. Many of these factors are interdependent in their prognostic effect and share their predictive influence, at least partly. This is notably the case for the cluster gathering gender, age at onset of MS, initial symptoms, and initial course of the disease: older age at onset, dysfunction of long tract–related initial symptoms, progressive initial course, and male gender are associated with a worse outcome, whereas the combination of younger age at onset, optic neuritis as initial symptom, RR initial course, and female gender is associated with a better prognosis. Initial course of MS is the most influential factor on the prognosis. Age at onset of MS holds the second place. Initial symptoms and gender have a marginal or even a nil effect when initial course and age at onset are already taken into account. Although highly significant at the statistical level, the prognostic effect of these variables is moderate, at best, even when combined. Although its interest is undeniable for a general population of patients with MS, this is not the case at an individual level.

There has been an intense search for paraclinical factors predictive of the outcome of MS. Abnormalities on the baseline brain MR image have a predictive value. In a study involving 84 patients with an initial monofocal episode suggestive of MS, the T2 lesion load on baseline MR image was strongly correlated to the disability level 5 years later.[73] Similar results have been obtained in Barcelona for 156 patients with a clinically isolated syndrome followed for a median of 7 years: the EDSS score at 5 years correlated with the number of lesions and of Barkhof criteria at baseline.[133] The Queen Square prospective observational study of 71 patients presenting with clinically monofocal episodes and followed up to 14 years[109] demonstrated that the EDSS assessed at the end of the follow-up was significantly correlated with the T2 lesion volume at baseline and the increase in T2 lesion volume at all time points (baseline and 5, 10, and 14 years of follow-up). The correlation was the highest, although moderate, for MR imaging at 5 years ($r = 0.60$) and the increase over the first 5 years of the disease ($r = 0.61$). The same group has been able to reassess 107 patients after a mean of 20.2 years among the initial group of 140 patients admitted for a first neurologic episode suggestive of MS.[134] This led to confirmatory results of the previous study: baseline brain MR imaging findings are predictive for the development of CDMS and T2 lesion volume and its changes at earlier time points are predictive of later disability. This study also brought about that, among patients with an initial RR course of MS, the rate of increase in the T2 lesion volume was three times higher in those who converted to SPMS than in those who remained in the RR stage during the follow-up. Interestingly, this study clearly showed a linear correlation between the number of T2 lesions on the baseline MR image and the likelihood of reaching a score of DSS 6 during the follow-up: it ranged from 6% for patients with no lesion to 45% for patients with at least 10 lesions on the baseline MR image. Noticeably, however, among patients with at least 10 lesions on baseline MR image, still 35% had an EDSS score not higher than 3 and 18% had not converted to CDMS.

The search for other paraclinical factors that could be predictive of the outcome has not been rewarding up to now.[3] This is the case for the presence of oligoclonal bands in the cerebrospinal fluid and for prolonged latencies on the visual evoked potentials at onset of MS. The presence of the HLA-DR15 allele does not significantly influence the course and severity of the disease.[135–139] The influence of the apolipoprotein E alleles is still a matter of controversy. According to several large series of patients with MS, the epsilon 4 allele is associated with a rapid accumulation of disability[140–142] and an accelerated evolution of brain MR imaging abnormalities.[143-145] For others, this allele is not influential.[146]

Currently, only MR imaging can provide useful adjuncts to the clinical evaluation for improving outcome predictions in MS. Unfortunately, as precise and reliable clinical and MR imaging predictors may be at the level of a population of patients, they are still too imprecise and unreliable for individual predictions. To conclude, two considerations deserve emphasis. First, the predictive factors of the disability accumulation in MS are

Box 1
Clinical predictors of a worse prognosis

1. Male gender, but this influence, when present, is weak.
2. Older age at onset of MS. This effect has been considered by most authors as strong.
3. An initial symptomatology consisting of a spinal cord syndrome, or motor-balance-pyramidal-cerebellar symptoms, or long-tracts dysfunction as compared with optic neuritis and, in some series, brainstem syndrome. This effect has usually been found to be mild to moderate.
4. A progressive initial course, as compared with cases with an initial RR course. This is considered as the strongest clinical predictor of the time course of disability. An illustration is shown in **Fig. 9** using the Kaplan-Meier method for the 1844 patients with MS of the Lyon cohort.[31,32] The differences in the median times between cases with an RR onset and cases with a progressive onset to reach the DSS scores of 4, 6, and 7, could be estimated 11, 16, and 20 years, respectively. All these differences were highly significant.
5. An incomplete recovery of the initial neurologic episode.
6. A shorter time to the second neurologic episode. This criterion has received much attention and delaying the time to the second neurologic episode has become a key outcome for the approval of DMAs when administered after a first neurologic episode suggestive of MS. This time-dependent parameter has been considered as not influential, however, when the survival estimates were calculated from the date of occurrence of the second episode as starting point in the Gothenburg[36,37] and in the Lyon series (Renoux and colleagues, personal communication, 2008).
7. A higher frequency and number of relapses during the first 2 to 5 years of MS. This effect, however, has usually been found to be quite weak. In some series, it was nil.[19,21,65,118,127] There was also no effect in the Gothenburg study[36,37] when the time-dependency of the variable was accounted for and the survival analysis estimates of the time to DSS 6 were calculated using 5 years after onset of MS as the starting point.
8. A greater DSS score, or the presence of pyramidal or cerebellar signs, or a greater number of affected functional systems, as assessed at 2 or 5 years of disease duration. Kurtzke and colleagues[127] is to be credited as being the first to demonstrate this association. Moreover, the Gothenburg study[36,37] has demonstrated that the effect was still present when the time to the disability end point (DSS 6 in this series) was estimated by the survival analysis using 5 years after onset of MS as the starting point.
9. A shorter time to reaching DSS 3[38–40] or DSS 4.[32] In the Lyon series, however, this effect was present for reaching DSS 6 and DSS 7 when onset of MS was selected as the starting point. It was no longer present when the date of assignment of DSS 4 was selected.[32]
10. A shorter time to secondary progression.[30]

essentially the same as those that are predictive of SPMS, which is not really surprising. Second, two phenomena seem to be operating: a weak interplay between relapses and prognosis contrasting with a strong interplay between age and prognosis. This is further discussed later.

Benign Multiple Sclerosis

As for many of the currently acknowledged clinico-pathologic distinguishing features of MS, Charcot[147] was the first to envision that the disease could become completely quiescent or even recover. Six decades later, Brain[148] endorsed the same opinion. But it is the seminal work of McAlpine[1,123] that has made popular the concept of benign MS (BMS). By studying an essentially hospital-based population of 241 patients with MS seen within 3 years of onset and followed-up until 15 years or more, McAlpine was able to demonstrate that 62 patients (26%) were still unrestricted, that is "without restriction of activity for normal employment and domestic purpose but not necessarily symptom-free," after a mean disease duration of 18.2 years.[2] All these patients were able to walk for more than 500 m without rest or support from a stick. This would qualify them nowadays for a DSS score of no more than 4. This figure of 26% is strikingly consistent with the results obtained with survival analysis techniques in long-term longitudinal follow-up studies of large natural history cohorts. For instance, in the Lyon cohort of 1844 patients with MS, patients with an initial progressive course included, 35%, 26%, and 13% of the patients had not reached the irreversible DSS 4 landmark at 15, 20, and 30 years of disease duration, respectively. The reassessment of the Gothenburg cohort after a 37- to 50-year follow-up allowed to estimate by a Kaplan-Meier analysis that the proportions of benign cases at 30 and 40 years of disease duration were 26% and 21%, respectively.[149] To be classified as benign in this study, patients had to be free of

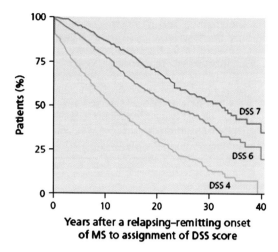

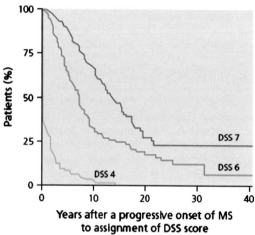

Fig. 9. Kaplan-Meier estimates for the time (years) from the onset of MS to the assignment of an irreversible score of 4, 6, and 7 on the Kurtzke Disability Status Scale (DSS), among the 1844 patients in the Lyon, France, MS cohort. Influence of the initial course of the disease. (*A*) Estimates for the 1562 patients with an exacerbating-remitting initial course. The median times (95% confidence interval) for reaching a score of 4, 6, and 7 were 11.4 (10.5–12.3), 23.1 (20.1–26.1), and 33.1 (29.2–37.0) years, respectively. (*B*) Estimates for the 282 patients with a progressive initial course of MS. The median times for reaching a score of 4, 6, and 7 were 0.0, 7.1 (6.3–7.9), and 13.4 (11.0–15.9) years, respectively. (*From* Confavreux C, Compston A. The natural history of multiple sclerosis. In: Compston A, editor. McAlpine's multiple sclerosis. 4th edition. London: Churchill Livingstone Elsevier; 2006. p. 183–272; with permission.)

secondary progression and have an EDSS score of no more than 4 at follow-up.

Presently, any physician agrees on the existence of BMS. The reality of the concept is reinforced by the well-known incidental findings of MS at autopsy[6–10] or at neuroimaging examinations.[11,12] There is also a strong consensus about the archetypal clinical phenotype of BMS, which recruits mainly among young women and usually follows an initial RR course.[1,3,7,30,123,124,150–152]

Several issues regarding BMS, however, are still debated. The first deals with the criteria qualifying for BMS. According to the results of the international survey undertaken by the United Sates National Multiple Sclerosis Society,[51] the consensus definition is "disease in which the patient remains fully functional in all neurologic systems 15 years after disease onset." There is still some imprecision in this definition about the boundaries of "fully functional." Furthermore, somewhat different definitions are used by different authors depending on the upper limit allowed for the disability score (usually DSS 3 or DSS 4) and on the minimum duration of the disease required (varying from 10–20 years, usually). In about half of the patients with a so-called BMS, inapparent symptoms, such as fatigue, pain, depression, and cognitive dysfunction, can be identified interfering with activities of daily life in otherwise fully ambulatory patients.[153,154] It is difficult to compare results between studies.

Another difficulty comes from the fact that patients with BMS often escape neurologic attention.[13] The authors analyzed the group of all suspected patients with MS in the geographic area of Southern Lower Saxony, amounting to 221 patients. They compared this group with the 1837 cases collected throughout Germany mainly in the hospitals taking part in a national epidemiologic program devoted to MS. In the geographically based series, there were many cases that had never attended any hospital or any outpatient department. Although the mean disease duration was longer in the Saxony cohort (12.1 years) than in the hospital cohort (10.5 years), the percentage of patients unrestricted or minimally restricted at the time of the survey was 52% in the Saxony cohort compared with 26% in the nation-wide hospital cohort.

Another point deserves comment: it is always difficult, if not risky, to be confident that an individual classified in the BMS category will remain so thereafter. This is illustrated by the survival curves, which show a steady decrease in the proportion of individuals still free of the disability end point with increasing disease duration. This is also illustrated by comparative serial analyses in the long-term of a given population of patients with MS:[1,121,155–158] about half of the patients classified as "benign MS" at some time point of the disease no longer fall in this category when reassessed 10 years later. Altogether it may be considered that the figure of 30% is a reasonable estimate of the proportion of benign forms in MS.

Multiple Sclerosis with Childhood Onset

After being denied and then neglected for several decades, childhood-onset MS has received great attention recently and, as the number of studies devoted to childhood-onset MS increases, knowledge becomes more complete.[69,159–166] This has been notably the case since the publication of the results of the Kids with MS (KIDMUS) study, an observational multicenter study of 394 patients who had MS with an onset at 16 years of age or younger and who were compared with a group of 1775 patients who had MS with an onset after 16 years of age.[167] Onset of MS in childhood is rare, around 2% of the total cases with the disease. It has a female preponderance and most studies have found a gender ratio (female/male) ranging from 2.2 to 3, higher than in adult-onset MS. The cases with a very early onset, however, tend to show a higher number of males affected. The diagnosis in children is challenged by the differential diagnosis with acute disseminated encephalomyelitis.[168] Among 296 patients with a first demyelinating event of the CNS before the age of 16, with a mean follow-up of 3 years, 20% of the 168 patients with a final diagnosis of MS had been initially diagnosed as acute disseminated encephalomyelitis.[165] It can roughly be estimated that isolated optic neuritis occurs in approximately 20% to 25% of the patients with childhood-onset MS, isolated brainstem dysfunction in 10% to 25%, and isolated long-tract dysfunction in 40% to 50%. In a small proportion of cases, neurologic symptoms may be accompanied by various encephalitic manifestations.[165–167] An RR course is by far the most common form at onset in all published studies with a relapse as the first manifestation of the disease in 85.7% to 97.7% of cases.[162,167,169] According to the KIDMUS study,[167] the Kaplan-Meier estimates for the median time from the onset of MS to the second neurologic episode was 2 years, with no difference with adult-onset MS (2.2 years). By contrast, patients with childhood-onset MS converted to SPMS on average 10 years later than patients with adult-onset MS but reached this phase of the disease on average 10 years younger. The same observation could be made for the reaching of disability landmarks of DSS 4, DSS 6, and DSS 7 (**Fig. 10**). Once a certain threshold of irreversible disability had been reached, further accumulation of disability developed at a similar pace in childhood- and adult-onset MS patients.[167]

SURVIVAL IN MULTIPLE SCLEROSIS

For a long time, knowledge on survival in MS has been fragmentary. Indeed, it had been restricted to US Army veterans[126,170] or observational cohorts of patients but with a limited proportion of deceased individuals.[30,35–39,42,65,68,69,85,119,131,132,171–177] The national Danish study made an especially important contribution to the issue of survival in MS.[178–180] At the most recent update, 9881 patients with MS were registered among whom 4254 (43%) had died during follow-up.[181] The cohort takes advantage of the Danish MS Registry established on the back of a prevalence survey completed in 1956, and includes information about patients in Denmark with onset of MS from 1949. Virtually all Danish inhabitants with MS are registered on the database, and information is systematically validated and updated. The study is also linked to the Danish Civil Registration System established in 1968 and the Cause of Death Registry comprising data on all deaths since 1943. These two official registers gather data on emigration, death, and cause of death for the patients with MS, and for the general Danish population. The recent reassessment included patients whose initial symptoms began in the period 1949 to 1996, and were logged before January 1, 1997. Median survival time from onset of MS to death was estimated to be 31 years (**Fig. 11**). It was significantly longer in females than males. It was about 10 years shorter for patients with MS than for the age-matched general population. Survival improved significantly during the 50-year period of observation, the median 10-year shorter life expectancy being almost halved during that period. This change was independent of the general decline in mortality experienced by Danes since the 1950s and presumably related to improved medical management. According to available certificates, 56% of deaths were related to MS. Those unrelated were mainly attributable to cardiovascular diseases (15%); cancer (10%); infectious and respiratory diseases (5%); and accidents and suicide (5%). Compared with the general population, there was excess mortality caused by cardiovascular disease, infections, and respiratory causes, and to accidents and suicide, but a lower risk of death from cancer. MS is essentially chronic and disabling but not fatal per se.

MECHANISMS UNDERLYING THE CLINICAL COURSE

Understanding the mechanisms underlying the course and prognosis of MS deserves most

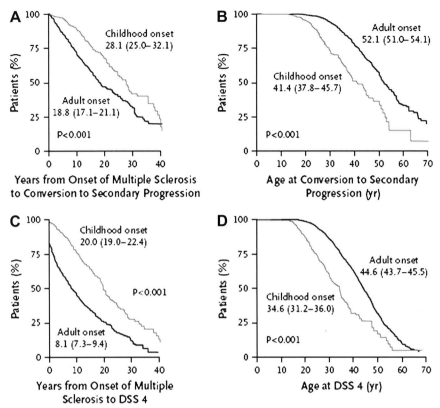

Fig. 10. Kaplan-Meier estimates of the time to (*A*) and the age at (*B*) conversion to secondary progression and of the time to (*C*) and the age at (*D*) assignment of an irreversible score of 4 on the Kurtzke Disability Status Scale (DSS), among the 394 patients with childhood-onset and the 1775 patients with adult-onset MS in the Kids with MS (KIDMUS) study. Panels *A* and *C* include median number of years and 95% confidence intervals; and panels *B* and *D* include median age and 95% confidence intervals. (*From* Renoux C, Vukusic S, Mikaeloff Y, et al. Natural history of multiple sclerosis with childhood onset. N Engl J Med 2007;356:2603–13; with permission.)

interest because it may result in major pathogenetic and therapeutic conclusions. The course of MS may be considered as an interplay between two clinical phenomena: relapses and progression. Both of them can lead to irreversible disability. This brings into question which of them is the most important in the disability accumulation process. The classical view is to consider that the succession of relapses could eventually lead to accumulation of disability and clinical progression could result from infraclinical relapses. A series of observations, however, tend to challenge this view.

Relapses and Accumulation of Irreversible Disability

At first glance, relapses are the major player. This has been somewhat a dogma for decades. As far as in the 1950s, renowned authorities in the field could write: "The main aim of any treatment should be to reduce the frequency of relapses … Influencing disability is a secondary aim in treatment trials, mainly because this depends absolutely on relapse rate."[182] Indeed, any clinician is familiar with definitive neurologic deficit caused by a relapse in MS. Among the 1562 patients of the Lyon cohort with an RR onset, 274 (18%) did suffer from an initial relapse with irreversible incomplete recovery. Among the 1288 patients making a complete recovery after the initial relapse, 391 (30%) later experienced incomplete recovery from a subsequent episode.[32] A detailed analysis of pooled data from 224 patients with RRMS enrolled in the placebo arms of several randomized controlled trials allowed comparisons between EDSS assessments before, at the time of, and after a relapse.[183] The net increase in the EDSS score was 0.27 (± 1.04), as measured at a median of 63 days after the relapse This corresponded to 42% of the patients with greater than or equal to 0.5, and 28% with greater than or equal to 1 point increase in EDSS scores. Furthermore, many relapse-related factors are associated with

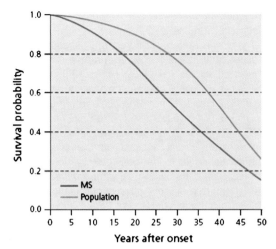

Fig. 11. Actuarial probability of survival among 9881 patients with MS, of whom 4254 had died before the end of follow-up on January 1, 2000, and the matched general population in Denmark. (*From* Bronnum-Hansen H, Koch-Henriksen N, Stenager E. Trends in survival and cause of death in Danish patients with multiple sclerosis. Brain 2004;127:844–50; with permission.)

rapid accumulation of irreversible disability: an incomplete recovery from the initial neurologic episode, a short interval between the first two episodes, and a high number or rate of relapses during the first years of the illness.[30,32,39,40]

The real contribution of relapses to disability accumulation, however, is not that simple. There are an increasing number of arguments for considering that relapses are not the major player. Evidence from the PP form of MS indicates that irreversible disability may occur without superimposed relapses. The rate of disability accumulation in these forms of the disease is similar to that seen in RP form.[30,42,44] Other evidence comes from a prospective analysis of the individual course of the disease among 73 patients in Denmark (see **Fig. 8**),[19] and where it was concluded that the two components of the clinical course of MS are mutually independent. Relapses occur in an unpredictable way. Their frequency varies between individuals but also within a given individual. By contrast, the clinical progression of the neurologic deficits can be subjected to mathematical analysis. It is often very constant in degree in an individual patient but its slope, which is decisive for the prognosis, varies between individuals. Relapses can be superimposed above the process of progression, but progression apparently pursues its course independent of the individual relapses. "To me at least, it seems strange that such a [steady progression] [...] could be explained solely by the summation of single attacks. [...] It seems therefore reasonable to believe that the phase of progression represents another biological process than the attack."[19]

Further evidence comes from the analysis of pooled data from 289 patients with RRMS enrolled in the placebo arms of two randomized controlled trials and assessed at 3-month intervals with a 2-year follow-up.[184] In these series, disability progression was defined as significant if the increase in the EDSS score was greater than or equal to 1 point for cases with a baseline EDSS score within the 0 to 5 range, or greater than or equal to 0.5 point for cases with a baseline EDSS score greater than or equal to 5.5. According to the observed course of EDSS scores throughout the 2 years of follow-up, 29% of the patients could be classified as showing progression in the trial with confirmation at 3 months. Among those who progressed, however, the EDSS increase was still present at the end of the follow-up period in about half of the participants. The probability of misclassification at the end of the trial regarding the progression status was 0.52. Applying the more stringent definitions of greater than or equal to 2 EDSS increase or a confirmation at 6 months led to essentially the same estimation for the probability of misclassification. These results clearly show that an increase in disability confirmed at 3 or even 6 months must not be considered as equivalent to an irreversible increase in disability. Interestingly, as discussed previously using similar resources, Lublin and colleagues[183] also found a greater than or equal to 1 point EDSS increase relative to baseline in 28% of patients at a median of 63 days after a relapse. This suggests that, in the available placebo cohorts of patients with RRMS, the confirmed disability increases are mainly relapse-driven. It seems logical to conclude that, in RRMS, short-term confirmed increase in disability depends primarily on relapses and is often reversible.

Systematic studies of long-term accumulation of irreversible disability have also been instructive in this respect. Among the 1844 patients in the Lyon MS cohort, the well-known difference between the cases with an RR onset and those with a progressive onset could be observed: median times from the onset of MS to assignment of irreversible scores of DSS 4, DSS 6, and DSS 7 were significantly longer in the RR- than progressive-onset cases (**Fig. 12**).[31] This is in agreement with former analyses of this cohort[30] and with results from many other series (**Fig. 13**).[36,37, 39,40,42,44,45,78,82,119,121,135] By contrast, accumulation of irreversible disability from the assignment of DSS 4 to DSS 6 was similar in cases

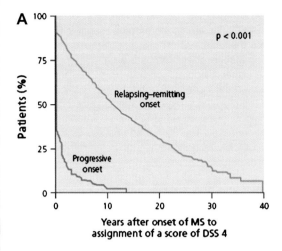

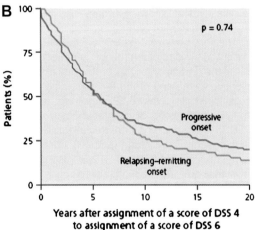

Fig. 12. Kaplan-Meier estimates for (A) the time from the onset of MS to the assignment of an irreversible score of 4, and (B) the time from the assignment of an irreversible score of 4 to the assignment of an irreversible score of 6 on the Kurtzke Disability Status Scale (DSS), depending on the initial course of the disease, among the 1844 patients in the Lyon, France, MS cohort. (*From* Confavreux C, Vukusic S, Moreau T, et al. Relapses and progression of disability in multiple sclerosis. N Engl J Med 2000;343:1430–38; with permission.)

with an RR onset and a progressive onset (see **Fig. 12**). This was also true for the accumulation of disability from DSS 4 to DSS 7, and from DSS 6 to DSS 7.[31] The rate of accumulation of irreversible disability from the assignment of DSS 4 is not affected by the presence or the absence of relapses preceding the onset of the SP phase of the disease. Confirmation can be found by looking at the influence of current age on the course of MS: age at onset of the progressive phase is similar in PPMS and SPMS (see later). It is unaffected by the

presence or the absence of relapses preceding disease progression.

The same material allowed the assessment of the possible influence of superimposed relapses during either the PP or SP phase (**Fig. 14**).[31] In the cases with a PP course, the accumulation of irreversible disability from the assignment of DSS 4 to DSS 6, but also from DSS 4 to DSS 7 and from DSS 6 to DSS 7, was similar whether or not relapses were superimposed on the progressive phase. Essentially, identical observations could be made on cases with a SP course. It seems as though the rate of irreversible accumulation of disability from the assignment of DSS 4 is unaffected by relapses occurring during the progressive phase. These results match and extend those from other large studies on the natural history of MS. In the London, Ontario, cohort, the survival curves were almost identical when PRMS patients were compared with those with PPMS stricto sensu with respect to the time from onset of MS to the assignment of DSS 6, DSS 8, and death.[44] Similar conclusions have been reached by others studying forms of MS with a progressive onset for the time to DSS 6.[185] Accumulation of irreversible disability in MS is essentially dissociated from relapses.

These results from the Lyon cohort have been reached by dichotomizing the status of relapses as present or not present. Similar results were obtained when analyzing the possible influence of relapses at onset and during the early years of the disease. Noticeably, an incomplete recovery of the first neurologic episode, a shorter time to the second neurologic episode (**Fig. 15**), and a higher number of relapses during the first 5 years of the disease were associated with a shorter time from onset of MS to the assignment of DSS 4, DSS 6, and DSS 7.[32] Similar observations have been made in many other series.[5,19,30,36,38–41,64,68,71,77,78,82,119,123,127,129,132,176,186–188] The originality of the French study is that it assessed the possible influence of the same clinical variables on the accumulation of irreversible disability from the time of assignment of DSS 4 to DSS 6, and also from DSS 4 to DSS 7 and DSS 6 to DSS 7.[32] None of the variables remained predictive of the time course of disability past the DSS 4 point (see **Fig. 15**). Accumulation of irreversible disability is seemingly amnesic with respect to the clinical characteristics of relapses that occurred during the initial stages of the disease. More generally, long-term progression of irreversible disability is mainly relapse-dissociated and progression-driven. These observations are reminiscent of those regarding gender and age at onset of MS in the Gothenburg series: both variables showed

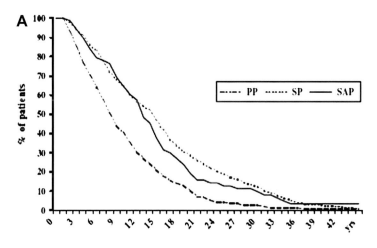

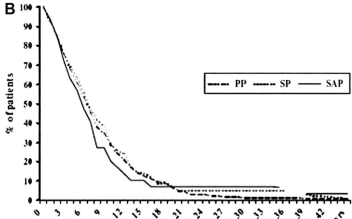

Fig. 13. Kaplan-Meier estimates for the time (years) from (A) the onset of MS and (B) the onset of progression to the assignment of a score of 6 on the Kurtzke Disability Status Scale (DSS) in patients with primary-progressive (N = 219), single-attack progressive (N = 140), and secondary-progressive (N = 146) MS among the patients in the London, Ontario, MS cohort. PP, primary progressive; SAP, single-attack progressive; SP, secondary progressive. (*From* Kremenchutzky M, Rice GP, Baskerville J, et al. The natural history of multiple sclerosis: a geographically based study. 9: Observations on the progressive phase of the disease. Brain 2006;129:584–94; with permission.)

a correlation with prognosis when analyzed from the onset of MS, but not when the analyses were repeated taking 5 years after onset as the starting point.[36]

Although beyond the scope of this article, another argument against the prominent role of relapses in the accumulation of disability comes from the experience gathered with the use of DMAs in MS. Schematically, dramatically reducing the frequency of relapses is far from always resulting in an arrest of the progression of disability.

Course and Prognosis: An Age-Dependent Process

The influence of age on the course and the prognosis of MS has received attention for long. Pioneer studies[2,68,69,189] already pointed out that MS patients with a late onset of the disease tend to show a PP course, whereas most patients with an early onset tend to follow an initial RR course. McAlpine and Compston[2] also observed

a constant rate of conversion from the RR to the SP stage of the disease throughout the course of MS. Other classic but more recent studies have suggested that onset of the RR and of the progressive phase of MS are age-related, independently of the overall course of the disease.[19,29,30,42,44,64,71,80]

This issue has recently been readdressed in the Lyon cohort.[33,34] Among the 1562 patients with an initial RR course of the disease, the median age at onset of the disease was 29 years, with no difference in the 1066 patients who continued to experience relapses (28.7 years) and in the 496 patients who converted to SPMS (29.5 years) (Fig. 16). For the 778 patients who entered the progressive phase of the disease, either from the onset of MS or secondary to an earlier RR phase, the median age at the onset of the progressive phase was 39.1 years, with no significant difference in the 496 patients with a SP course (39.1 years) and the 282 patients with an overall course progressive from onset (40.1 years) (see Fig. 16).

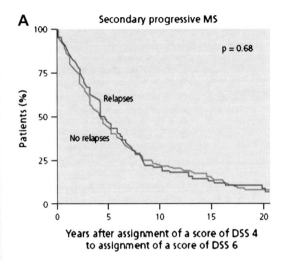

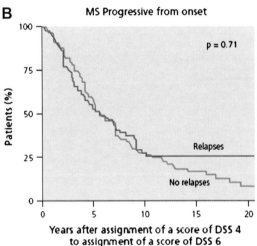

Fig. 14. Kaplan-Meier estimates for the time from the assignment of an irreversible score of 4 to the assignment of an irreversible score of 6 on the Kurtzke Disability Status Scale (DSS) among the 1844 patients in the Lyon, France, MS cohort. (A) Estimates for the 496 patients with secondary-progressive MS. (B) Estimates for the 282 patients with primary-progressive MS. Both graphs are according to the presence or absence of superimposed relapses during progression. (From Confavreux C, Vukusic S, Moreau T, et al. Relapses and progression of disability in multiple sclerosis. N Engl J Med 2000;343:1430–38; with permission.)

From the same series, Kaplan-Meier estimates were calculated for the age of the patients at the time of assignment of an irreversible score of disability. Median age was 44.3 years for a score of DSS 4, 54.7 years for a score of DSS 6, and 63.1 years for a score of DSS 7.[33] The 1562 patients with an initial RR course were compared with the

282 patients having a progressive course from onset with respect to age at the time of reaching irreversible scores of disability. Patients with an RR onset were older than those progressing from onset, for assignment of DSS 4 and DSS 6. Ages were similar for assignment of DSS 7 (Fig. 17). Noticeably, the differences were only 2.7 and 2.3 years for median ages at assignment of DSS 4 and 6, respectively, for a disease usually encompassing several decades of life. There was overlap in the 95% confidence intervals of these medians for both assignments. Furthermore, when the subgroup of patients with SPMS was selected among the group of patients with RR onset, those patients were found to be younger at the time of reaching DSS 4, DSS 6, and DSS 7 than those with a course progressive from onset (see Fig. 17). Conversion from the initial RR phase to SPMS occurs at a constant rate throughout the course of the disease. Considering a cohort of patients with MS studied at a given time, patients with the SP course are likely to represent a subgroup of more rapidly worsening forms of MS within the entire group of patients with RR disease at onset. The actual age at assignment of irreversible disability in patients with an initial RR course lies between boundaries for this whole group of patients and for patients with the SP course, and closer to ages found for patients with a progressive course from onset.[33] Taken together, it could be concluded that age at time of reaching disability landmarks is not substantially influenced by the initial course of MS.

It is an oversimplification, however, to consider disability in MS as strictly age dependent. Age at disease onset also influences prognosis: the earlier the onset of the disease, the younger the age at disability landmarks.[30,33,120] This is well illustrated in Fig. 18 drawn from the analysis of the Lyon, France, cohort[33] and Fig. 19 drawn from that of the British Columbia cohort.[120] It must also be reminded that age at onset is influential on the time from onset of MS to disability landmarks, but not from one step of disability to another (Fig. 20).[32] A complex interaction between age at onset of MS and current age of the individual does operate. In a hospital-based study of 1463 Italian patients with MS,[190] age at onset and current age of the patients were found both to correlate with disease severity, the effect of the former being smaller by comparison.

It is another oversimplification to consider that the course of the disease is uniform across individuals with MS. The clear-cut homogeneity that can be observed for a group of patients does not contradict the high variability in age at onset of the RR and progressive phases, and times of reaching

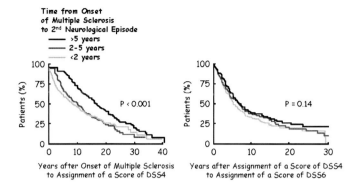

Fig. 15. Kaplan-Meier estimates for (*left*) the time from the onset of MS to the assignment of an irreversible score of 4, and (*right*) the time from the assignment of an irreversible score of 4 to the assignment of an irreversible score of 6 on the Kurtzke Disability Status Scale (DSS), depending on the time from onset of MS to the second neurologic episode, among the 1562 patients with an exacerbating-remitting initial course in the Lyon, France, MS cohort. (*Adapted from* Confavreux C, Vukusic S, Adeleine P. Early clinical predictors and progression of irreversible disability in multiple sclerosis: an amnesic process. Brain 2003;126:770–82; with permission.)

disability landmarks, observed among individuals with MS. The age dependency phenomenon surmounts this variability, however, showing no influence of the initial course on age at disability milestones.

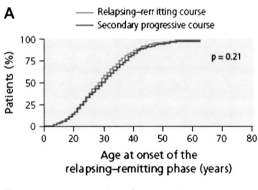

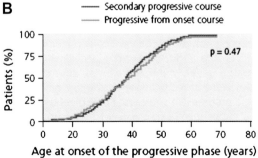

Fig. 16. Kaplan-Meier estimates for (*A*) the age at onset of the relapsing-remitting phase of MS, and (*B*) the age at onset of the progressive phase of MS, depending on the overall course of the disease, among the 1844 patients in the Lyon cohort. (*From* Confavreux C, Vukusic S. Natural history of multiple sclerosis: a unifying concept. Brain 2006;129:606–16; with permission.)

Primary and Secondary Progression: Differences and Similarities

The reasons why progression may start de novo or after a period of episodes remains largely unexplained. This has led many neurologists to consider PPMS as a separate entity from other forms of the disease. Recent analysis of the Lyon cohort[34] and available data from other sources has allowed the clinical evidence for and against this hypothesis to be reconsidered.[3]

Secondary-progressive multiple sclerosis and relapsing-remitting multiple sclerosis

In the Lyon cohort, the two populations were similar in the distribution of initial symptoms during the RR phase, the degree of recovery from the first relapse, and the time from onset to the second neurologic episode. Distribution according to age at onset of the RR phase was also strikingly similar (see **Fig. 16**) and in agreement with other series.[19,64,71,80] By contrast, the two populations in the Lyon cohort clearly differed in duration of the disease, which was twice as long in the SPMS compared with the RRMS group. Others have reached the same conclusions.[78,80] It must be reminded that patients with an initial RR course of MS naturally convert to the SP phase at a rate of around 2% to 3% per annum, following an essentially linear curve (see **Fig. 6**). The longer the disease duration at the time of the survey, the higher the proportion of cases classified as SPMS compared with those classified as having RR disease. Although the RR and SP phases clearly represent two clinical stages of the disease, these data altogether are in favor of the hypothesis that SPMS is RRMS that has had "time to grow older."[29,30]

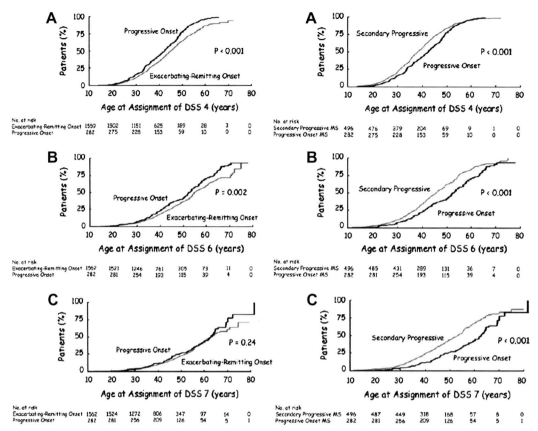

Fig. 17. Kaplan-Meier estimates for the age at assignment of an irreversible score of 4 (*A*), 6 (*B*), and 7 (*C*) on the Kurtzke Disability Status Scale (DSS), depending on the initial course of the disease, among the 1844 patients in the Lyon cohort. Left panel, estimates for the 1562 patients with an exacerbating-remitting initial course and the 282 patients with a progressive onset of MS. Right panel, estimates for the 496 patients with secondary-progressive MS and the 282 patients with a progressive onset of MS. (*From* Confavreux C, Vukusic S. Age at disability milestones in multiple sclerosis. Brain 2006;129:595–605; with permission.)

Primary-progressive and progressive-relapsing multiple sclerosis

By definition, these apparently distinct forms of MS share the progressive onset but differ in that superimposed relapses accompany PRMS but not PPMS.[51] Among the 218 patients of the London, Ontario, series with an initial progressive course,[42,44] 28% exhibited superimposed relapses during progression. The corresponding figure was 39% among the 282 patients with a progressive initial course of MS from the Lyon series.[30,34] In this Lyon series, median age at onset was earlier in PR (37 years) than in PP cases (41 years), although this is the only difference that could be observed when comparing these two forms of MS according to demographic and clinical characteristics, such as gender and initial symptoms of the disease.[34] A similar trend for age at onset was found in the London, Ontario, series.[44] The rates at which irreversible disability

progresses, calculated from the onset of MS or from assignment of a given disability score, were essentially similar in PRMS and PPMS in both series[30,34,42,44] and in a smaller Californian cross-sectional study.[135] These results indicate that PRMS and PPMS are, from a clinical point of view, essentially the same. It is appropriate to pool these cases in a single category initially having a progressive course, the only difference being the subsequent experience of superimposed relapses. The occasional confusion between PRMS and SPMS might account for the slightly earlier onset in PRMS than in PPMS.

Secondary-progressive multiple sclerosis and multiple sclerosis with progressive onset

Most clinicians consider MS with progressive onset to be distinct from SP disease. The female preponderance is much reduced in cases with an initial progressive course, compared with those

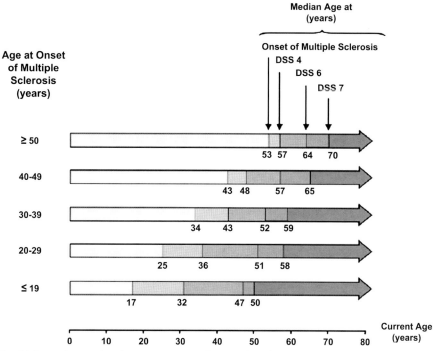

Fig. 18. Kaplan-Meier estimates for the age at onset of MS and at the times of assignment of an irreversible disability score of 4, 6, and 7 on the Kurtzke Disability Status Scale (DSS) among the 1844 patients in the Lyon, France, MS cohort. Each horizontal arrow represents a category of patients by age at onset of MS. For each category, the digits below the corresponding horizontal arrow indicate the median ages (years) at the onset of MS (*left*), and the assignment of DSS 4 (*middle left*), of DSS 6 (*middle right*), and of DSS 7 (*right*). (*From* Confavreux C, Vukusic S. Age at disability milestones in multiple sclerosis. Brain 2006;129:595–605; with permission.)

with SPMS.[42,44,50,191,192] In the Lyon cohort there was only a trend in that direction, however, which did not reach statistical significance.[34] As compared with SP disease, MS with progressive onset stands for its very different initial clinical course, its initial symptoms being more often related to dysfunction of long tracts, its older age at disease onset, and its shorter time from disease onset to reaching disability milestones.

The distinction, however, is not necessarily so clear-cut. Comparing cases from the time that progression becomes manifest (at onset or after a period of episodes) reveals many similarities. In the Lyon cohort, age and initial symptoms at onset of the progressive phase were similar in the 496 cases with SPMS and the 282 cases with progressive disease from onset. The proportion of cases with superimposed relapses during progression was around 40% in both categories. The time course of disability accumulation during the progressive phase of the disease was more rapid and occurred at a younger age in SPMS than individuals with a progressive onset. For instance, median survival from DSS 4 to DSS 6 was 4 years in

SPMS and 5.4 years in MS with progression from onset. Similarly, median age at reaching DSS 4 was 37.6 and 42.1 years in these two groups, respectively.[31,34] In the London, Ontario, cohort,[42,44] the median survival time from onset of progression to reach DSS 6 was 5.5 years in the 538 patients with SPMS and 9.5 years in the 218 patients with an initial progressive course. When this cohort was reassessed later on with a longer disease duration, however, although restricted to the cases where onset of progression was identifiable at DSS of 2 or less, this estimated median time was around 6 years, similar in SP, single-attack progressive, and PPMS.[45] In the Gothenburg cohort,[36] median survival time from the onset of progression to DSS 6 was 5.2 years for the 162 cases with SPMS and 6 years for the 36 with progression from onset, a not significant difference (**Fig. 21**). Interestingly, in this cohort, the proportion of SPMS (77% of the cases with an RR onset) and the duration of the disease (>25 years) were both high. The conclusion that, once clinical progression has started, the rate at which disability accumulates is faster in SPMS than cases with

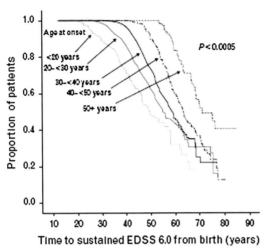

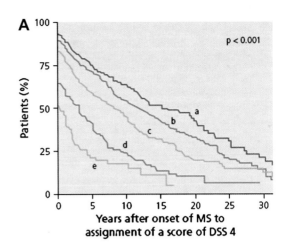

Fig. 19. Kaplan-Meier estimates for the age at assignment of an irreversible score of 6 on the Kurtzke Expanded Disability Status Scale (EDSS), depending on the age at onset of the disease, among the 2837 patients in the British Columbia, Canada, MS cohort. (*From* Tremlett H, Paty D, Devonshire V. Disability progression in multiple sclerosis is slower than previously reported. Neurology 2006;66:172–7; with permission.)

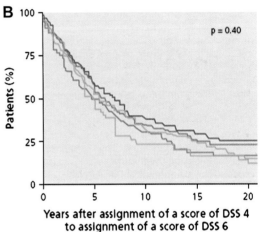

Fig. 20. Kaplan-Meier estimates for (*A*) the time from the onset of MS to the assignment of an irreversible score of 4, and (*B*) the time from the assignment of an irreversible score of 4 to the assignment of an irreversible score of 6 on the Kurtzke Disability Status Scale (DSS), among the 1844 patients in the Lyon, France, MS cohort, according to the age of the patient at disease onset. *A*, 0–19 years; *B*, 20–29 years; *C*, 30–39 years; *D*, 40–49 years; *E*, ≥50 years. (*From* Tremlett H, Paty D, Devonshire V. Disability progression in multiple sclerosis is slower than previously reported. Neurology 2006;66:172–7; with permission.)

progression from onset probably reflects limited disease duration at the time of the survey. It is indeed likely that, with sufficient follow-up for allowing a sufficient proportion of RR onset cases to convert to SP, analyses will lead to the observation in most series that the rate of accumulation of irreversible disability during the progressive phase of the disease is similar in PPMS and SPMS.

Multiple sclerosis with relapsing-remitting onset and multiple sclerosis with progressive onset

It serves little purpose to restate the differences regarding gender ratio, age, and symptoms at onset or survival times from onset because these are essentially similar to what has already been discussed. The objective here is to compare, within a general cohort of patients having MS, all cases with an RR onset (ie, RRMS and SPMS) and those with a progressive onset (ie, PRMS and PPMS) with respect to the time course of disability. It is enough to remind here that, in the Lyon cohort, survival times between disability landmarks seemed strikingly similar for the 1562 patients with an RR onset and the 282 patients with a progressive onset (see **Fig. 12**).[31,34] Furthermore, as already discussed, age at time of assigning disability landmarks can be viewed as not substantially influenced by the initial course, be that RR or progressive.

Altogether, available data from currently available natural history series provide strong arguments for concluding that, from a clinical and statistical perspective, secondary and primary progression share much more than they differ.

INTERCURRENT LIFE EVENTS

The person with MS is not less exposed to intercurrent life events than any other member of the society. These events may be natural, such as

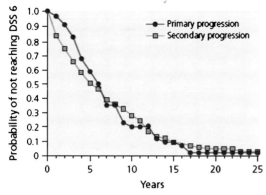

Fig. 21. Kaplan-Meier estimates for the time (years) from onset of progression to the assignment of a score of 6 on the Kurtzke Disability Status Scale (DSS) among 162 patients with secondary-progressive and 36 patients with primary-progressive MS. Primary-progressive MS denotes here the pooling of cases with primary-progressive MS and cases with progressive-relapsing MS according to the classification of Lublin and Reingold (1996). (*From* Runmarker B, Andersen O. Prognostic factors in a multiple sclerosis incidence cohort with twenty five years of follow-up. Brain 1993;116:117–34; with permission.)

pregnancy; accidental, as in stress, trauma, and infection; or interventional, such as anesthesia, surgery, and vaccinations. Most intercurrent life events are suspected of triggering relapses or even the onset of MS. This raises the issue of coincidence versus causality (for a more detailed review see.[3])

Pregnancy and Puerperium

MS mainly affects women in their childbearing years, and the issue of pregnancy is a major concern. For many years, women with MS were actively discouraged from contemplating pregnancy because of the possible deleterious effect of pregnancy on the disease. Since 1998, the European Pregnancy In Multiple Sclerosis study has provided robust and reassuring epidemiologic information on this topic.[193,194] The study concerned 227 women with MS contemplating pregnancy and followed them up until 2 years after delivery. As compared with the year before pregnancy, the relapse rate decreased by two thirds during pregnancy, especially during the third trimester, before increasing by two thirds during the first 3 months after delivery and thereafter returning to the prepregnancy level (**Fig. 22**). Overall, the relapse rate during the pregnancy year (encompassing the 9 months of pregnancy and the first 3 months after delivery) was not different from that observed during the year before pregnancy. One third of women suffered from a relapse during the whole pregnancy period. A similar proportion suffered from a relapse during the first 3 months after delivery. Pregnancy and puerperium had no significant effect on the residual disability. Epidural analgesia and breast-feeding had no specific effect on the relapse rate or the time course of disability. The patients who suffered from one or more relapses before and during pregnancy were at increased risk of a relapse during the first 3 months after delivery but no reliable algorithm could be found for predicting which patient will

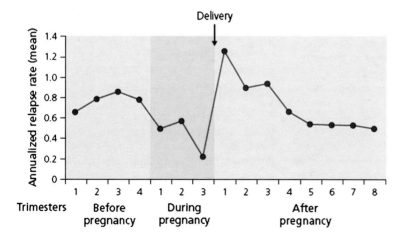

Fig. 22. Mean annualized relapse rate during the year before pregnancy, the pregnancy, and the 2 years after delivery, among the 227 women with MS in the Pregnancy In Multiple Sclerosis (PRIMS) study. (*Data from* Confavreux C, Hutchinson M, Hours MM, et al. Rate of pregnancy-related relapse in multiple sclerosis: pregnancy in multiple sclerosis group. N Engl J Med 1998;339:285–91; and Vukusic S, Hutchinson M, Hours M, et al. Pregnancy and multiple sclerosis (the PRIMS study): clinical predictors of post-partum relapse. Brain 2004;127:1353–60. [Epub 2004 May 6. Erratum in: Brain 2004;127:1912].)

experience a relapse postpartum.[194] MS did not alter the course of the pregnancy and the delivery or the health of the newborn. Eventually, the decision to contemplate childbearing in women with MS is most likely to hinge on perceptions of present and future disability, impairment, and participation. These are not so easy to predict.

Psychologic Stress

The possibility that psychologic stress may trigger the onset or subsequent activity in MS has been repeatedly proposed, but hard to prove, because the definition of a stressful event is particularly difficult and the personal impact of a stressful event cannot be easily standardized. The numerous epidemiologic studies addressing the issue provide conflicting results. Despite consistent and confident statements in the literature that psychologic stress and disease activity in MS are linked, a more critical reading suggests that the association is, at best, weak and the effect size modest.

Physical Trauma

The pathophysiologic and medicolegal importance of this question is obvious. A complete reading of the currently available literature provides no epidemiologic evidence in favor of an association and a causal link between physical trauma and MS.

Anesthesia and Surgery

No epidemiologically robust studies on MS and anesthesia or surgery have been performed yet and evidence is mostly anecdotal. Anesthesia is considered to be safe in persons with MS and the same is true for surgical procedures. There is no rationale to let potential effects on disease activity influence decisions on the need for anesthesia or surgery.

Infections

Anecdotal evidence suggests the possibility of an increased risk of relapse following infection, although it is difficult to establish. Indeed, the boundaries are often unclear between genuine relapse and pseudorelapse, notably the worsening of pre-existing symptoms or the reappearance of previous symptoms caused by an increase in the body temperature (Uhthoff's phenomenon). With the availability of epidemiologic studies specifically designed to address this issue, the current consensus is that infections do trigger relapses in MS.

Vaccinations

The concern of an association between vaccinations and MS has been revived, notably in France in the 1990s, on the occasion of the extensive immunization program against hepatitis B. Two issues have been raised: are vaccinations in general and hepatitis B vaccination in particular a risk factor for the onset of MS in the general population; and are they associated with an increased risk of relapse in patients with CDMS. Currently available data from epidemiologic studies provide an essentially negative answer to the first question.[195] With only one exception from a study whose results are disputable methodologically,[196] no association has been reported between hepatitis B vaccination and the clinical onset of MS. As for the second question, the Vaccines in MS European multicenter study has not observed any deleterious effect of vaccination among 643 patients with MS.[197] Indeed, the relative risk of a relapse associated with exposure to any vaccination during the previous 2 months was 0.71 (95% confidence interval, 0.40–1.26). Results were similar for specific vaccinations against tetanus alone, tetanus associated with poliomyelitis or diphtheria, influenza, and hepatitis B. The most plausible explanation for the reported examples of association between vaccinations and MS is coincidence not causality. Vaccines are not contraindicated in patients with MS. More specifically, there is currently no rationale to advise patients with MS to avoid vaccinations, including hepatitis B. It makes sense to wait for a relatively silent period of the disease, free from relapse for 12 months at least. Patients receiving immunosuppressive drugs should avoid vaccinations with live components. Similarly, there is no rationale to advise relatives of patients with MS, notably children, to avoid vaccinations, including hepatitis B, and the general population to avoid hepatitis B vaccination.[3]

SUMMARY

Knowledge of the natural history of MS has made steady progress during the past decades. Now, the overall course and prognosis of the disease are clearly delineated with consistent results available from the different representative cohorts, which have been set up worldwide since the 1970s. Several statements can be made with reasonable confidence (Box 2).

From a clinical and statistical point of view, the course and prognosis of MS are essentially age-dependent. RR disease can be regarded as MS in which insufficient time has elapsed for the conversion to SP; SP forms as RRMS that has "grown

Box 2
Course and prognosis: main features

1. The course of MS results from the interplay of two clinical processes, relapses and progression. Three main clinical forms may be identified as RR, SP, and PP.
2. The clinical onset occurs on average at the age of 30 years. It is characterized by an RR course in 85% of the patients contrasting with a progressive course in the remaining 15%. Initial symptoms are related to isolated optic neuritis, isolated brainstem dysfunction, isolated dysfunction of long tracts, or various combinations of these features in around 15%, 10%, 50%, and 25% of the cases, respectively.
3. The relapse rate is one relapse on average every other year.
4. With time, most cases with an RR onset convert to SPMS at a rate of 2% to 3% per year, and the median time interval for conversion is around 19 years.
5. Relapses persist in around 40% of the cases during the progressive phase, be this primary or secondary.
6. Clinically detectable relapses have only a marginal effect on the accumulation of irreversible disability.
7. For a representative population of patients with MS, it takes a median time of 8, 20, and 30 years to reach the irreversible disability levels of DSS 4 (limitation of ambulation), 6 (walking with a stick), and 7 (wheelchair dependency), respectively.
8. It takes much longer for cases with an RR onset than those with progressive onset to reach levels of irreversible disability, but median ages at assignment of the irreversible disability levels of DSS 4, 6, and 7 are around 42, 53, and 63 years of age, irrespective of the initial course.
9. Onset of the RR and progressive phases, like onset of irreversible disability levels, is essentially driven by current age.
10. Life expectancy is only marginally reduced by the disease.

considering MS as one disease with different clinical phenotypes rather than an entity encompassing several distinct diseases, each having a different etiology and mechanism. This is the position of complexity rather than true heterogeneity.

Contrasting with this well-delineated overall prognosis, MS stands out for its extreme variability in course and prognosis in individuals. A full spectrum does exist from silent cases to rapidly lethal forms. Unfortunately, it must be acknowledged that the dividend from studies of the natural history mainly relates to groups and not the individual patient. Despite intense research in this area, outcome predictions for the individual, notably for the long run, are still a "mission impossible" because of the weak (at best) predictive value of clinical and presently available paraclinical markers. Progress may come from the discovery of new markers or from methodologic developments, such as deterministic approaches or individually tailored mathematical models.

Lessons from studies of the natural history of MS have important implications for understanding disease mechanisms. They suggest that MS is a one-stage disorder, with a tight intermingling of acute focal recurrent inflammation and diffuse chronic progressive neurodegeneration from the very outset of the disease, despite the distinctive clinical course comprising a RR phase followed by progression. Diffuse neurodegeneration is operating from the outset although, at first, clinically not detectable. Given the marginal influence of the relapses on the overall accumulation of irreversible disability, acute inflammatory lesions are probably not the major player of diffuse neurodegeneration. This resonates with the evidence that currently available immunologically active treatments essentially do not affect neurodegeneration, despite suppressing acute inflammation. Presumably, treating the acute focal inflammation, as useful as it may be for the control of relapses, is not enough. The fight against MS must also address the chronic diffuse inflammation of the CNS that evolves silently beyond the blood-brain barrier.[198] This could represent a key-step in the development of more effective therapies for MS.

older;" and progressive from onset as MS "amputated" from the usual preceding RR phase. Times to reach disability milestones, and the ages at which these landmarks are met, follow a predefined schedule not obviously influenced by relapses, whenever they may occur, or by the initial course of the disease, whatever its phenotype. This leads to a unifying concept of the disease in which primary and secondary progression might be regarded as essentially similar. This favors

ACKNOWLEDGMENTS

The authors are indebted to Professor Alastair Compston for the many fruitful discussions during the writing of the chapter published in the McAlpine textbook,[3] which has served as a basis for this article; and to France-Isabelle Pairel for technical assistance in the preparation of the manuscript.

REFERENCES

1. McAlpine D. The benign form of multiple sclerosis: results of a long-term follow up. Br Med J 1964;2: 1029–32.
2. McAlpine D, Compston ND. Some aspects of the natural history of disseminated sclerosis: incidence, course and prognosis; factors affecting onset and course. Q J Med 1952;21:135–67.
3. Confavreux C, Compston A. The natural history of multiple sclerosis. In: Compston A, editor. McAlpine's multiple sclerosis. 4th edition. London: Churchill Livingstone Elsevier; 2006. p. 183–272.
4. Sackett DL, Haynes RB, Tugwell P. Clinical epidemiology: a basic science for clinical medicine. Boston: Little, Brown; 1985. p. 161–2.
5. Ebers GC. Natural history of multiple sclerosis. In: Compston A, Ebers G, Lassmann H, et al, editors. McAlpine's multiple sclerosis. 3rd Edition. London: Churchill Livingstone; 1998. p. 191–221.
6. Georgi W. Multiple sklerose: pathologisch-anatomische Befund multipler sklerose bei klinisch nicht diagnostizierten Krankheiten. Schweiz Med Wochenschr 1961;91:605–7.
7. McKay RP, Hirano A. Forms of benign multiple sclerosis: report of two clinically silent cases discovered at autopsy. Arch Neurol 1967;17:588–600.
8. Gilbert JJ, Sadler M. Unsuspected multiple sclerosis. Arch Neurol 1983;40:533–6.
9. Engell T. A clinical patho-anatomical study of clinically silent multiple sclerosis. Acta Neurol Scand 1989;79:428–30.
10. Mews I, Bergmann M, Bunkowski S, et al. Oligodendrocyte and axon pathology in clinically silent multiple sclerosis lesions. Mult Scler 1998;4:55–62.
11. McDonnell GV, Cabrera-Gomez J, Calne DB, et al. Clinical presentation of primary progressive multiple sclerosis 10 years after the incidental finding of typical magnetic resonance imaging brain lesions: the subclinical stage of primary progressive multiple sclerosis may last 10 years. Mult Scler 2003;9:210–2.
12. Lebrun C, Bensa C, Debouverie M, et al. On behalf of CFSEP. Unexpected multiple sclerosis: follow-up of 30 patients with magnetic resonance imaging and clinical conversion profile. J Neurol Neurosurg Psychiatr 2008;79:195–8.
13. Poser S, Bauer HJ, Poser W. Prognosis of multiple sclerosis: results from an epidemiological area in Germany. Acta Neurol Scand 1982;65:347–54.
14. Weinshenker BG, Ebers GC. The natural history of multiple sclerosis. Can J Neurol Sci 1987;14:255–61.
15. Poser CM, Paty DW, Scheinberg L, et al. New diagnostic criteria for multiple sclerosis: guidelines for research protocols. Ann Neurol 1983;13:227–31.
16. McDonald WI, Compston A, Edan G, et al. Recommended diagnostic criteria for multiple sclerosis: guidelines from the international panel on the diagnosis of multiple sclerosis. Ann Neurol 2001;50:121–7.
17. Confavreux C, Compston DAS, Hommes OR, et al. EDMUS, a European database for multiple sclerosis. J Neurol Neurosurg Psychiatr 1992;55:671–6.
18. Amato MP, Grimaud J, Achiti I, et al. European validation of a standardized clinical description of multiple sclerosis. J Neurol 2004;251:1472–80.
19. Fog T, Linnemann F. The course of multiple sclerosis: in 73 cases with computer designed curves. Acta Neurol Scand 1970;46(Suppl):1–175.
20. Lhermitte F, Marteau R, Gazengel J, et al. The frequency of relapse in multiple sclerosis: a study based on 245 cases. J Neurol 1973;205:47–59.
21. Patzold U, Pocklington PR. Course of multiple sclerosis: first results of a prospective study carried out of 102 MS patients from 1976–1980. Acta Neurol Scand 1982;65:248–66.
22. Confavreux C. Establishment and use of multiple sclerosis registers: EDMUS. Ann Neurol 1994;36(Suppl):136–9.
23. Confavreux C, Paty DW. Current status of computerization of multiple sclerosis clinical data for research in Europe and North America: the EDMUS/MS - COSTAR connection. Neurology 1995;45:573–6.
24. Confavreux C, Hours M, Moreau T, et al. Clinical databasing in multiple sclerosis: EDMUS and the European effort. In: Abramsky O, editor. Frontiers in multiple sclerosis: clinical research and therapy. London: Martin Dunitz Ltd; 1996. p. 299–312.
25. Weinshenker BG. Databases in MS research: pitfalls and promises. Mult Scler 1999;5:206–11.
26. Kaplan EL, Meier P. Non-parametric estimation from incomplete observations. J Am Stat Assoc 1958;53:457–81.
27. Cox DR. Regression models and life tables. J R Stat Soc Series B 1972;Series B 34:187–220.
28. Confavreux C, Ritleng C, Debouverie M, et al. Defining the natural history of multiple sclerosis: the need for complete data and rigorous definitions. Answer to Tremlett, et al Mult Scler 2008;14:1144–7.
29. Confavreux C. L'histoire naturelle de la sclérose en plaques. Etude par informatique de 349 observations. Thèse de médecine. Lyon: Université Claude Bernard; 1977. 184 pages.
30. Confavreux C, Aimard G, Devic M. Course and prognosis of multiple sclerosis assessed by the computerized data processing of 349 patients. Brain 1980;103:281–300.
31. Confavreux C, Vukusic S, Moreau T, et al. Relapses and progression of disability in multiple sclerosis. N Engl J Med 2000;343:1430–8.

32. Confavreux C, Vukusic S, Adeleine P. Early clinical predictors and progression of irreversible disability in multiple sclerosis: an amnesic process. Brain 2003;126:770–82.

33. Confavreux C, Vukusic S. Age at disability milestones in multiple sclerosis. Brain 2006;129:595–605.

34. Confavreux C, Vukusic S. Natural history of multiple sclerosis: a unifying concept. Brain 2006;129:606–16.

35. Broman T, Andersen O, Bergmann L. Clinical studies on multiple sclerosis. I. Presentation of an incidence material from Gothenburg. Acta Neurol Scand 1981;63:6–33.

36. Runmarker B, Andersen O. Prognostic factors in a multiple sclerosis incidence cohort with twenty five years of follow-up. Brain 1993;116:117–34.

37. Eriksson M, Andersen O, Runmarker B. Long-term follow-up of patients with clinically isolated syndromes, relapsing-remitting and secondary progressive multiple sclerosis. Mult Scler 2003;9:260–74.

38. Weinshenker BG, Bass B, Rice GPA, et al. The natural history of multiple sclerosis: a geographically based study. 1. Clinical course and disability. Brain 1989;112:133–46.

39. Weinshenker BG, Bass B, Rice GPA, et al. The natural history of multiple sclerosis: a geographically based study. 2. Predictive value of the early clinical course. Brain 1989;112:1419–28.

40. Weinshenker BG, Rice GPA, Noseworthy JH, et al. The natural history of multiple sclerosis: a geographically based study. 3. Multivariate analysis of predictive factors and models of outcome. Brain 1991;114:1045–56.

41. Weinshenker BG, Rice GPA, Noseworthy JH, et al. The natural history of multiple sclerosis: a geographically based study. 4. Applications to planning and interpretation of clinical trials. Brain 1991;114:1057–67.

42. Cottrell DA, Kremenchutzky M, Rice GPA, et al. The natural history of multiple sclerosis: a geographically based study. 5. The clinical features and natural history of primary progressive multiple sclerosis. Brain 1999;122:625–39.

43. Cottrell DA, Kremenchutzky M, Rice GPA, et al. The natural history of multiple sclerosis: a geographically based study. 6. Applications to planning and interpretation of clinical therapeutic trials in primary progressive multiple sclerosis. Brain 1999;122:641–7.

44. Kremenchutzky M, Cottrell D, Rice G, et al. The natural history of multiple sclerosis: a geographically based study. 7. Progressive-relapsing and relapsing-progressive multiple sclerosis: a re-evaluation. Brain 1999;122:1941–9.

45. Kremenchutzky M, Rice GP, Baskerville J, et al. The natural history of multiple sclerosis: a geographically based study. 9: Observations on the progressive phase of the disease. Brain 2006;129:584–94.

46. Charcot M. Leçons sur les maladies chroniques du système nerveux. I - Des scléroses de la mœlle épinière. Gaz Hôp 1868;41:405–6, 409.

47. Marie P. Sclórose en plaques et maladies infectieuses. Progr Méd 1884;12:287–9, 305–7, 349–51.

48. Youl BD, Turano G, Miller DH, et al. The pathophysiology of acute optic neuritis: an association of gadolinium leakage with clinical and electrophysiological deficits. Brain 1991;114:2437–50.

49. Schumacher GA, Beebe G, Kibler RF, et al. Problems of experimental trials of therapy in MS: report by the panel on the evaluation of experimental trials of therapy in MS. Ann N Y Acad Sci 1965;122:552–68.

50. Thompson AJ, Polman CH, Miller DH, et al. Primary progressive multiple sclerosis. Brain 1997;120:1085–96.

51. Lublin FD, Reingold SC. for the National Multiple Sclerosis Society (USA) Advisory Committee on Clinical Trials of New Agents in Multiple Sclerosis. Defining the clinical course of multiple sclerosis: results of an international survey. Neurology 1996;46:907–11.

52. Kurtzke JF. On the evaluation of disability in multiple sclerosis. Neurology 1961;11:686–94.

53. Kurtzke JF. Further notes on disability evaluation in multiple sclerosis, with scale modifications. Neurology 1965;15:654–61.

54. Kurtzke JF. Rating neurological impairment in multiple sclerosis: an expanded disability status scale (EDSS). Neurology 1983;33:1444–52.

55. Hobart J, Lamping DL, Thompson A. Evaluating neurological outcome measures: the bare essentials. J Neurol Neurosurg Psychiatr 1996;60:127–30.

56. Rudick R, Antel J, Confavreux C, et al. Clinical outcomes assessment in multiple sclerosis. Ann Neurol 1996;40:469–79.

57. Rudick R, Antel J, Confavreux C, et al. Recommendations from the national multiple sclerosis society clinical outcomes assessment task force. Ann Neurol 1997;42:379–82.

58. Amato MP, Fratiglioni L, Groppi C, et al. Interrater reliability in assessing functional systems and disability on Kurtzke scale in multiple sclerosis. Arch Neurol 1988;45:746–8.

59. Willoughby EW, Paty DW. Scales for rating impairment in multiple sclerosis: a critique. Neurology 1988;38:1793–8.

60. Noseworthy JH, Vandenvoort MK, Wong CJ, et al. Interrater variability with the Expanded Disability Status Scale (EDSS) and Functional Systems (FS) in a multiple sclerosis clinical trial. The Canadian

Cooperation MS Study Group. Neurology 1990;40: 971–5.

61. Francis DA, Bain P, Swan AV, et al. An assessment of disability rating scales used in multiple sclerosis. Arch Neurol 1991;48:299–301.

62. Goodkin DE, Cookfair D, Wende K, et al. Inter- and intra-rater scoring agreement using grades 1.0 to 3.5 of the Kurtzke Expanded Disability Status Scale (EDSS). Multiple Sclerosis Collaborative Research Group. Neurology 1992;42:859–63.

63. Hobart J, Lamping D, Fitzpatrick R, et al. The Multiple Sclerosis Impact Scale (MSIS-29): a new patient-based outcome measure. Brain 2001;124: 962–73.

64. Minderhoud JM, Van der Hoeven JH, Prange AJA. Course and prognosis of chronic progressive multiple sclerosis: results of an epidemiological study. Acta Neurol Scand 1988;78:10–5.

65. Miller DH, Hornabrook RW, Purdie G. The natural history of multiple sclerosis: a regional study with some longitudinal data. J Neurol Neurosurg Psychiatr 1992;55:341–6.

66. Sharrack B, Hughes RAC, Soudain S, et al. The psychometric properties of clinical rating scales used in multiple sclerosis. Brain 1999;122: 141–59.

67. Confavreux C. Defining the natural history of multiple sclerosis: the need for complete data and rigorous definitions. Mult Scler 2008;14:289–91.

68. Müller R. Studies on disseminated sclerosis: with special reference to symptomatology, course and prognosis. Acta Med Scand 1949;133(Suppl 222): 1–214.

69. Müller R. Course and prognosis of disseminated sclerosis in relation to age at onset. Arch Neurol Psychiatry 1951;66:561–70.

70. Leibowitz U, Halpern L, Alter M. Clinical studies of multiple sclerosis in Israel. I. A clinical analysis based on a country-wide survey. Arch Neurol 1964b;10:502–12.

71. Leibowitz U, Alter M. Multiple sclerosis: clues to its cause. Amsterdam and London: North-Holland Publishing Company; 1973. 1–373.

72. Morrissey SP, Miller DH, Kendall BE, et al. The significance of brain magnetic resonance imaging abnormalities at presentation with clinically isolated syndromes suggestive of multiple sclerosis: a 5-year follow-up study. Brain 1993;116: 135–46.

73. Filippi M, Horsfield MA, Morrissey SP, et al. Quantitative brain MRI lesion load predicts the course of clinically isolated syndromes suggestive of multiple sclerosis. Neurology 1994;44:635–41.

74. Barkhof F, Filippi M, Miller DH, et al. Comparison of MRI criteria at first presentation to predict conversion to clinically definite multiple sclerosis. Brain 1997;120:2059–69.

75. O'Riordan JI, Thompson AJ, Kingsley DPE, et al. The prognostic value of brain MRI in clinically isolated syndromes of the CNS: a 10-year follow-up. Brain 1998;121:495–503.

76. Tintoré M, Rovira A, Martinez MJ, et al. Isolated demyelinating syndromes: comparison of different MR imaging criteria to predict conversion to clinically definite multiple sclerosis. AJNR Am J Neuroradiol 2000;21:702–6.

77. Riise T, Gronning M, Fernandez O, et al. Early prognostic factors for disability in multiple sclerosis: a European multicenter study. Acta Neurol Scand 1992;85:212–8.

78. Trojano M, Avolio C, Manzari C, et al. Multivariate analysis of predictive factors of multiple sclerosis with a validated method to assess clinical events. J Neurol Neurosurg Psychiatr 1995;58:300–6.

79. Leibowitz U, Alter M, Halpern L. Clinical studies of multiple sclerosis in Israel. III. Clinical course and prognosis related to age at onset. Neurology 1964a;14:926–32.

80. Poser S. Multiple sclerosis: an analysis of 812 cases by means of electronic data processing. Berlin: Springer-Verlag; 1978.

81. Poser S, Raun NE, Poser W. Age at onset, initial symptomatology and the course of multiple sclerosis. Acta Neurol Scand 1982b;66:355–62.

82. Phadke JG. Clinical aspects of multiple sclerosis in north-east Scotland with particular reference to its course and prognosis. Brain 1990;113:1597–628.

83. Kurtzke JF. Course of exacerbations of multiple sclerosis hospitalised patients. Archives of Neurology and Psychiatry 1956;76:175–84.

84. Kurtzke JF, Beebe GW, Nagler B, et al. Studies on the natural history of multiple sclerosis. 7: correlates of clinical changes in an early bout. Acta Neurol Scand 1973;49:379–95.

85. Myhr KM, Riise T, Vedeler C, et al. Disability an prognosis in multiple sclerosis: demographic and clinical variables important for the ability to walk and awarding of disability pension. Mult Scler 2001;7:59–65.

86. Beck RW, Cleary PA, Anderson MM, et al. A randomized controlled trial of corticosteroids in the treatment of acute optic neuritis. N Engl J Med 1992;326:581–8.

87. Beck RW, Cleary PA, Trobe JD, et al. The effect of corticosteroids for acute optic neuritis on the subsequent development of multiple sclerosis. N Engl J Med 1993;329:1764–9.

88. Beck RW. The Optic Neuritis Treatment Trial: three-year follow-up results. Arch Ophthalmol 1995;113: 136–7.

89. Jacobs LD, Beck RW, Simon JH, et al. Intramuscular interferon beta-1a therapy initiated during a first demyelinating event in multiple sclerosis. N Engl J Med 2000;343:898–904.

90. Beck RW, Chandler DL, Cole SR, et al. Interferon ß-1a for early multiple sclerosis: CHAMPS trial subgroup analyses. Ann Neurol 2002;51:481–90.

91. Comi G, Filippi M, Barkhof F, et al. Effect of early interferon treatment on conversion to definite multiple sclerosis: a randomised study. Lancet 2001;357: 1576–82.

92. Kappos L, Polman CH, Freedman MS, et al. Treatment with interferon beta-1b delays conversion to clinically definite and McDonald MS in patients with clinically isolated syndromes. Neurology 2006;67:1242–9.

93. Hickman SJ, Dalton CM, Miller DH, et al. Management of acute optic neuritis. Lancet 2002;360: 1953–62.

94. Nilsson P, Larsson EM, Maly-Sundgren P, et al. Predicting the outcome of optic neuritis: evaluation of risk factors after 30 years of follow-up. J Neurol 2005;252:396–402.

95. Tintore M, Rovira A, Rio J, et al. Is optic neuritis more benign than other first attacks in multiple sclerosis? Ann Neurol 2005;57:210–5.

96. Korteweg T, Tintore M, Uitdehaag B, et al. MRI criteria for dissemination in space in patients with clinically isolated syndromes: a multicentre follow-up study. Lancet Neurol 2006;5:221–7.

97. Optic Neuritis Study Group. The 5-year risk of MS after optic neuritis: experience of the Optic Neuritis Treatment Trial. Neurology 1997;49:1404–13.

98. CHAMPS Study Group. MRI predictors of early conversion to clinically definite MS in the CHAMPS placebo group. Neurology 2002;59:998–1005.

99. Miller DH, Ormerod IEC, McDonald WI, et al. The early risk of multiple sclerosis after optic neuritis. J Neurol Neurosurg Psychiatr 1988;51:1569–71.

100. Miller DH, Ormerod IEC, Rudge P, et al. The early risk of multiple sclerosis following acute syndromes of the brainstem and spinal cord. Ann Neurol 1989; 26:635–9.

101. Paty DW, Oger JJ, Kastrukoff LF, et al. MRI in the diagnosis of MS: a prospective study with comparison of clinical evaluation, evoked potentials, oligoclonal banding and CT. Neurology 1988;38: 180–5.

102. Frederiksen JL, Larsson HBW, Olesen J, et al. MRI, VEP, SEP and biothesiometry suggest monosymptomatic acute optic neuritis to be a first manifestation of multiple sclerosis. Acta Neurol Scand 1991; 83:343–50.

103. Lee KH, Hashimoto SA, Hooge JP, et al. Magnetic resonance imaging of the head in the diagnosis of multiple sclerosis: a prospective 2-year follow-up with comparison of clinical evaluation, evoked potentials, oligoclonal banding, and CT. Neurology 1991;41:657–60.

104. Martinelli V, Comi G, Filippi M, et al. Paraclinical tests in acute-onset optic neuritis: basal data and results of a short follow-up. Acta Neurol Scand 1991;84:231–6.

105. Ford B, Tampieri D, Francis G. Long-term follow-up of acute partial transverse myelopathy. Neurology 1992;42:250–2.

106. Soderstrom M, Ya-Ping, Hillert J, et al. Optic neuritis: prognosis for multiple sclerosis from MRI, CSF, and HLA findings. Neurology 1998;50:708–14.

107. Brex PA, Miszkiel KA, O'Riordan JI, et al. Assessing the risk of early multiple sclerosis in patients with clinically isolated syndromes: the role of a follow-up MRI. J Neurol Neurosurg Psychiatr 2001;70: 390–3.

108. Tintoré M, Rovira A, Rio J, et al. New diagnostic criteria for multiple sclerosis: application in first demyelinating episode. Neurology 2003;60:27–30.

109. Brex PA, Ciccarelli O, O'Riordan JI, et al. A longitudinal study of abnormalities on MRI and disability from multiple sclerosis. N Engl J Med 2002;346: 158–64.

110. Polman CH, Reingold SC, Edan G, et al. Diagnostic criteria for multiple sclerosis: 2005 revisions to the McDonald criteria. Ann Neurol 2005;58:840–6.

111. Berger T, Rubner P, Schautzer F, et al. Antimyelin antibodies as a predictor of clinically definite multiple sclerosis after a first demyelinating event. N Engl J Med 2003;349:139–45.

112. Kuhle J, Pohl C, Mehling M, et al. Lack of association between antimyelin antibodies and progression to multiple sclerosis. N Engl J Med 2007; 356:371–8.

113. Panelius M. Studies on epidemiological, clinical and etiological aspects of multiple sclerosis. Acta Neurol Sand 1969;45(Suppl 39):1–82.

114. Goodkin DE, Hertsgaard D, Rudick RA. Exacerbation rates and adherence to disease type in a prospective followed-up population with multiple sclerosis: implications for clinical trials. Arch Neurol 1989;46:1107–12.

115. Vukusic S, Confavreux C. Prognostic factors for progression of disability in the secondary progressive phase of multiple sclerosis. J Neurol Sci 2003; 206:135–7.

116. Tremlett H, Zhao Y, Devonshire V. The natural history of secondary progressive multiple sclerosis. Mult Scler 2008;14:314–24.

117. Amato MP, Ponziani G, Bartolozzi ML, et al. A prospective study on the natural history of multiple sclerosis: clues to the conduct and interpretation of clinical trials. J Neurol Sci 1999;168: 96–106.

118. Amato MP, Ponziani G. A prospective study on the prognosis of multiple sclerosis. Neurol Sci 2000; 21(Suppl):831–8.

119. Kantarci O, Siva A, Eraksoy M, et al. Survival and predictors of disability in Turkish MS patients. Neurology 1998;51:765–72.

120. Tremlett H, Paty D, Devonshire V. Disability progression in multiple sclerosis is slower than previously reported. Neurology 2006;66:172–7.

121. Pittock SJ, Mayr WT, McClelland RL, et al. Disability profile of MS did not change over 10 years in a population-based prevalence cohort. Neurology 2004; 62:601–6.

122. Thygesen P. Disseminated sclerosis: influence of age on the different modes of progression. Acta Psychiatr Neurolo Scand 1955;30:365–74.

123. McAlpine D. The benign form of multiple sclerosis: a study based on 241 cases seen within three years of onset and followed up until the tenth year or more of the disease. Brain 1961;84: 186–203.

124. Bonduelle M. Les formes bénignes de la sclérose en plaques. Press Méd 1967;75:2023–6.

125. Kurtzke JF, Beebe GW, Nagler B, et al. 1968 Studies on natural history of multiple sclerosis. 4: Clinical features of the onset bout. Acta Neurol Scand 1968;44:467–94.

126. Kurtzke JF, Beebe GW, Nagler B, et al. 1970 Studies on the natural history of multiple sclerosis. V. Long-term survival in young men. Arch Neurol 1970;22:215–25.

127. Kurtzke JF, Beebe GW, Nagler B, et al. 1977 Studies on the natural history of multiple sclerosis. 8: Early prognostic features of the later course of the illness. J Chronic Dis 1977;30:819–30.

128. Leibowitz U, Alter M. Clinical factors associated with increased disability in multiple sclerosis. Acta Neurol Scand 1970;46:53–70.

129. Clark VA, Detels R, Visscher BR, et al. Factors associated with a malignant or benign course of multiple sclerosis. JAMA 1982;248:856–60.

130. Detels R, Clark VA, Valdiviezo NL, et al. Factors associated with a rapid course of multiple sclerosis. Arch Neurol 1982;39:337–41.

131. Visscher BR, Liu KS, Clark VA, et al. Onset symptoms as predictors of mortality and disability in multiple sclerosis. Acta Neurol Scand 1984;70:321–8.

132. Phadke JG. Survival pattern and cause of death in patients with multiple sclerosis: results from an epidemiological survey in north-east Scotland. J Neurol Neurosurg Psychiatr 1987;50:523–31.

133. Tintoré M, Rovira A, Rio J, et al. Baseline MRI predicts future attacks and disability in clinically isolated syndromes. Neurology 2006;67:968–72.

134. Fisniku LK, Brex PA, Altmann DR, et al. Disability and T2 MRI lesions: a 20-year follow-up of patients with relapse onset of multiple sclerosis. Brain 2008; 31:808–17.

135. Runmarker B, Andersson C, Oden A, et al. Prediction of outcome in multiple sclerosis based on multivariate models. J Neurol 1994;241:597–604.

136. Celius EG, Harbo HF, Egeland T, et al. Sex and age at diagnosis are correlated with the HLA-DR2, DQ6 haplotype in multiple sclerosis. Neurol Sci 2000; 178:132–5.

137. Masterman T, Ligers A, Olsson T, et al. HLA-DR15 is associated with lower age at onset in multiple sclerosis. Ann Neurol 2000;48:211–9.

138. Weatherby SJ, Thomson W, Pepper L, et al. HLA-DRB1 and disease outcome in multiple sclerosis. J Neurol 2001;248:304–10.

139. Hensiek AE, Sawcer SJ, Feakes R, et al. HLA-DR 15 is associated with female sex and younger age at diagnosis in multiple sclerosis. J Neurol Neurosurg Psychiatr 2002;72:184–7.

140. Evangelou N, Jackson M, Beeson D, et al. Association of the APOE epsilon4 allele with disease activity in multiple sclerosis. J Neurol Neurosurg Psychiatr 1999;67:203–5.

141. Chapman J, Vinokurov S, Achiron A, et al. APOE genotype is a major predictor of long-term progression of disability in MS. Neurology 2001;56: 312–6.

142. Fazekas F, Strasser-Fuchs S, Kollegger H, et al. Apolipoprotein E epsilon 4 is associated with rapid progression of multiple sclerosis. Neurology 2001; 57:853–7.

143. Fazekas F, Strasser-Fuchs S, Schmidt H, et al. Apolipoprotein E genotype related differences in brain lesions of multiple sclerosis. J Neurol Neurosurg Psychiatr 2000;69:25–8.

144. Enzinger C, Ropele S, Smith S, et al., Accelerated evolution of brain atrophy and black holes in MS patients with APOE-epsilon 4. Arch Neurol 2004a;55:563–9.

145. Enzinger C, Ropele S, Strasser-Fuchs S, et al. Lower levels of N-acetylaspartate in multiple sclerosis patients with the apolipoprotein E epsilon 4-allele. Arch Neurol 2004b;61:296.

146. Kantarci OH, Hebrink DD, Achenbach SJ, et al. Association of APOE polymorphisms with disease severity in MS is limited to women. Neurology 2004;62:811–4.

147. Charcot JM. Leçons sur les maladies du système nerveux. Paris: Delahaye; 1872.

148. Brain WR. Prognosis of disseminated sclerosis. Lancet 1936;2:866–7.

149. Skoog B, Runmarker B, Andersen O. A 37–50 year follow-up of the Gothenburg multiple sclerosis cohort. Mult Scler 2004;10(Suppl):S156.

150. Lehoczky T, Halasy-Lehoczky M. Forme bénigne de la sclérose en plaques. La Presse Médicale 1963;1:2294–6.

151. Thompson AJ, Hutchinson M, Brazil J, et al. A clinical and laboratory study of benign multiple sclerosis. Q J Med 1986;58:69–80.

152. Rodriguez M, Siva A, Ward J, et al. Impairment, disability, and handicap in multiple sclerosis: a population-based study in Olmsted County, Minnesota. Neurology 1994;44:28–33.

153. Amato MP, Zipoli V, Goretti B, et al. Benign multiple sclerosis: cognitive, psychological and social aspects in a clinical cohort. J Neurol 2006;253: 1054–9.

154. Glad S, Nyland H, Myhr KM. Benign multiple sclerosis. Acta Neurol Scand 2006;183(Suppl): 55–7.

155. Hawkins SA, McDonnel GV. Benign multiple sclerosis? Clinical course, long term follow up, and assessment of prognostic factors. J Neurol Neurosurg Psychiatr 1999;67:148–52.

156. Pittock SJ, Mayr WT, McClelland RL, et al. Change in MS-related disability in a population-based cohort: a 10-year follow-up study. Neurology 2004; 62:51–9.

157. Pittock SJ, McClelland RL, Mayr WT, et al. Clinical implications of benign multiple sclerosis: a 20-year population-based follow-up study. Ann Neurol 2004;56:303–6.

158. Sayao AL, Devonshire V, Tremlett H. Longitudinal follow-up of benign multiple sclerosis at 20 years. Neurology 2007;68:496–500.

159. Duquette P, Murray TJ, Pleines J, et al. Multiple sclerosis in childhood: clinical profile in 125 patients. J Pediatr 1987;111:359–63.

160. Sindern E, Haas J, Stark E, et al. Early onset MS under the age of 16: clinical and paraclinical features. Acta Neurol Scand 1992;86:280–4.

161. Ghezzi A, Deplano V, Faroni J, et al. Multiple sclerosis in childhood: clinical features of 149 cases. Mult Scler 1997;3:43–6.

162. Boiko A, Vorobeychik G, Paty D, et al. Early onset multiple sclerosis: a longitudinal study. Neurology 2002;59:1006–10.

163. Ghezzi A, Pozzilli C, Liguori M, et al. Prospective study of multiple sclerosis with early onset. Mult Scler 2002;8:115–8.

164. Simone IL, Carrara D, Tortorella C, et al. Course and prognosis in early-onset MS: comparison with adult-onset forms. Neurology 2002;59:1922–8.

165. Mikaeloff Y, Suissa S, Vallée L, et al. First episode of acute CNS inflammatory demyelination in childhood: prognostic factors for multiple sclerosis and disability. J Pediatr 2004;144:246–52.

166. Mikaeloff Y, Caridade G, Assi S, et al. Prognostic factors for early severity in a childhood multiple sclerosis cohort. Pediatrics 2006;118:1133–9.

167. Renoux C, Vukusic S, Mikaeloff Y, et al. Natural history of multiple sclerosis with childhood onset. N Engl J Med 2007;356:2603–13.

168. Hynson JL, Kornberg AJ, Coleman LT, et al. Clinical and neuroradiologic features of acute disseminated encephalomyelitis in children. Neurology 2001;56:1308–12.

169. Cole GF, Stuart CA. A long perspective on childhood multiple sclerosis. Dev Med Child Neurol 1995;37:661–6.

170. Wallin MT, Page WF, Kurtzke JF. Epidemiology of multiple sclerosis in US veterans. VIII. Long-term survival after onset of multiple sclerosis. Brain 2000;123:1677–87.

171. Leibowitz U, Kahana E, Alter M. Survival and death in multiple sclerosis. Brain 1969;92:115–30.

172. Poser S, Poser W, Schlaf G, et al. Prognostic indicators in multiple sclerosis. Acta Neurol Scand 1986;74:387–92.

173. Riise T, Gronning M, Aarli JA, et al. Prognostic factors for life expectancy in multiple sclerosis analised by Cox-models. J Clin Epidemiol 1988;41: 1031–6.

174. Wynn DR, Rodriguez M, O'Fallon WM, et al. A reappraisal of the epidemiology of multiple sclerosis in Olmsted Country, Minnesota. Neurology 1990;40: 780–6.

175. Sadovnick AD, Eisen RN, Ebers GC, et al. Cause of death in patients attending multiple sclerosis clinics. Neurology 1991;41:1193–6.

176. Midgard R, Albrektsen G, Riise T, et al. Prognostic factors for survival in multiple sclerosis: a longitudinal, population-based study in More and Romsdal, Norway. J Neurol Neurosurg Psychiatr 1995;58: 417–21.

177. Sumelahti ML, Tienari PJ, Wikström J, et al. Survival of multiple sclerosis in Finland between 1964 and 1993. Mult Scler 2002;8:350–5.

178. Stenager EN, Stenager E, Koch-Henriksen N, et al. Suicide and multiple sclerosis: an epidemiological investigation. J Neurol Neurosurg Psychiatr 1992; 55:542–5.

179. Bronnum-Hansen H, Koch-Henriksen N, Hyllested K. Survival of patients with multiple sclerosis in Denmark: a nationwide, long-term epidemiologic survey. Neurology 1994;44:1901–7.

180. Koch-Henriksen N, Bronnum-Hansen H, Stenager E. Underlying cause of death in Danish patients with multiple sclerosis: results from the Danish Multiple Sclerosis Registry. J Neurol Neurosurg Psychiatr 1998;65:56–9.

181. Bronnum-Hansen H, Koch-Henriksen N, Stenager E. Trends in survival and cause of death in Danish patients with multiple sclerosis. Brain 2004;127: 844–50.

182. McAlpine D, Compston ND, Lumsden CE. Multiple sclerosis. Edinburgh: Livingstone; 1955.

183. Lublin FD, Baier M, Cutter G. Effect of relapses on development of residual deficit in multiple sclerosis. Neurology 2003;61:1528–32.

184. Liu C, Blumhardt LD. Disability outcome measures in therapeutic trials of relapsing-remitting multiple sclerosis: effects of heterogeneity of disease course in placebo cohorts. J Neurol Neurosurg Psychiatr 2000;68:450–7.

185. Andersson PB, Waubant E, Gee L, et al. Multiple sclerosis that is progressive from the time of onset:

clinical characteristics and progression of disability. Arch Neurol 1999;56:1138–42.

186. Hyllested K. Lethality, duration, and mortality of disseminated sclerosis in Denmark. Acta Psychiatr Scand 1961;36:553–64.

187. Poser S, Hauptvogel H. Clinical data from 418 MS patients in relation to the diagnosis: first experiences with an optical mark reader documentation system. Acta Neurol Scand 1973;49:473–9.

188. Thygesen P. Prognosis in initial stage of disseminated primary demyelinating disease of central nervous system. Arch Neurol Psychiatry 1949;61:339–51.

189. McLean AR, Berkson J. Mortality and disability in multiple sclerosis: a statistical estimate of prognosis. JAMA 1951;146:1367–9.

190. Trojano M, Liguori M, Bosco Zimatore G, et al. Age-related disability in multiple sclerosis. Ann Neurol 2002;51:475–80.

191. McDonnell GV, Hawkins SA. Primary progressive multiple sclerosis: a distinct syndrome? Mult Scler 1996;2:137–41.

192. McDonnel GV, Hawkins SA. Clinical study of primary progressive multiple sclerosis in Northern Ireland, UK. J Neurol Neurosurg Psychiatr 1998; 64:451–4.

193. Confavreux C, Hutchinson M, Hours MM, et al. Rate of pregnancy-related relapse in multiple sclerosis: pregnancy in multiple sclerosis group. N Engl J Med 1998;339:285–91.

194. Vukusic S, Hutchinson M, Hours M, et al. Pregnancy and multiple sclerosis (the PRIMS study): clinical predictors of post-partum relapse. Brain 2004;127:1353–60 [Epub 2004 May 6. Erratum in: Brain 2004;127:1912].

195. Confavreux C. Vaccination contre l'hépatite B et sclérose en plaques. Presse Med 2005;34:1205–8.

196. Hernan MA, Jick SS, Olek MJ, et al. Recombinant hepatitis B vaccine and the risk of multiple sclerosis: a prospective study. Neurology 2004;63: 838–42.

197. Confavreux C, Suissa S, Saddier P, et al. Vaccinations and the risk of relapse in multiple sclerosis. N Engl J Med 2001;344:319–26.

198. Kutzelnigg A, Lucchinetti CF, Stadelmann C, et al. Cortical demyelination and diffuse white matter injury in multiple sclerosis. Brain 2005;128:2705–12.

Basic Principles of Magnetic Resonance Imaging

Joseph C. McGowan, PhD, PE[a,b,*]

KEYWORDS

- MR imaging • MR physics
- Magnetic resonance • Spin echo • Gradient echo
- K-space • Fast spin echo

Magnetic resonance (MR) imaging has become the dominant clinical imaging modality with widespread, primarily noninvasive, applicability throughout the body and across many disease processes. This progress of MR imaging has been rapid compared with other imaging technologies and it can be attributed in part to physics and in part to the timing of the development of MR imaging, which corresponded to an important period of advances in computing technology. The history of MR imaging dates from the experiments of Paul Lauterbur[1] in the 1970s and includes the work that resulted in his being awarded the Nobel Prize. Compared to radiography, which develops contrast based upon density, MR imaging probes at least three fundamental parameters and a number of derivative ones. For this reason, exquisite soft tissue differentiation is possible. The flexibility of MR imaging enables the development of purpose-built optimized applications. Concurrent developments in digital image processing, microprocessor power, storage, and computer-aided design have spurred and enabled further growth in capability. Although MR imaging may be viewed as "mature" in some respects, the field is rich with new proposals and applications that hold great promise for future research health care uses.

MR imaging is a modality that richly rewards the clinical practitioner who understands the underlying physics. Compared to other imaging techniques, there are many degrees of freedom in the acquisition parameters for MR imaging. There are opportunities for standardization and also opportunities to tailor protocols to specific disease manifestations and even to specific patients. A variety of artifacts can potentially compromise image quality and their presence can be mitigated or addressed with choices of technique. In MR imaging, there is always an opportunity to trade speed for quality (or vice versa), and the balance point of this compromise may yield an optimum study that maximizes benefit to the patient. The interested reader is encouraged to investigate these topics further in any of several more comprehensive texts.[2–4]

SPIN PHYSICS

When the physics of MR imaging is discussed in the classical sense, the fundamental concept is that of "spin" or of "a spin." Spin refers to a magnetic moment that results from or is associated with a "current loop" created by a spinning charged particle, where the charge resides on the outer surface of the particle. This current can be quantified as

$$I = q*v/2\pi r$$

with q the charge on the particle, r the radius of the particle, and v the tangential velocity of a point on the surface of the particle. For clinical MR imaging, the spin of interest is most often that associated with a proton of water.

The magnetic dipole moment that results is the product of the area of the particle and the current. It is a vector quantity and has direction that is

[a] Drexel University, School of Biomedical Engineering, 3141 Chestnut Street, Philadelphia, PA 19104, USA
[b] Exponent, Inc., 3401 Market Street, Suite 300, Philadelphia, PA 19104, USA
* Drexel University, School of Biomedical Engineering, 3141 Chestnut Street, Philadelphia, PA 19104.
E-mail address: jmcgowan@exponent.com

Neuroimag Clin N Am 18 (2008) 623–636
doi:10.1016/j.nic.2008.06.004

parallel to the angular momentum of the spinning particle. The equation

$$\mu = q/2m * J$$

quantifies the dipole moment with J the angular momentum, q the charge and m the mass of the particle.

Spins tend to align with an external magnetic field, in the same way that iron filings align with a magnetic field in free space. There are two preferred alignments for spins, referred to as "up" and "down" relative to the direction of the applied field. A slight energy difference exists between the two orientations, and thus a system of many spins can be characterized by its energy state. Over time, when spins experience an external field, they will align to a lower energy, or equilibrium, state, characterized by the distribution between the up and down states. A stronger field will develop stronger polarization between the two states, and when the external field changes for a given system of spins a process of "relaxation" to the new equilibrium state will transpire. When a large number of spins are considered as a system, the effect described is observed as that of a single magnetic moment with a direction that can vary in three dimensions. The energy transfer processes that underlie this effect are exploited by MR imaging techniques to gain information about the relevant spins.

When spins are "polarized" or aligned by a static external magnetic field, they can be excited as an ensemble by the application of radiofrequency energy and, given a large enough number of spins, the effects can be detected. The size of the ensemble required for detection is also related to the strength of the external field- giving rise to some fundamental tenets of MR imaging: a larger sample gives a better signal, and a larger (stronger) magnet will do the same, all else equal.

The excitation of the spin ensemble is achieved via resonance, which is the familiar phenomenon by which certain systems can be most effectively excited at a certain frequency. A common example of this is experienced when pushing a child on a swing. If every sequential push is performed with a constant force there is a certain frequency of pushing that will result in the largest effective energy transfer and consequently a higher arc for the child/swing system. Pushing faster or slower has a diminished effect. In magnetic resonance, the characteristic frequency depends upon the characteristics of the spin under investigation and the strength of the applied magnetic field as:

$$f = \gamma B$$

where gamma is the gyromagnetic ratio, a fundamental constant for a given spin, and B the field strength. This famous relationship is known as the Larmor equation. Excitation of the spin system through application of energy at the resonance frequency can be shown to be equivalent to exposing the system to an altered magnetic field, eg, one that is perpendicular to the applied external field. The spins respond, as given above, by relaxing toward the (new) equilibrium state that is associated with the altered field. Thus they relax or move toward an axis that is not parallel to the (large) applied static field.

The motion of the vector representation of a spin ensemble toward an equilibrium position is essential to understanding the basis of MR imaging. That motion is precession, analogous to that observed in a gyroscope (**Fig. 1**). Precession is characterized by the path taken by a spinning object under the influence of an external force, eg, in the case of a gyroscope: gravity. A spinning gyroscope does not behave as it would were it stationary. Instead of falling over in response to gravity, it "spins down" toward a final rest position at a rate related to its mass and spin velocity. Similarly, when a spin system, aligned with the main magnetic field, is exposed through resonance radiofrequency irradiation to an effectively altered field, it will pass from rotation about the axis of the external field to precession around the axis of the effective field. Upon removal of the resonance excitation, the spin system will again experience only the external field and will precess toward its former equilibrium position.

The motions of spins, or, more correctly, ensembles of spins, were elucidated by Bloch and Purcell who for this work shared the Nobel Prize in 1952. Bloch[5] described this motion with a series of coupled differential equations (Bloch equations) that when solved give rise to two exponential relaxation constants known as T1 and T2. The T1 constant is associated with spin–lattice relaxation and describes the exchange of energy between the spin system and the environment. T1 also (or equivalently) describes the longitudinal relaxation along the z-axis. The state of z-magnetization can be normalized to between 1 (equilibrium) and -1. The T2 constant describes the coherence of the spin system, a measure of how "together" the spins are as they rotate. This can be normalized to 1 for the situation where all of the spins are aligned, and to zero when describing a completely random orientation between spins within the system.

A special case of motion of the effective spin vector is seen when the vector rotates perpendicular to the main magnetic field. If the main field is assumed to be oriented in the z-direction as is conventional, this spin rotation is said to be in the x–y plane. With the spins rotating in this

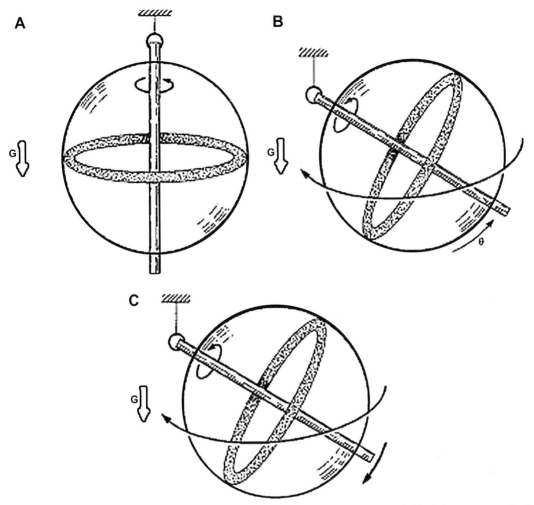

Fig. 1. (A) A spinning gyroscope is suspended in alignment with the gravitational field. If the gyroscope is displaced by the application of a force, it will continue to rotate about its physical axis but will also precess about the direction of gravity (B). As the rotational velocity of the gyroscope decreases, the angle θ approaches zero (C). (From McGowan JC. Magnetic Resonance. In: Brans, Hay, editors. Physiological monitoring and instrument diagnosis in perinatal and neonatal medicine. New York: Cambridge University Press; 1995. p. 67; with permission, Cambridge University Press.)

manner, it is possible to introduce a coil of wire such that the spins effectively serve as magnets whose lines of flux cut the coil, giving rise to Faraday induction and an induced voltage in the coil. This principle is exploited to obtain the signal associated with the spin behavior at a given time, resulting in data from which an image can be reconstructed.

MR IMAGING HARDWARE

Principal components that comprise an MR imaging system include: a main magnet, gradient magnets, radiofrequency coils to transmit and/or receive the MR imaging signal, and associated signal processing equipment.

State of the art clinical MR imaging systems typically incorporate a superconducting magnet to produce a relatively large static magnetic field. The function of this magnet is to produce a stable, spatially homogeneous magnetic field over a prescribed volume. Such a magnet may operate at 1.5 Tesla (T), or 15,000 Gauss, which can be compared with the earth's magnetic field at approximately 0.5 Gauss. Modern magnet systems can also be obtained at 3T and higher fields, and there are also lower-field magnets available, typically at lower cost or for special purposes. Superconducting magnets are cooled by cryogens such as liquid nitrogen and liquid helium and, after the static field is established, they require no electric power to maintain it. Cost, weight, and siting are often important considerations when installing a magnet system. Increased field strength is desirable from the standpoint of signal to noise ratio (SNR) (ie, signal quality) but carries the disadvantages of increased cost largely because of the need for more wire to carry the high current as well as the increased size of the cryostat. In addition, fringe fields must be designed for and the footprint of the device may be large relative to other imaging equipment.

The main magnet will typically incorporate the capability of making small adjustments to the field to achieve the homogeneity necessary for MR imaging. This may be accomplished with secondary magnetic fields known as "shims," which add to the main field in a spatially inhomogeneous way to correct errors and compensate for engineering factors.

Another kind of secondary magnetic field incorporated for MR imaging is known as a gradient. Gradient coils are electromagnets installed so that when energized, they predictably perturb the main magnetic field along an axis. Thus, in the z-direction, the effective (net) field in the presence of a gradient can be given as

$$B_{net} = B_0 + \Delta B_0 = B_0 + G_z Z$$

where B_0 is the strength of the main magnetic field, ΔB_0 is the contribution to the effective field from the gradient, G_z is the strength of the gradient in the z-direction, and Z is the distance along the z-axis (**Fig. 2**). The value G is usually given in mT/m. Referring to the Larmor equation given above, it is seen that in the presence of a gradient, the resonance frequency associated with the sensitive volume of the main magnet varies along the gradient axis. Assuming that the variation of the field along that axis is linear, the frequency variation will also be linear. This observation will form the basis for the MR imaging techniques discussed below.

To obtain three-dimensional images, it is required that at least three gradients be present. An additional practical requirement is that they must be able to be switched on and off very rapidly. The isocenter of the three gradients should be co-located with the isocenter of the main magnet.

Radiofrequency coils are used to excite a particular volume of interest by adding energy to the tissue or material within that volume. They also serve to detect the eventual MR imaging signal. In some applications, both transmit and receive functions are performed by the same coil; in other systems, it is advantageous to employ separate transmit and receive coils. Analogous to the swing example given above, the radiofrequency coils are tuned to the resonance frequency of the spins and thus

A

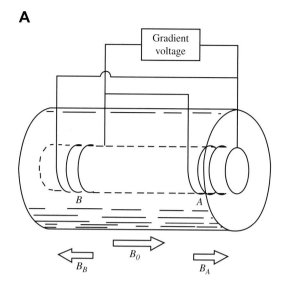

B

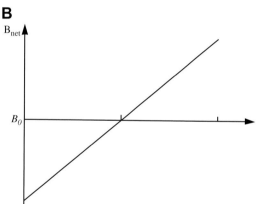

Fig. 2. (*A*) Application of gradient voltage produces gradient magnetic fields B_A and B_B. The effective magnetic field B_{net} is obtained by adding, at each location along the z-axis, the contribution from all three fields. As shown in the graph (*B*) B_{net} increases with increasing z and is equal to B_0 at the magnet center. The effective combination of B_a and B_b is equal to the ΔB_0 term given in the text. (*From* McGowan JC. Magnetic Resonance. In: Brans, Hay, editors. Physiological monitoring and instrument diagnosis in perinatal and neonatal medicine. New York: Cambridge University Press; 1995. p. 75; with permission, Cambridge University Press.)

they are able to add energy in an effective manner to the spin systems. Radiofrequency coils can be constructed with a variety of geometries and they are increasingly built for specific applications. They vary from the large "body coil" that is supplied with many magnet systems and still used for imaging of larger portions of the body, to coils designed for a single finger or perhaps an internal organ. There is a substantial advantage to tailoring the size of the coil to the tissue being examined because the signal in the image must only come from the tissue of interest, whereas the noise associated with that image will originate in the entirety of the coil. Because the image quality is related to the SNR, it is apparent that the highest quality will in general be achieved with coil size optimized to the tissue of interest. It is not only possible but also ubiquitous to "trade" speed for quality in MR imaging. Whenever sufficient quality exists in the acquisition, one can opt to image faster while sacrificing a predictable amount of quality, measured as the SNR.

Radiofrequency coils are increasingly provided as arrays of individual coils that are used sequentially during the imaging sequence. This design can be used to increase quality by redundant or semiredundant acquisition of data, or to increase coverage of an area by establishing a coil array with a predominant linear dimension, for example, to image the spine. This is a way of increasing SNR, which can be used to produce images with higher quality or, alternatively, to increase the speed of acquisition.

When voltage is induced in the radiofrequency coil, the voltage is amplified by a receiver and sent through a signal processing train to be stored in a computer. The computer will carry out the reconstruction of an image when sufficient data is obtained. When phased arrays of coils are used, each must be connected to a separate channel for signal processing.

RELAXATION AND THE MAGNETIC RESONANCE SIGNAL

The state of a spin system can be described in terms of the amount of longitudinal magnetization (z-direction) and the amount of transverse magnetization (x–y direction). The equilibrium position of the magnetization is fully aligned with the z-direction. When energy is added to the spins, the magnetization is "tipped" or "flipped" such that there can be a component of transverse, or x–y magnetization. The largest amount of transverse magnetization is achieved by tipping the spins ninety degrees. The state of the spin systems can be described by or decomposed into two vectors, one constantly pointing along the z-axis and one representing the projection of the total magnetization in the x–y plane. A spin system that is not at equilibrium energy will tend to relax to equilibrium as predicted by the Bloch equations. This relaxation is governed by the two exponential relaxation constants T1 and T2. T1 relaxation, also known as spin–lattice relaxation, describes the motion of the z-magnetization vector as it proceeds to its equilibrium state. To understand T2 relaxation, one must recognize that when the spins are tipped

into the transverse plane, they can get out of phase with one another because of the presence of small variations in resonance frequency arising from differences in the spatial environment, chemical environment, or random processes. As the spins in the transverse plane tend to be less aligned, they begin to cancel each other out so that the net transverse vector gets progressively smaller. The time constant for this process is T2 and this is called spin–spin relaxation. The composite relaxation process can be envisioned as precession, which is analogous to a gyroscope relaxing to an equilibrium state in the presence of gravity.

The presence of transverse magnetization (and only transverse magnetization) induces voltage in the radiofrequency coil. This is illustrated by a simple coil design whereby a loop of wire is placed within the static magnetic field and aligned as shown in **Fig. 3**. Faraday's Law provides the requirements for inducing a voltage: a conductor, a magnetic field, and relative motion between the two. These requirements are met by the coil (serving as the conductor), spin system (as the magnetic field), and the motion of the transverse magnetization serving to make the lines of flux associated with the spin magnetization cut through the conductor of the coil (**Fig. 4**).

Assuming that energy has been added to a spin system via excitation at the resonance frequency, a coil in position to detect a signal will have induced in it a decaying sinusoidal voltage that is known as a "free induction decay" (FID). Note that a FID begins immediately after the excitation

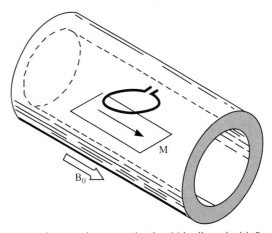

Fig. 3. The sample magnetization M is aligned with B_0 and in proximity to a conducting coil. (*From* McGowan JC. Magnetic Resonance. In: Brans, Hay, editors. Physiological monitoring and instrument diagnosis in perinatal and neonatal medicine. New York: Cambridge University Press; 1995. p. 69; with permission, Cambridge University Press.)

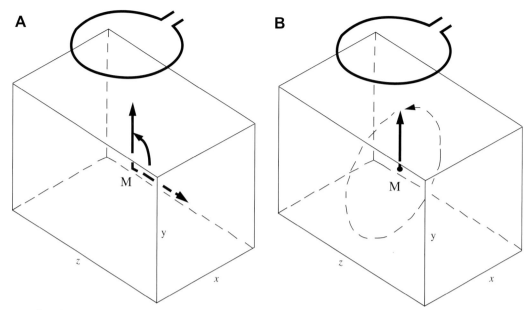

Fig. 4. After the magnetization M is tipped from the z-direction by ninety degrees (*A*) it begins to precess in the x–y plane (*B*) and satisfies the requirements for Faraday induction. (*From* McGowan JC. Magnetic Resonance. In: Brans, Hay, editors. Physiological monitoring and instrument diagnosis in perinatal and neonatal medicine. New York: Cambridge University Press; 1995. p. 69; with permission, Cambridge University Press.)

ceases. This signal can be useful, particularly in the area of spectroscopy. However, to perform imaging it is often desirable to separate the signal in time from the excitation pulse. To do this, one can manipulate the phase state of the spins in the transverse plane. As stated above, the spins dephase through a combination of random (or irreversible) and nonrandom (potentially reversible) processes; dephasing is directly related to the magnitude of signal. The spins can be caused to dephase (and subsequently rephase) by the application of a gradient along one axis. Recalling the Larmor relationship, the spins experience a decrease or increase in frequency that is proportional to the change in applied local field compared with the static field. Thus, the spins begin to get out of alignment with one another and they are said to acquire a phase difference or to dephase. To rephase the spins, the gradient amplitude is at some point in the sequence simply reversed. Immediately, the frequency differences between spins are reversed and the spins begin to acquire phase in the opposite direction. As the spins are rephased, the signal will reflect a buildup to a maximum magnitude followed by a decay in magnitude, and this "gradient echo" can be positioned as desired, in time, through the timing of the gradient application.

A different dephasing/rephasing process results from the small inhomogeneities present in the static field. These are not aligned with an axis like the variations a field gradient would impose, but they are spatially invariant. This dephasing, which occurs naturally following excitation, is most effectively reversed via the application of a radiofrequency pulse corresponding to a 180-degree flip angle, and the resulting signal is called a spin echo (or Hahn echo, after Erwin Hahn, the discoverer of the effect).[6] The spin echo signal is displaced from the initial excitation by a time called "TE" (echo time) (with the second RF pulse at time TE/2) and also builds up and decays in a similar manner to that described above. Two depictions of the effects of rephasing the reversible dephasing are given in **Fig. 5**. In these examples, one can see the effects of the inversion pulse on a simple two-spin system with the phase position tracked in time (see **Fig. 5**), and, equivalently, in the time-domain representation of sinusoids with different frequencies corresponding to several spins (see **Fig. 5**). In a system with many spins, the effect is more dramatic because the signal essentially vanishes for a period of time, and then reappears at the predicted time of the spin echo.

GRADIENT ECHO IMAGING

Through the application of field gradients, it is possible to change the magnetic field of each point inside the MR imaging machine. Similarly, it is possible to establish a single point in the magnet that has a particular resonance frequency through

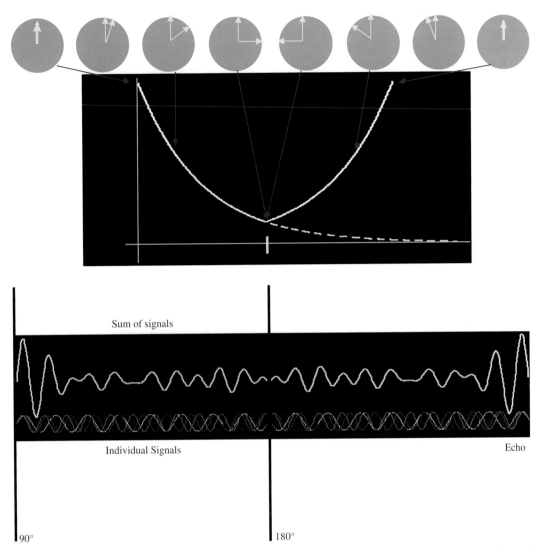

Fig. 5. A two-spin system is depicted following excitation whereby the spins are tipped into the transverse plane. The signal, consisting of the addition of the two spins, is maximized when the spins are in phase. As one spin gains phase relative to the other, the total signal decreases (left to right on the figure) until a 180-degree pulse is given (yellow tick on the signal graph) and the phase difference now tends to rephase the spins (top). When the signals are viewed as sinusoids in the time domain, their individual magnitudes are constant but their sum varies with the state of phase. Three sinusoids are shown to dephase, experience a 180-degree pulse, and rephase to an echo.

manipulation of the gradients in all three dimensions. If excitation is performed at that frequency, the information gathered from the single point in space can be stored and later combined with others to form an image. This method of imaging was dubbed the "sensitive point" method and represented an early attempt to exploit MR imaging.[7] However, this method is impractical for clinical imaging because of the time required for data acquisition. Modern imaging employs the field gradients to encode spatial information and, using the Fourier transform, allow the simultaneous acquisition of data from many points along an axis.

The first step in the formation of a 2D magnetic resonance image is to "select" a slice of the tissue under examination. This is done by establishing a gradient in one direction, for example, the z-direction, and applying a radiofrequency pulse that will add energy to the spins. However, the frequency of this pulse is adjusted such that the only spins that have a corresponding frequency (and thus will experience the resonance effect) are those that lie within the "selected" slice by being in the correct position along the z-axis (**Fig. 6**).

Recall the general premise that the application of a field gradient along an axis establishes

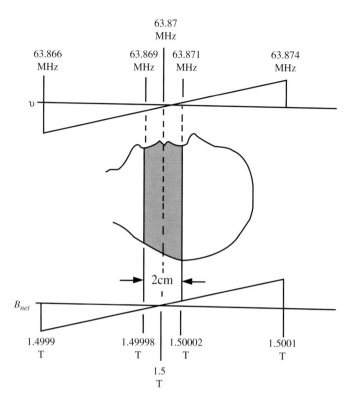

Fig. 6. Application of rf excitation over a range of frequencies in conjunction with a field gradient is used for slice selection. The example depicts a 2-kHz-wide excitation bandwidth, applied with a gradient that changes the B_{net} field by 0.2 G/cm. The rf excitation corresponds to the resonance frequencies of protons experiencing fields of 1.49998–1.50002 T, or a range of 0.4 G. This results in excitation of a slice 2 cm thick that is centered on the magnet center. (*From McGowan JC. Magnetic Resonance. In: Brans, Hay, editors. Physiological monitoring and instrument diagnosis in perinatal and neonatal medicine. New York: Cambridge University Press; 1995. p. 76; with permission, Cambridge University Press.*)

a correspondence between frequency and spatial position. If the signal in the coil is recorded during the gradient application, the spins along the gradient axis will effectively rotate with characteristic frequencies that reflect their position. In fact, the gradient application in one direction, for example, the x-direction, is applied such that it encompasses in time the gradient echo. Thus, the signal in the coil will consist of an effective summation of many signals at different frequencies. The "encoded" information is recovered via the mathematical process of Fourier transformation.

The process of forming and recovering such a gradient echo can be repeated after the application of an orthogonal gradient that establishes a phase relationship along the remaining axis, in the previous example, the y-direction. The mathematics involved in the reconstruction of this data is a two-dimensional Fourier transformation, the details of which are beyond the scope of this article. Applying both phase encoding in the y-direction before the acquisition of signal and frequency encoding in the x-direction during the signal acquisition makes each point in the image plane have a particular and unique history regarding the resonance frequency during the precession of the spins.

The gradient echo pulse sequence diagram is presented as **Fig. 7**. Gradient echo imaging is

more demanding with respect to the scanner than spin–echo techniques, because the dephasing that results from inhomogeneities within the static field (but not because of field gradients that are under the operator's control) is not rephased and thus, any signal that is lost on that time scale is not recovered. However, improvements in magnet design and construction have made it possible to acquire good quality gradient echo images and, in fact, at higher fields where spin echo inversion pulses are limited because of power deposition, gradient echo imaging can be the best option.

SPIN ECHO IMAGING

Spin echo imaging has been the workhorse pulse sequence during the history of MR imaging. One reason for this is the excellent signal quality that is achieved when the reversible dephasing is completely rephased. Specifically, in the spin echo method, all dephasing associated with magnetic field inhomogeneities that are stationary, is rephased at the time of the spin echo. Simultaneously, because of frequency encoding gradients that are applied in a manner identical to that explained above, a gradient echo also occurs. The pulse sequence is almost identical to the gradient echo pulse sequence, with the exception of

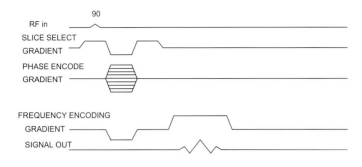

Fig. 7. In a gradient echo pulse sequence a single excitation is applied (90 degrees is shown here) The slice-select gradient is turned on when the rf excitation is applied such that only the desired slice is affected by the rf. The phase encode gradient is turned on between the excitation and inversion pulses, with a different magnitude for each TR. The frequency encode gradient is applied during phase encoding (dephase) and signal acquisition (rephase). As time passes from left to right, when the area under the frequency-encode gradient curve sums to zero all of the dephasing effects of the gradient have been reversed and a gradient echo is formed.

adding the inversion pulse that creates a spin echo at time TE. It is depicted in **Fig. 8**. Slice selection, frequency and phase encoding, and reconstruction of the image are achieved in the same manner as for the gradient echo. Instead of slice selection, yet another phase encoding gradient may be incorporated into the pulse sequence, and the reconstruction of the image performed with a three-dimensional Fourier transform. The result of such a process is three-dimensional MR imaging and it offers advantages that include the ability to obtain smaller slices.

MR IMAGING CONTRAST

Referring to the spin–echo pulse sequence (see **Fig. 8**), one can see that there are two principal timing variables: repetition time (TR) and TE. The TR can be thought of as the time spacing between phase encode pulses, or alternatively and equivalently, as the time to play out one complete pulse train. The TE represents the time between the initial RF excitation and the acquisition of the signal. It has been noted that the spin echo methodology rephases spins that were dephased by spatially invariant magnetic field inhomogeneities. There

are other mechanisms of dephasing that are random in nature and thus cannot be reversed. The irreversible dephasing leads to a loss of signal that is described by the T2 time constant. The reversible dephasing that is refocused by the spin echo can be combined with the T2 processes and the composite time constant is known as T2*. T2 decay is thus always slower than T2* decay, and usually markedly so. The effects of T2 and T2* can be further understood by considering that the decay of a FID reflects T2*, while the difference in signal strength in spin echo acquisitions with differing TE reflects T2.

The effect of changing TR can be understood by considering two spin systems with equal equilibrium magnetization but differing T1 decay constants. An example in the brain would be the lateral ventricles, more water-like with long T1, and brain parenchyma, with shorter T1. Both tissues can be excited by a 90-degree radiofrequency pulse and allowed to return to equilibrium during a long repetition period (TR) after which the process is repeated. In this example, after each excitation, the magnetization is at its maximum value, and after each excitation, the signals from short and long T1 regions are identical. If

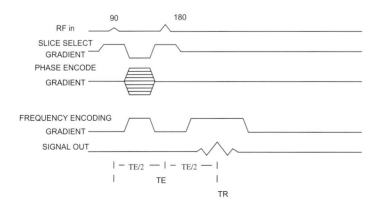

Fig. 8. In a spin–echo pulse sequence the rf excitation can take the form of a 90-degree pulse followed at time TE/2 by a 180-degree inversion pulse. Slice select and phase-encode gradients are applied as discussed above. The first positive lobe of the frequency encode gradient (coincident with the phase-encode gradient) is effectively reversed by the 180 degree pulse and so the point of the gradient echo (where the effects of the frequency encode gradient sum to zero) corresponds to the spin echo at time TE.

the equilibrium magnetizations from the spin systems were not equal, the signal from each would reflect the number of spins or the spin density. In MR imaging, an image reflecting these differences is called a proton-density image and is analogous to an x-ray image. Proton-density images are less often prescribed compared with relaxation-time-weighted images, but there are examples where their use is preferred. On the other hand, if the TR is shortened, the situation can arise where one spin system relaxed back to equilibrium but the other, experiencing longer decay times, did not. In this instance, the subsequent excitation pulse will cause the fully relaxed spin system to attain full transverse magnetization (and signal strength), but the partially relaxed system will attain less than full transverse magnetization. This can be understood by imagining that the short T1 spins are at a longitudinal magnetization of 1, but the long T1 spins, having not fully relaxed, might be at a longitudinal magnetization of 0.5. A subsequent excitation would result in high transverse magnetization for the short T1 spins, but low for the long T1 spins. The system with the longer T1 is said to be partially saturated in this case. If imaging is performed in this way, the spins with longer T1 (for example, those from fluid as opposed to tissue) will appear hypointense on the image. Since the image demonstrates differences in T1, this is called T1-weighted imaging. T1-weighted imaging is often excellent for demonstrating anatomy. Note that although longitudinal magnetization is not detected directly, the maximum transverse magnetization (and thus signal) that can be achieved directly reflects the state of longitudinal magnetization immediately before the excitation pulse. This gives rise to another imaging option, known as inversion recovery.

The longitudinal magnetization of a spin system reaches a maximum value at equilibrium, and the magnitude of this is often called M_0. A composite spin pointing along the z-axis with magnitude M_0 can be rotated through any number of degrees about any axis via the proper excitation radio-frequency pulse. It is possible to rotate that magnetization ninety degrees and, in essence, convert all of the longitudinal magnetization to signal-producing transverse magnetization. In another special case example, the longitudinal magnetization is rotated 45 degrees and at that point the transverse and longitudinal magnetization values are equal. In general, up to ninety degrees, each increase in rotation of the spin vector results in more transverse magnetization and less longitudinal magnetization following the rotation. It is also possible to rotate the spin

vector greater than ninety degrees, and as the rotation increases the amount of transverse magnetization now decreases, but the longitudinal magnetization following excitation continues to be farther from equilibrium up to a maximum of a 180-degree excitation. In this final special case, the transverse magnetization following the excitation is zero, and the longitudinal magnetization is M_0. The spin system is said to be inverted. Relaxation proceeds, then, without any transverse magnetization being developed, however, at any time a second excitation pulse can be applied to convert the present state of longitudinal magnetization to transverse and produce a signal. A very interesting and useful case is possible whereby the second excitation pulse is given when the spins associated with a tissue or substance of interest (typically fat or water) pass through the null state where their z-magnetization is equal to zero. When this is done the rest of the tissue (having differing T1) will develop transverse magnetization and produce signal, but the tissue that is going through the null will produce no signal. The image reconstructed from this data will have areas of zero intensity corresponding to the nulled tissue. When the sequence is designed to null water (including cerebrospinal fluid), the technique is called FLuid Attenuated Inversion Recovery (FLAIR).[8]

Returning the TR to a (long) value that minimizes T1-weighting, one can consider the effects of changing the TE. In particular, lengthening the TE allows the signal from some spin systems to completely dephase before it is acquired and thus, upon acquisition, there is no signal. On the other hand, other spin systems (with long T2) will demonstrate substantial signal at the time of acquisition. Thus, the resulting image will demonstrate hyperintensity corresponding to regions of long T2 and hyperintensity corresponding to regions of short T2. This is, of course, T2-weighting.

Summarizing, if TE is short on the T2 time scale of the tissue, a TR that is short on the T1 time scale of the tissue of interest will produce T1-weighting, and a TR that is relatively long will produce proton-density weighting. The combination of a long TR and a relatively long TE is used to obtain T2-weighting. These timing variables can be optimized to develop specific contrast that is relevant to the tissue of interest. In general, the time to acquire an image is equal to the repetition time multiplied by the number of repetitions, equivalent to the number of phase–encode steps. In clinical imaging, it is typical to use 256 repetitions of the sequence, but 512 is not uncommon, and 128 or fewer repetitions is sometimes used in the interest of obtaining a faster examination.

A BRIEF INTRODUCTION TO K-SPACE AND FAST SPIN ECHO IMAGING

Since the first magnetic resonance images were obtained there was interest in acquiring images faster, and with higher quality. During the intervening time, there have been concomitant advances in the technologies of computing and of mechanical design and construction such that current MR imaging scanners offer significantly advanced capabilities. A limitation that was soon observed with the rise of T2-weighted diagnostic scanning was the need for long TR periods, to avoid saturating spin systems and thus adding T1 contrast when "pure" T2 contrast was desired. Additionally, it was observed that the process of T2-weighted imaging was relatively inefficient in that the largest part the time duration of the pulse sequence was spent simply waiting for relaxation to occur. At the same time, it was recognized that the process of refocusing spins with a spin echo technique could be repeated within a single TR period, causing multiple spin echoes to occur within one repetition. If these multiple echo signals are acquired and stored, multiple images can be reconstructed corresponding to different TEs within the same TR. A natural, yet profound, evolution of this technique led to a rapid method for acquiring T2-weighted diagnostic images. Understanding the idea of "k-space" is necessary to appreciate this development and quite helpful in the understanding of many modern MR imaging methods.

Consider that the signal acquired during an MR imaging sequence is recorded over time. Each spin echo (or gradient echo) that is sensed in the receiver coil requires a certain amount of time to play out and the echo is stored in the computer memory, to be combined with the rest of the echoes that comprise the pulse sequence. It was noted that via a Fourier transformation this echo data is converted, or reconstructed, into an image. The Fourier transformation is a mathematical tool that can be thought of as a decomposition of a complicated signal into component parts, each with a characteristic frequency and magnitude. This is a particularly useful tool for MR imaging because, as has been noted, the spatial position information is encoded into the signal via the function of gradient magnetic fields that establish a correspondence between frequency and spatial position. Thus, the signal detected in the receiver coil is a composite of many frequencies. The signal is referred to as a time–domain signal because it is simply a recording of signal strength in time. The Fourier transformation breaks this signal into component frequencies and magnitudes. If the result of this were plotted on a graph, the ordinate could be labeled frequency. Hence, this is a frequency–domain representation. The utility of this application in MR imaging is that frequency is related to space (again, via the gradients) and thus the frequency domain is equivalent to the spatial domain. Thus, for each component part of the signal, the Fourier transformation effectively establishes the source position (along the gradient axis). The number of spins at that location (effectively spin density) is preserved in the magnitude of the signal.

A mathematician would view an image as simply a matrix of numbers, each corresponding to a level of intensity on the scale from black to white. Each intensity number of course corresponds to a position in space. A matrix of data from the receiver coil can also be formed by essentially stacking the intensity values from the coil so that the first spin echo is depicted as a row across the matrix, and each successive spin echo (having a different phase encode gradient applied) forms another row. Each intensity value in this matrix, the k-space matrix, corresponds to a position in time, and represents the signal received by the coil at that time. To complete the theoretic picture, it was noted that the Fourier transformation is used to convert from spatial dimensions to time dimensions. This can be in one dimension, as discussed above, or in two dimensions as is related to image formation, or even in higher dimensions to achieve, for example, three-dimensional imaging. The matrix full of data, the k-space matrix, is acquired in time and then the matrix is transformed into the frequency, or spatial, domain where it can be displayed as an image. The two matrices — image space and k-space — have the same dimensions. Thus, one can see that to construct an image, k-space must be "filled" with data with the same number of points as there will be elements in the final image. There is a counterintuitive aspect of k-space and the Fourier transformation in that the signal acquired at a particular time (that is, at a point in k-space) does not directly transfer to the intensity of a single point in image space. Rather, each point in k-space influences all points in image space. Equivalently, each point in image space is contributed to by all points in k-space. This gives rise to the interesting phenomenon that the central region of k-space is highly influential over the contrast in the entire image, whereas the periphery of k-space determines the edge definition and fine structural quality of the image.

The reason that the center of k-space determines contrast is related to the fact that the signal strength corresponding to the central k-space is the strongest. This can be understood by considering the effect of gradients when turned on. That effect is to change the phase of spins and when spins start out in phase, the effect is to dephase them according to their position along the gradient axis. Considering the pattern of phase during a gradient echo, it can be seen that the spins will be most in phase (with strongest signal) at the center of the echo, which is also the center of k-space in the x-dimension. The center of k-space in the y-dimension corresponds to the zero magnitude of the phase-encode gradient, and thus is also the region of least dephasing.

If the k-space matrix is viewed as a blank slate on which the data points can be written, it is easy to understand the concept of "covering" k-space to acquire enough points to reconstruct an image. Turning on the frequency encoding gradient in the foregoing discussion can be envisioned as moving across k-space from left to right (to fill in one row) while the phase encode gradient has the effect of moving up and down so as to prepare to fill in another row. Depending on the design of the pulse sequence, gradients may be used to move in any direction within the k-space matrix.

Returning to the challenge of rapid acquisition of T2-weighted images, recall that it is possible to create multiple spin echoes within a single TR period by simply applying additional RF excitation pulses within the time period. Thus, there are several spin echoes, for example, four, within each TR, and they are grouped by TE. If the resulting spin echoes are recorded and stored as groups, there will eventually be enough data to construct four images: one corresponding to each TE for which spin echoes are collected (Fig. 9). Instead of filling up four groups of echoes, all of the echoes collected are kept together and used to reconstruct a single image (Fig. 10a). In this example, the matrix for that single image will be filled four times as fast compared with the conventional acquisition (see Fig. 10b). This is the premise of "turbo" or "fast" spin echo, first introduced as rapid acquisition with relaxation enhancement (RARE).[9]

The alert reader will have noted that there is a significant difference in the k-space makeup of a fast spin echo (FSE) image compared with a conventional T2-weighted image as discussed above. Specifically, the FSE image is composed of spin echoes that reflect, in this example, four different values of TE. Because the T2-weighted contrast is a function of the TE, this leads to the question of what the contrast in the FSE image means. The answer reflects the observation above that

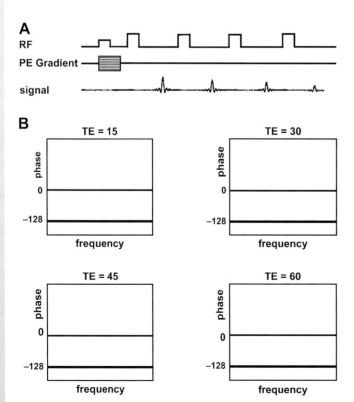

Fig. 9. In a multiple spin–echo sequence, one phase-encode gradient application per TR is used (top). Four images are acquired when the PE gradient is incremented through full range, and the contrast is each image reflects the TE of the echo associated with that image. K-space maps are shown (bottom) reflecting only the first TR period where the PE gradient is at maximum negative amplitude. Each echo signal decreases in magnitude according to T2* and the maximum amplitude decreases with each successive echo due to the effects of T2 decay. (*From* McGowan JC. Fast imaging with an introduction to k-space. In: Filippi, DeStefano, Dousset, et al, editors. MR imaging in white matter diseases of the brain and spinal cord. Berlin: Springer-Verlag; 2005. p. 48; with permission, Springer Science and Business Media.)

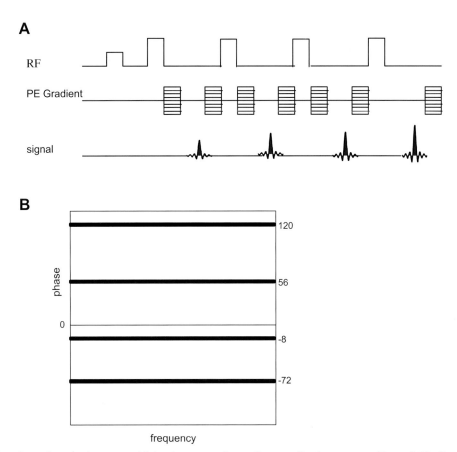

Fig. 10. In a fast spin–echo image, multiple phase-encode gradient applications are used in each TR. One image is acquired after all phase-encode values are applied (*A*). A k-space map for the first TR period is shown (*B*). As depicted, the normalized values of the phase-encode gradients are 120, −72, 56, −8. Ordering in this way makes the signal intensity of the echoes increase during the TR, as the signal gain from reduced dephasing exceeds the signal loss from T2. In this example, if the pattern is continued the contrast of the resultant image will reflect the later echo. (*From* McGowan JC. Fast imaging with an introduction to k-space. In: Filippi, DeStefano, Dousset, et al, editors. MR imaging in white matter diseases of the brain and spinal cord. Berlin: Springer-Verlag; 2005. p. 48; with permission, Springer Science and Business Media.)

the contrast in any image reflects the data in the central region of k-space. Thus, in this example, one can choose to have the central k-space data come exclusively from only one of the TE values. This value will be the effective TE for that image and the contrast in that image will closely resemble the contrast that would be obtained from a conventional acquisition with a single TE equivalent to the effective TE.

The time to acquire a FSE sequence is related to the time given above for a conventional acquisition by the number of spin echoes created and acquired during each repetition time (ie, between excitation pulses). Some manufacturers refer to this number as "echo train length" and others refer to it as the "turbo factor" and indeed the gain in speed is proportional to that number. Thus, the total acquisition time can be found by multiplying the number of phase encode steps by the repetition time and dividing that product by the number of echoes (echo train length, turbo factor) during each repetition.

OTHER RAPID IMAGING TECHNIQUES

One of the first rapid imaging techniques to be introduced followed the advance of magnet technology to the point where usable signal could be obtained without relying on a spin echo to refocus the large amount of reversible dephasing. The Fast Low Angle SHot or FLASH[10] technique exploited the observation that recovery of sufficient longitudinal magnetization to allow a subsequence excitation was much faster if an initial pulse much less than ninety degrees was used. With this imaging technique, it is also not necessary to wait for full relaxation of the longitudinal magnetization as a steady-state condition is achieved and exploited. This gradient echo technique is useful to acquire T1 or proton density contrast. Related techniques are also useful in the clinic as a means of identifying hemorrhage because the dephasing is associated with deposits of blood, a phenomenon that evolves over time.

More recent advances in rapid imaging have included a family of gradient echo techniques known as "echo–planar" imaging (EPI).[11] EPI makes use of very rapidly changing gradients to cover k-space completely following a single excitation pulse. In one variant of EPI, a spin echo is formed with an excitation pulse and a single inversion pulse. During the spin echo, the rapidly oscillating gradients effectively form many gradient echoes that are acquired during the span of milliseconds. EPI finds application whenever subsecond imaging times are required, for example, in the presence of physiologic motion that is too fast to capture with conventional or even FSE imaging. Functional imaging of the brain is also often performed with EPI pulse sequences. Hybrid forms incorporating aspects of both gradient echo imaging and spin echo imaging are increasingly common as MR imaging applications grow. Other newer techniques abandon the Cartesian (row and column) approach to covering k-space and substitute spiral or radial trajectories, each providing both advantages and disadvantages that have relevance to particular applications. Still newer techniques known collectively as parallel imaging[12,13] exploit the signals from an array of coils and combine them with sophisticated mathematics to effectively conduct, essentially, a number of imaging experiments at the same time. The increase in available signal can be used to improve quality or can be traded off for speed.

REFERENCES

1. Lauterbur PL. Image formation by induced local interactions: examples employing nuclear magnetic resonance. Nature 1973;242:190–1.
2. Filippi M, DeStefano N, Dousset V, et al, editors. MR imaging in white matter diseases of the brain and spinal cord. Berlin: Springer-Verlag; 2005.
3. Haake M, Brown RW, Thompson MR, et al, editors. Magnetic resonance imaging: physical principles and sequence design. New York: Wiley-Liss; 1999.
4. Atlas SW, editor. Magnetic resonance imaging of the brain and spine. New York: Raven Press; 1996.
5. Bloch F. Nuclear induction. Physical Review 1946; 70:460–74.
6. Hahn EL. Spin echoes. Physical Review 1950;80: 580–94.
7. Hinshaw WS. Image formation by nuclear magnetic resonance: the sensitive point method. J Appl Phys 1976;47:3709–21.
8. Hajnal JV, Bryant DJ, Kasuboski L, et al. Use of fluid attenuated inversion recovery (FLAIR) pulse sequences in MRI of the brain. J Comput Assist Tomogr 1992;16:841–4.
9. Hennig J, Friedburg H. RARE imaging: a fast imaging method for clinical MR. Magn Reson Imaging 1986;3:823–33.
10. Hasse A, Frahm J, Mattaei D, et al. FLASH imaging: rapid NMR imaging using low flip angle pulses. J Magn Reson 1989;67:388–97.
11. Mansfield P, Pykett IL. Biological and medical imaging by NMR. J Magn Reson 1978;29:355–73.
12. Pruessman KP, Weiger M, Sheidegger MB, et al. SENSE: sensitivity encoding for fast MRI. Magn Reson Med 1999;42:952–62.
13. Sodickson DK, Manning WI. Simultaneous acquisition of spatial harmonics (SMASH): fast imaging with radiofrequency coil arrays. Magn Reson Med 1997;38:591–603.

MR Image Postprocessing for Multiple Sclerosis Research

Mark A. Horsfield, PhD

KEYWORDS

- MR imaging • Image analysis • Postprocessing
- Multiple sclerosis • Visualization

Standard T1-and T2-weighting have formed the basis of contrast in most MR images since the clinical utility of these types of scan was demonstrated by showing abnormal morphology or pathology.[1,2] For diagnostic purposes, a simple dual-echo image allows the radiologist or clinician to assess the number, position, and shape of tissue abnormalities in the brain and spinal cord, all of which are factors in making a differential diagnosis of multiple sclerosis (MS). Lesions that enhance with injectable contrast agents, such as gadolinium diethylenetriamine penta-acetic acid (Gd-DTPA), are most easily seen on T1-weighted images.[3]

The need to make quantitative measurements of factors that are more subtle, or open to subjective interpretation, has long been recognized, however; for this, computerized analysis makes these sorts of measurement feasible or can assist in reducing any operator bias in the measurement, or even remove it completely. This review summarizes the tasks that are commonly applied in the analysis of MR images so that quantitative results can be presented.

UNIFORMITY (BIAS) CORRECTION

MR images have an arbitrary intensity scale, in which the actual intensity values depend on such factors as the receiver gain setting, sequence parameters (repetition time [TR], echo time [TE]), and tissue type. Furthermore, the intensity of a certain tissue type varies according to its position in the radiofrequency (RF) transmitter and receiver coils, because the RF field and reception properties vary spatially. This intensity nonuniformity (or bias) is most obvious in images acquired using surface receiver coils, such as those used for spinal cord imaging, but it is present in all MR scans.[4]

For quantitative image analysis, which relies on relative intensities, this bias is obviously a problem, and several methods for its correction have been put forward. Ideally, the bias field can be measured at the time of scanning by running extra pulse sequences and then corrected in situ. However, retrospective correction has been investigated by several groups (for a review, see the article by Belaroussi and colleagues[5]). A basic assumption behind all the retrospective correction methods is that the bias field varies only slowly in space, which is a reasonable assumption, given that the bias field comes mainly from nonuniformities in the RF field. Some methods model the bias field as a sum of smooth polynomial or trigonometric functions,[6,7] whereas others assume that the bias field is (spatially) piecewise uniform.[8] Other methods integrate the classification of tissue types (eg, white matter, gray matter, cerebrospinal fluid [CSF]) with bias field correction by making the assumption that all tissues in the same class should have a similar intensity.[9]

Accurate uniformity correction becomes more important as the number of high-field scanners

Medical Physics Section, Department of Cardiovascular Sciences, University of Leicester, Leicester Royal Infirmary, Leicester LE1 5WW, UK
E-mail address: mah5@le.ac.uk

Neuroimag Clin N Am 18 (2008) 637–649
doi:10.1016/j.nic.2008.06.006

increases and with the greater use of phased-array receiver coils for head imaging (**Fig. 1**). Whatever the correction method, uniformity correction is used as a preprocessing step in several applications, particularly in image registration and segmentation.

REGISTRATION

Another common task that forms a part of many aspects of image analysis is registration, whereby scans performed at different times are aligned so that the same anatomic locations can be superimposed.[10] The time between scans may be on the order of a second or so, as is seen with functional MR imaging (fMRI), where the registration corrects small amounts of patient movement. The time could be several years, however, in long-term follow-up studies of brain change. The scans may be performed with essentially the same type of contrast (eg, serial T1-weighted images used to assess atrophy[11]), or they may have a different contrast or even be collected using a different imaging modality (eg, to integrate data about glucose metabolism using positron emission tomography [PET] scans with high-resolution structural MR imaging scans[12]).

The process of registering images generally follows a common framework: by an iterative process, a transform is calculated that distorts one scan (the "floating image") so that it overlays another image (the "base image") accurately. The parameters of the transform are adjusted to obtain a good match between the two images, and the goodness of the match is evaluated using a "cost function." The cost function is evaluated over the whole image (sometimes after background removal), and the choice of cost function is dictated by the types of image that are to be aligned. In cases in which the images have similar

brightness and contrast (eg, in fMRI time series), the root-mean-square difference or cross-correlation is most appropriate.[13] When images have similar contrast but different absolute intensity ranges (as can occur in images acquired with the same pulse sequence with a long time interval between acquisitions, or on different scanners), the standard deviation of the intensity ratio can be useful.[14]

When images are acquired with different contrast or with different modalities, another class of cost function should be used. These rely on the assumption that although the intensities at the same anatomic location may not be similar across modalities, the intensities are consistent, such that a certain tissue type has a fairly constant intensity for any one modality. When the two images are closely aligned, a two-dimensional (joint) histogram of intensities formed from the images therefore shows sharp peaks, and any misalignment causes a blurring of the histogram, because tissues of different types overlap. Woods and mutual information are among these types of cost function, and they are a measure of this blurring of the joint histogram.[15]

To compare images from different patients, it is necessary to transform them into a standard anatomic space. One such space is based on the brain atlas from the Montreal Neurological Institute (MNI). This was composed by registering the scans from a large sample of control subjects to an average brain that was previously created by transforming a large number of other scans to the standard space of Talairach and Tournoux.[13] The original atlas of Talairach and Tournoux[16] was created from a single rather unrepresentative subject postmortem, which has resulted in some differences between the MNI atlas and the Talairach and Tournoux atlas.[16] Nevertheless, for the purposes of identifying gross anatomic features, the MNI atlas serves well, and the disparity can

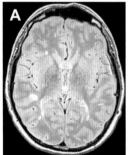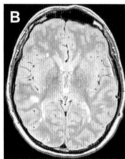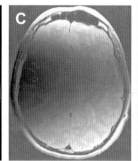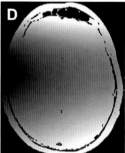

Fig. 1. Bias field correction of a proton density image collected at 3 T. (*A*) Uncorrected image. (*B*) Nonuniformity corrected using the method by Horsfield and colleagues[6] that models the bias field using a 3-dimensional polynomial surface of order 3. (*C*) Difference between (*A*) and (*B*). (*D*) Representation of the polynomial surface model of the bias field.

largely be corrected by applying an additional transform.[17] Therefore, after registering a set of scans to the MNI atlas, it is possible to compare image features across subjects in anatomic space.

One use of this type of registration to standard space is so-called "voxel-based morphometry" (VBM) analysis, such as that built into the a statistical parametric mapping (SPM) package from the Wellcome Trust Centre for Neuroimaging, London.[18] The goal of VBM is to allow the identification of significant differences in brain tissue across groups of subjects, and it allows the regional and anatomic variation to be visualized,[19] revealing the subtle changes that can occur and the differences among the different MS phenotypes.

Most registration is done using a simple distortion to transform the image to be registered, such as the affine transform, a property of which is that it always preserves the straightness of straight lines when the transform is applied. This type of linear transform cannot therefore account for the complex differences in the shapes of the brain that occur among individuals; more complex general transforms are needed in this case. Registration using nonlinear transforms is now becoming a much more mature procedure, although it is still compute-intensive. The deformation required to bring about registration is normally modeled as a sum of polynomial, trigonometric, or radially symmetric basis functions.[20] It is used for intersubject registration or for assessing atrophy within a subject.[21] **Fig. 2** shows an attempt to register a patient who has MS and a severely atrophied brain to a control subject, first using a simple affine transform and then, with nonlinear registration, using radial basis functions to model the deformation field.[20] Considering the severity of the atrophy, the nonlinear registration produces quite a good anatomic match between the patient and the control.

IMAGE SEGMENTATION

Image segmentation refers to the process of splitting an image into multiple regions (sets of pixels). Segmentation of MRI scans is typically used to identify different types of tissue and their boundaries, such that the volumes or shapes of the individual tissues can be quantified or analyzed further.

Image segmentation can result in a set of regions that, when combined, cover the entire image or a set of object boundaries, such that each of the pixels in a region has some similarity to the others in that object. The similarity may be a simple intensity similarity, may contain information about connectivity within regions, or may be based on some collective shape property. The objective is usually to determine regions that form a set of tissue types, such as white matter, gray matter, or MS lesion.

Measurement of Lesion Volumes

The first and most straightforward use of segmentation in the field of MS research was probably to determine the volume of hyperintense lesions on *T*2-weighted images. The segmentation of MS lesions can be done by manually drawing around the boundary of the lesions while showing the scans, slice-by-slice, on a computer display. Using this process, it is quite possible to achieve reasonable reproducibility, but it is labor-intensive. Changes in lesion volumes are used as secondary outcomes measures in clinical trials of new putative treatments for MS, and the lesions may be hyperintense[22] on *T*2-weighted images or hypointense on *T*1-weighted images ("black

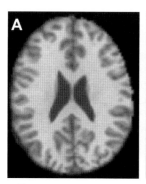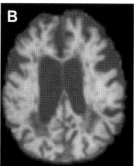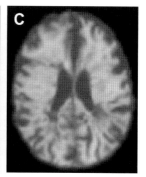

Fig. 2. Linear (affine) and nonlinear registration. (*A*) Normal control subject to which a patient who has MS with severe cerebral atrophy has been registered. (*B*) Patient registered using an affine transform. (*C*) Same patient but registered using the nonlinear registration algorithm by Rohde and Aldroubi.[20] (*Courtesy of* E. Pagani, MPhil, Milan, Italy.)

holes").[23] Black hole lesions are thought to represent tissues with more severe cellular damage.[24]

Many workers have addressed the problem of reducing the amount of operator time and improving the reproducibility of the measurement of MS lesion volumes using computer-assisted or fully automated computerized methods. Methods include edge detection and contour following,[25,26] multiparametric image analysis,[27–29] template-driven segmentation,[30–32] and fuzzy connectedness.[33] Of these, the one that is probably most commonly used in clinical trials is one that still relies on operator judgment to identify the individual lesions, but uses an edge detector to find the border of the lesion.[26] The operator visually determines a fairly well-defined portion of the lesion boundary and clicks on it with the computer mouse, an edge detector selects the sharpest part of the boundary, and a contour surrounding the lesion is generated by following a level of isointensity from the initial edge point. This simple method has been shown to improve reproducibility considerably compared to manual outlining.[25]

Many other methods are used by individual research groups for their own clinical and MR imaging research programs. The reproducibilities are often shown to be better than manual identification and outlining, but they are often tested using data from only one MR imaging scanner with specific pulse sequence parameters. It may be that some of these methods do not transfer to the context of multicenter clinical trials because they are sensitive to the subtle differences in images seen between different manufacturers for what are nominally the same pulse sequence parameters.

The most promising approaches are probably based on multiparametric segmentation, whereby information from several scans (eg, the two echoes of a dual-echo sequence and fluid-attenuated inversion recovery [FLAIR]) are combined to segment the lesions based on the position of pixels in an N-dimensional intensity space.[34] The number of dimensions is equal to the number of images and, in principle, the greater the number of images used, the higher is the discriminating power that allows the lesion to be distinguished from other tissues. Fuzzy connectedness can be regarded as an extension of multiparametric methods, but it is a general method for image segmentation in which the object membership of pixels depends on the way they "hang together" spatially in spite of gradual variations in their intensity. For the task of measuring lesion volumes, Udupa and colleagues[33] adopted a three-part procedure. First was the manual identification by the operator of a few typical tissue types on the scan, including MS lesion, normal white matter, normal gray matter, and CSF. Next, the fuzzy connectedness algorithm automatically identified "candidate" MS lesions, and in the final stage, these candidate lesions were presented to the operator, who reviewed them and accepted, rejected, or modified them. Thus, the method implicitly recognized that human operators are good at identifying image features but do not perform well when attempting to delineate the poorly defined borders of the lesions. The operator time required to assess typical image sets from patients who had MS was between 2 and 20 minutes, depending on the number and complexity of the lesions. Another approach based on fuzzy connectedness principles incorporated "domain knowledge" in the form of probability maps, which showed the probability of finding MS lesion tissue at any given anatomic location.[35] This allowed the number of "false-positive" lesions to be greatly reduced, eliminating the need for review. Nevertheless, it was still necessary for the operator to identify each MS lesion manually with a mouse click.

Atrophy

Brain and spinal cord atrophy measures are becoming standard in MS clinical trials, where the loss of neuronal tissue is thought to be an indicator of long-term irreversible tissue damage.[36] This is slightly complicated by the phenomenon of "pseudoatrophy," whereby the anti-inflammatory effect of some treatments causes a rapid initial loss of brain volume because of a reduction in the amount of excess fluid in the brain. Brain atrophy is a normal feature of aging, with progressive loss of tissue starting in early adulthood.[37] The brain volume is highly variable among individuals, however.

Brain atrophy can be measured cross-sectionally or longitudinally. Cross-sectional measures estimate the total volume of brain tissue. Because the cranial volume and brain size are so variable, however, the results are not easily compared, except in studies of large populations. One way to standardize the measures is to provide a "normalized" brain volume, and there are really two ways to do this. The first is to divide the brain parenchymal volume by the cranial volume, because the cranial volume remains largely fixed throughout adult life.[38] The second is to divide it by the sum of the parenchymal and CSF volumes to form what is known as the brain parenchymal fraction (BPF).[39] As atrophy occurs, the CSF-filled ventricles and sulci enlarge and the BPF reduces; therefore, the BPF is a highly effective measure of the state of atrophy and can be compared across individuals. In longitudinal studies, it is, of course, possible simply to measure the reduction in normalized brain volume over time. More sophisticated approaches first register the scans made at different time points, however; it then becomes possible not only to assess the gross change in tissue volume but to visualize the anatomic location of tissue loss.[40]

Although there are several software packages that can be used to assess atrophy, it is necessary that they have a scan-rescan coefficient of variation (CoV) of around 0.5% or better if they are to be useful for MS research. This allows differences in atrophy rates among groups of subjects to be assessed with relatively small groups (typically 25–50 patients).[41] Virtually all methods use high-resolution T1-weighted images (multislice spin-echo or three-dimensional [3-D] gradient-echo) as input, wherein the timing parameters are optimized to maximize contrast between the low-intensity CSF and the parenchyma. As a preprocessing step, it is necessary to separate the cranial contents from other tissues, such as scalp, eyes, and facial tissues; this can be achieved in a variety of ways, but one of the most popular is the brain extraction tool,[42] which uses an expanding triangulated surface model that "sticks" to the brain-CSF boundary as it expands from the center of the brain. With sufficient image contrast, segmentation can then be achieved using an intensity threshold to separate brain from CSF.[39] More sophisticated approaches assess gray matter, white matter, and CSF volumes separately, allowing loss of different types of tissue to be assessed;[37] however, this method is prone to errors because of the misclassification of MS lesions as gray matter. Taking this a stage further, a VBM approach allows the identification of the individual brain structures that are particularly subject to atrophy.[19]

It has also been shown that the spinal cord is subject to atrophy, and that the degree of atrophy is related to disability.[43] The cord is, of course, a much smaller structure; because of this, cord atrophy measurements have a much lower reproducibility (larger CoV) than those for the whole brain. A typical approach is to measure the cord area over a fairly limited portion of the cervical region. The cord can be segmented using methods similar to those used in the brain, with a threshold to separate the CSF from the cord parenchyma[44] or using edge detection.[43]

MAGNETIZATION TRANSFER

Standard MR imaging detects signal only from hydrogen nuclei (protons) that are "mobile" (contained within a liquid)—if a hydrogen atom is part of a molecule that is large and cannot move about freely, the signal from that hydrogen atom decays too quickly to be seen using a clinical MR imaging scanner. Such protons are found in large molecules (macromolecules), such as those of cell membranes and myelin. The mobile protons are in constant motion, however, and come into regular and intimate contact with the macromolecular protons, and the spin state (the proton magnetization state, which is measured with MR imaging) of the mobile protons can exchange with that of the macromolecular protons. This exchange of magnetization forms the basis of magnetization transfer imaging (MTI).[45]

A magnetization transfer ratio (MTR) image is calculated from a pair of images acquired in an identical way, except that one has extra off-resonance RF pulses applied, which saturates the macromolecular magnetization pool. The MTR is calculated for every corresponding pair of pixels in the two images. If the intensity of the pixel in the image without saturation pulses is $M0$ and the corresponding intensity in the image with saturation pulses is Ms, the MTR is as follows:

$$MTR = \frac{(M0 - Ms)}{M0} \cdot 100\%$$

The application of formulae, such as the previous one, on a pixel-by-pixel basis is a straightforward procedure of image processing and is generally referred to as "image algebra."

Misregistration can occur if the subject moves between the two scans, but the $M0$ and Ms images must be in register; otherwise, artifacts appear at the edges of features in the calculated MTR image, with false MTR values. It is best to acquire the two images in an interleaved way,[46,47] although it is possible to register them after acquisition.

Two forms of data analysis have been used extensively for MTR images: region of interest (ROI) and histogram analysis. ROI analysis may be useful for elucidating the degree of tissue damage within individual lesions seen on T2-weighted scans or within anatomic regions associated with particular symptoms. ROI analysis, however, can be subject to operator bias, because the placement of regions is normally done manually. This could be overcome by first registering scans to an anatomic template and using ROIs defined on the template image. With MTR histogram analysis, a histogram of pixel MTR values is formed from the whole of the brain parenchyma; thus, focal damage and more widespread diffuse tissue damage are reflected in changes to the shape of the histogram, with a general shift toward lower MTR values as the density of macromolecules is reduced with demyelination or axonal loss. Extraction of the brain parenchyma, using the same procedures that are used in atrophy measurements, is a necessary preprocessing step. After normalization (to remove any effect of the absolute brain size), the MTR histogram can be characterized by several simple statistics, such as the histogram peak position, the peak height, and the average MTR.

LEAST-SQUARES FITTING AND RELAXOMETRY

The calculated MTR images noted in the previous section allow a quantitative approach to the assessment of tissue damage. Although T1- and T2-weighted images show, qualitatively, the burden of tissue damaged by MS, a quantitative approach to relaxation time measurements is more rigorous. The mapping of T1, T2, and T2* (or their inverses: R1, R2, and R2*) is possible if images are acquired with more than one set of timing parameters: T1 maps can be produced from a series of images with varying TR, inversion time (TI), or flip angle (for gradient-echo sequences);[48] T2 can be produced from maps from spin-echo images; and T2* images can be produced from gradient-echo images with varying TEs.[49]

In a way that is similar to pixel-by-pixel MTR calculation, the relaxation time constants are calculated for every image pixel, normally by least-squares fitting to the different images. At least two images are needed to estimate simple T1 or T2 maps, because the fitted variables include the proton density and the relaxation time: the number of images acquired must be at least as many as the number of fit variables. Increasing the number of acquired images reduces the sensitivity to noise, reducing errors in the estimates of the fit variables. **Fig. 3** shows relaxation time and rate maps created from data collected using a dual–spin-echo sequence (T2) and a 16-echo gradient-echo sequence (T2*).

Simple least-squares fitting can reliably fit a single exponential decay curve, and possibly even a couple of isolated exponential components.[50] Because of noise in the data, however, fitting multiple relaxation components, representing different tissue water components, is notoriously unreliable. To make fitting stable, it is common to "regularize" the procedure by using a smooth distribution of exponential components.[51] This approach has been taken by the group of MacKay and his colleagues[52] in Vancouver to produce T2 distributions from brain tissue. Three peaks in the white

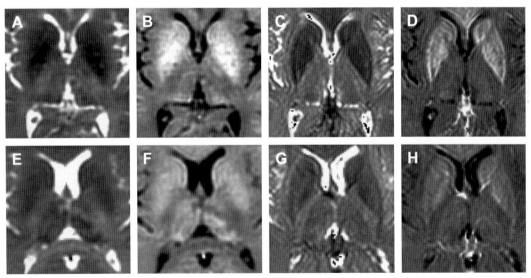

Fig. 3. Relaxometry maps: T2 (A, E), R2 (B, F), T2* (C, G), and R2* (D, H) Maps obtained at 3 T are shown from a patient who has relapsing-remitting MS (disease duration of 7 years, moderate disability [expanded disability status scale score = 5]) (A–D) and a healthy control (E–H). Marked hypointensity is seen in the caudate, putamen, and globus pallidus on T2 and T2* maps from the patient who has MS (A, C) compared with the normal control (E, G). Similarly, marked hyperintensity is seen in the caudate, putamen, and globus pallidus on R2 and R2* maps from the patient who has MS (B, D) compared with the normal control (F, H). The hypointensity seen on T2 and T2* maps and hyperintensity seen on R2 and R2* in the gray matter areas of patients who have MS likely represent excessive iron deposition. (*From* Neema M, Stankiewicz J, Arora A, et al. T1-and T2-based MRI measures of diffuse gray matter and white matter damage in patients with multiple sclerosis. J Neuroimaging 2007;17:16S–21S; with permission.)

matter *T2* distribution are attributed to the following: water between the myelin lipid bilayers (*T2* between 10 and 50 milliseconds), intracellular water (*T2* of approximately 70 milliseconds), and CSF (*T2* > 1 second) (**Fig. 4**). In recent studies, maps of the short *T2* component have been shown to correlate strongly with myelin staining in postmortem samples (**Fig. 5**).[53]

DIFFUSION TENSOR IMAGING

Diffusion-weighted (DW) MR imaging has been used in the human brain for almost 20 years to investigate numerous conditions, including MS.[54,55] The contrast in DW MR imaging is based on the diffusional displacement of water molecules, which, in the presence of a strong magnetic field gradient, causes the signal intensity to be attenuated. In simple anisotropic systems, diffusion in three dimensions can be represented mathematically by the diffusion tensor, a 3×3 matrix that specifies the root mean square diffusional displacements in any direction.[56] It is common to display images of properties of tensor rather than the tensor itself (**Fig. 6**).

Echo-planar imaging (EPI)[57] is normally used for DW applications because of the technique's insensitivity to bulk patient motion. Because of scanner hardware limitations, however, DW gradient pulses usually induce some distortions in DW EPI images, characterized by a shear, shift, and scaling of the images in the phase-encoded direction. The postprocessing correction of these distortions has been subjected to a good deal of work; the most successful methods exploit the relation between the type and magnitude of distortion and the magnetic field gradient vector direction and amplitude.[58,59] One approach is also capable of including a model of patient motion, such that gradient-induced distortion and patient motion can be corrected simultaneously.[60]

After distortion correction, calculation of the tensor is a relatively straightforward problem in multivariate regression.[56] Diagonalization of the tensor to extract the principal axes allows images showing the direction of greatest diffusivity, the degree of anisotropy, and the directionally averaged diffusivity (mean diffusivity, equivalent to one third of the trace of the diffusion tensor) to be synthesized (see **Fig. 6**). All these properties of the tensor reflect the diffusional behavior of water in the tissue and, given similar acquisition parameters, should be comparable across sites and at different field strengths.

Once the tensor is computed, it is possible to reconstruct the spatial path of the major white matter axonal bundles in "fiber tracking" applications.[61] Tractography is performed by following the direction of largest diffusivity to reconstruct a pathway corresponding to the underlying axonal fiber bundle. This allows the study of human white matter anatomy that could previously only be accessed by post-mortem dissection. Tissue damage along the reconstructed tracts can then be assessed by evaluating other parameters, such as the fractional anisotropy or mean diffusivity, along the tract.[62,63]

One problem with performing tractography on patients who have MS is that diffusion anisotropy is reduced in MS lesions, and a reduction in anisotropy leads to a greater uncertainty in the estimated principal diffusion direction (see **Fig. 6; Fig. 7**).[64] Tracking through lesions is therefore problematic, and it may be necessary to use an "atlas-based"

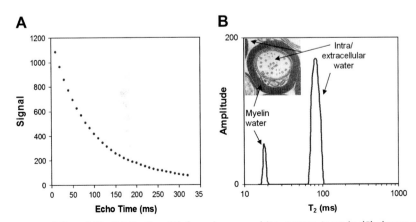

Fig. 4. *T2* decay curve (*A*) and *T2* distribution (*B*) from human white matter. Inset in (*B*) shows a cross section through an axon with the locations of the intra- and extracellular water and myelin water. (*From* Laule C, Vavasour IM, Kolind SH, et al. Magnetic resonance imaging of myelin. Neurotherapeutics 2007;4:463; with permission.)

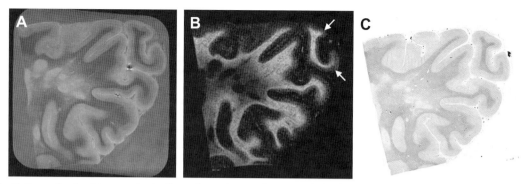

Fig. 5. Formalin-fixed human brain tissue from the partieto-occipital lobe of a patient who had MS. Magnetic resonance images acquired at 7 T: short echo image (TE = 20.1 milliseconds) (*A*), and myelin water map corresponding to that part of the *T*2 distribution with values less than 20 milliseconds (*B*). (*C*) Corresponding Luxol fast blue histology image. A good qualitative correspondence is observed between the myelin water map and histology stain for myelin. The normal prominent myelination of the deeper cortical layers (*arrows*) is also visible on the myelin water image. (*From* Laule C, Kozlowski P, Leung E, et al. Myelin water imaging of multiple sclerosis at 7 T: correlations with histopathology. Neuroimage 2008;40(4):1577; with permission.)

approach to determining the tissue characteristics within specific tracts, having first localized the tracts by performing fiber tracking on a large population.[65]

The simple model of diffusion that is provided by the diffusion tensor cannot capture the details of diffusion in complex white matter regions; these occur in brain areas in which fibers merge and cross. MR imaging does not have the spatial resolution to depict individual fiber bundles, but the MR imaging methods are sensitive to the diffusion of water over distances of a few microns; detailed analysis of the diffusion behavior can reveal more about white matter architecture on a smaller scale, in which an individual image voxel contains a mixed population of fibers. Such approaches as q-ball imaging[66] and determining the fiber orientation density function (ODF)[67] can resolve more details about these regions of mixed fiber orientations.

PERFUSION

Abnormalities of cerebral blood flow (CBF) have long been recognized in MS, and MR imaging can be used to assess perfusion in vivo. Perfusion can be measured in one of two ways: using standard injectable MR imaging contrast agents as a bolus (bolus tracking) or by using blood as an endogenous contrast agent, an experiment that is known as arterial spin labeling (ASL).

For bolus tracking, images are acquired rapidly and continuously as the contrast agent is injected over a short time (normally around 5 seconds) into the antecubital vein. From there, the bolus is carried to the heart, through the lungs, back to the heart, and then to the arterial system, where it can be measured in the carotid arteries, circle of Willis, or cerebral arteries. The images are normally acquired using an echo-planar sequence to give good time resolution (on the order of 1 or 2 seconds) and to give a large signal reduction

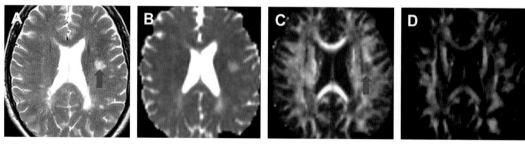

Fig. 6. *T*2-weighted image (*A*), diffusion tensor trace (*B*), fractional anisotropy (*C*), and color-coded direction maps (*D*) calculated from DW images of a patient who has multiple sclerosis. Hyperintense lesions (*arrows*) show high diffusivity and low anisotropy. In fiber-tracking applications,[61] this causes greater uncertainty in the orientation of the axonal fibers, and tracking errors. In the direction map, axonal fibers that have a left-right orientation are colored red, anterior superior fibers are green, and superior-inferior fibers are blue.

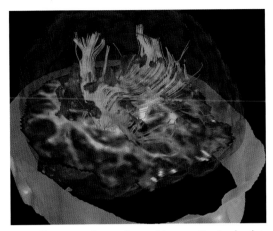

Fig. 7. Tractography performed in a patient who has MS. The MS lesions have been segmented from T2-weighted images and are rendered in red. Fiber tracking was initiated in the patient's right internal capsule, and the tracts pass through tissue affected by MS lesions. As they do so, the path spuriously deviates from the known motor tract and across the corpus callosum.

as the contrast agent passes through. This signal reduction is used to estimate the concentration of contrast agent for every voxel from the relaxivity and TE of the sequence.

By the time the contrast agent arrives in the feeding arteries, considerable dispersion has occurred, and the arterial input into the brain is no longer a short sharp bolus as would be required for straightforward analysis. An important part of the processing of bolus tracking data is therefore to account for this dispersion by a process of "deconvolution."[68] This mathematical process examines the real dispersed contrast agent input and the real passage through the brain tissue, and it reconstitutes what would have been the response to an ideal sharp "impulse" of contrast agent. This reconstructed impulse response is used to calculate the mean transit time (MTT) for contrast passage, and the cerebral blood volume (CBV) can be assessed by measuring the degree of signal change in the brain tissue compared with that in an artery. The CBF can then be calculated from the ratio:

$$CBF = \frac{CBV}{MTT}$$

Bolus tracking experiments are not normally considered to give accurate quantitative CBF values, mainly because of the difficulty of obtaining accurate estimates of the contrast agent concentration in the arteries and in the capillary bed: the relaxivity in T2-and T2*-weighted pulse sequences depends on the size of the vessels that contain the blood.

Furthermore, estimation depends on the contrast agent remaining within the vessels, and where disease is present, the blood-brain barrier may not be intact and the contrast agent leaks into tissue; however, it is possible to correct for this.[69] In spite of these problems, bolus tracking is considered to give good qualitative CBF maps, which can be used to make relative comparisons across regions within a single patient.

The basic idea of ASL is to acquire two images: in the first, the blood is "labeled" before it moves into the imaged slice, usually by inverting the magnetization; the second is a control image in which no labeling takes place. If carefully performed, the difference between the two images is then solely attributable to the labeled blood that has perfused the tissue volume imaged. Because the brain-blood volume fraction is small, however, the signal difference is also small (on the order of 1%); thus, this technique has inherently poor signal-to-noise ratio (SNR). Acquisition over a long period, with signal averaging, is usually necessary, and the method is of most use at higher field strength. The advantage of ASL over bolus tracking methods is that repeated measures can be made and the response to various interventions monitored as long as changes in blood flow occur and can be sustained over time scales longer than the acquisition time for a single measurement (typically 5 minutes). It is also totally noninvasive, because no contrast agent injection is needed.

There are many variants of the ASL experiment, which are designed to permit more complex assessment of the confounding factors that inhibit quantitative measurement of perfusion. One of the most common variants introduces a variable transit time between the inversion and the image readout in the brain; the impact of variable transit times should then be taken into account.[70] The details of processing of ASL data depend, of course, on the exact form of experiment and vary in complexity from a simple subtraction to a least-squares fitting to extract the various model parameters, including CBF (for a review, see the article by Petersen and colleagues[71]).

Bolus tracking[72] and ASL[73] methods have been used to map the regional changes in CBF that develop with MS, with reduced perfusion being seen in white and gray matter. Correlations have been seen between white matter perfusion and disability[72] and between gray matter perfusion and neuropsychologic impairment.[74]

VISUALIZATION

The mainstay of MR image computerized visualization is still the common multislice viewing system, analogous to a conventional light box, where image slices can be viewed singly, with arrays of slices, or, preferably, with images of different contrast being viewable side-by-side. For manual analysis (eg, counting the numbers of lesions), semiautomated analysis (semiautomatically outlining lesions),[26] or reviewing the output of fully automated methods,[75] this sort of presentation tool is efficient, enabling rapid throughput.

3-D visualization tools are popular for data exploration and presentation, however.[76,77] These generally allow surface models and cut-planes to be viewed simultaneously, such that the spatial relations among the various anatomic elements can be better appreciated (**Fig. 8**). Although these tools are established as valuable aids in other medical settings, such as surgical planning,[78] they are difficult to integrate into quantitative analysis procedures for MS research in a useful way.

DATA HANDLING

In the context of multicenter clinical trials, central analysis of image data is essential for improving the quality of data acquisition, consistency of processing, achieving validation of processing methods, and data archiving to the standards required for clinical trials of new therapeutic agents.[79] Basic transfer of image data has been greatly facilitated in the past few years by the adoption of the Digital Imaging and Communication in Medicine (DICOM) standards for image exchange by all mainstream manufacturers of medical equipment.[80] This allows data to be sent for analysis by fairly conventional means (by sending an archive compact disk read-only memory [CD-ROM] in the mail) or by transfer using standard protocols over the Internet.

Having received the image data, some groups have adopted a "pipeline" processing approach to ensure efficiency, consistency, and quality control of the analysis procedure.[75,81] By integrating the analysis pipeline with a database of patients enrolled in a trial and the trial scanning schedules, quality can be improved and the tasks streamlined. The sorts of task that can be automated by the pipeline include sending out automatic reminders to participating sites about scans that are due or not received; automatically implementing pre- and postprocessing steps; prioritizing and presenting tasks to be performed by neurologists, technologists and technicians; generating and collating reports; and archive of data.

SUMMARY

Image analysis methods have become much more mainstream over the past 5 years or so, and there are now many excellent tools available to enable the nonspecialist to participate in the sorts of tasks that were once considered to be only for those with expert knowledge and large computing resources. The resources required were not only specialist and expensive computer equipment but technical personnel who would implement and integrate the necessary processing steps. With the advent of powerful and inexpensive personal computers and mature software applications that have been designed for the general user, postprocessing of MRI data for quantitative analysis of the scans of patients who have MS is becoming much more mainstream. Over time, it is likely that some of these methods may become integrated into routine clinical practice so that, for example, individual patients' disease progression can be monitored and treatment plans designed accordingly.

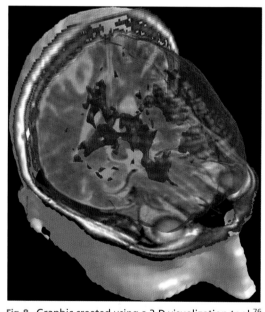

Fig. 8. Graphic created using a 3-D visualization tool.[76] The composite picture shows the surface-rendered skin surface in pink and a transparent extracted brain surface; the MS lesions' surface is rendered in red, and there is a backdrop of orthogonal planes from a T2-weighted image. The brain surface and lesions were found using preprocessing steps to extract them automatically.[6,35]

REFERENCES

1. Bydder GM, Steiner RE, Young IR, et al. Clinical NMR imaging of the brain: 140 cases. AJR Am J Roentgenol 1982;139(2):215–36.

2. Rinck PA, Bielke G, Meves M. Modified spin-echo sequence in tumor diagnosis. Proceedings of the Society of Magnetic Resonance in Medicine. Magn Reson Med 1984;1(2):236.

3. Miller DH, Rudge P, Johnson G, et al. Serial gadolinium enhanced magnetic resonance imaging in multiple sclerosis. Brain 1988;111(4):927–39.

4. Wicks DAG, Barker GJ, Tofts PS. Correction of intensity nonuniformity in MR images of any orientation. Magn Reson Imaging 1993;11(2):183–96.

5. Belaroussi B, Milles J, Carme S, et al. Intensity nonuniformity correction in MRI: existing methods and their validation. Med Image Anal 2006;10(2):234–46.

6. Horsfield MA, Rovaris M, Rocca MA, et al. Whole-brain atrophy in multiple sclerosis measured by two segmentation processes from various MRI sequences. J Neurol Sci 2003;216(1):169–77.

7. Brechbuhler C, Gerig G, Szekely GS. Compensation of spatial inhomogeneity in MRI based on a parametric bias estimate. Visualization in Biomedical Computing 1996;1131:141–6.

8. Sled JG, Zijdenbos AP, Evans AC. A nonparametric method for automatic correction of intensity nonuniformity in MRI data. IEEE Trans Med Imaging 1998; 17(1):87–97.

9. Gispert JD, Reig S, Pascau J, et al. Method for bias field correction of brain T1 weighted magnetic resonance images minimizing segmentation error. Hum Brain Mapp 2004;22(2):133–44.

10. Hill DLG, Batchelor PG, Holden M, et al. Medical image registration. Phys Med Biol 2001;46(3):R1–R45.

11. Fox NC, Freeborough PA. Brain atrophy progression measured from registered serial MRI: validation and application to Alzheimer's disease. J Magn Reson Imaging 1997;7(6):1069–75.

12. Studholme C, Hill DLG, Hawkes DJ. Automated three-dimensional registration of magnetic resonance and positron emission tomography brain images by multiresolution optimization of voxel similarity measures. Med Phys 1997;24(1):25–35.

13. Collins DL, Neelin P, Peters TM, et al. Automatic 3D intersubject registration of MR volumetric data in standardized Talairach space. J Comput Assist Tomogr 1994;18(2):192–205.

14. Woods RP, Grafton ST, Holmes CJ, et al. Automated image registration: I. General methods and intrasubject, intramodality validation. J Comput Assist Tomogr 1998;22(1):139–52.

15. Pluim JPW, Maintz JBA, Viergever MA. Mutual-information-based registration of medical images: a survey. IEEE Trans Med Imaging 2003;22(8): 986–1004.

16. Talairach J, Tournoux P. Co-planar stereotaxic atlas of the human brain. New York: Thieme Medical Publishers; 1988.

17. Lancaster JL, Tordesillas-Gutierrez D, Martinez M, et al. Bias between MNI and Talairach coordinates analyzed using the ICBM-152 brain template. Hum Brain Mapp 2007;28(11):1194–205.

18. Mechelli A, Price CJ, Friston KJ, et al. Voxel-based morphometry of the human brain: methods and applications. Current Medical Imaging Reviews 2005;1(2):105–13.

19. Sepulcre J, Sastre-Garriga J, Cercignani M, et al. Regional gray matter atrophy in early primary progressive multiple sclerosis—a voxel-based morphometry study. Arch Neurol 2006;63(8):1175–80.

20. Rohde GK, Aldroubi A, Dawant BM, et al. The adaptive bases algorithm for intensity-based nonrigid image registration. IEEE Trans Med Imaging 2003; 22(11):1470–9.

21. Pagani E, Horsfield MA, Rocca MA, et al. Assessing atrophy of the major white matter fiber bundles of the brain from diffusion tensor MRI data. Magn Reson Med 2007;58(3):527–34.

22. Filippi M, Horsfield MA, Ader HJ, et al. Guidelines for using quantitative measures of brain magnetic resonance imaging abnormalities in monitoring the treatment of multiple sclerosis. Ann Neurol 1998;43(4): 499–506.

23. Tomassini V, Paolillo A, Russo P, et al. Predictors of long-term clinical response to interferon beta therapy in relapsing multiple sclerosis. J Neurol 2006; 253(3):287–93.

24. Barkhof F, Karas GB, van Walderveen MAA. T1 hypointensities and axonal loss. Neuroimaging Clin N Am 2000;10(4):739–52.

25. Grimaud J, Lai M, Thorpe J, et al. Quantification of MRI lesion load in multiple sclerosis: a comparison of three computer-assisted techniques. Magn Reson Imaging 1996;14(5):495–505.

26. Cader S, Cifelli A, Abu-Omar Y, et al. Reduced brain functional reserve and altered functional connectivity in patients with multiple sclerosis. Brain 2006; 129(2):527–37.

27. Kikinis R, Shenton ME, Gerig G, et al. Routine quantitative analysis of brain and cerebrospinal fluid spaces with MR imaging. J Magn Reson Imaging 1992;2(2):619–29.

28. Bedell BJ, Narayana PA, Wolinsky JS. A dual approach for minimizing false lesion classifications on magnetic resonance images. Magn Reson Med 1997;37(1):94–102.

29. Zijdenbos A, Forghani R, Evans A. Automatic quantification of MS lesions in 3D MRI brain data sets: validation of INSECT. Lect Notes Comput Sci 1998; 1496:439–48.

30. Anbeek P, Vincken KL, van Osch MJP, et al. Probabilistic segmentation of white lesions in MR imaging. Neuroimage 2004;21(3):1037–44.

31. van Leemput K, Maes F, Vandermeulen D, et al. Automated segmentation of multiple sclerosis lesions by model outlier detection. IEEE Trans Med Imaging 2001;20(8):677–88.

32. Warfield S, Dengler J, Zaers J, et al. Automatic identification of gray matter structures from MRI to improve the segmentation of white matter lesions. J Image Guid Surg 1995;1(6):326–38.

33. Udupa JK, Wei L, Samarasekera S, et al. Multiple sclerosis lesion quantification using fuzzy-connectedness principles. IEEE Trans Med Imaging 1997; 16:598–609.

34. Sajja BR, Datta S, He RJ, et al. Unified approach for multiple sclerosis lesion segmentation on brain MRI. Ann Biomed Eng 2006;442(1):142–51.

35. Horsfield MA, Bakshi R, Rovaris M, et al. Incorporating domain knowledge into the fuzzy connectedness framework: application to brain lesion volume estimation in multiple sclerosis. IEEE Trans Med Imaging 2007;26(12):1670–80.

36. Fisher E, Rudick RA, Simon JH, et al. Eight-year follow-up study of brain atrophy in patients with MS. Neurology 2002;59(9):1412–20.

37. Good CD, Johnsrude IS, Ashburner J, et al. A voxel-based morphometric study of ageing in 465 normal adult human brains. Neuroimage 2001;14(1):21–36.

38. Smith SM, Zhang YY, Jenkinson M, et al. Accurate, robust, and automated longitudinal and cross-sectional brain change analysis. Neuroimage 2002; 17(1):479–89.

39. Rudick RA, Fisher E, Lee JC, et al. Use of the brain parenchymal fraction to measure whole brain atrophy in relapsing-remitting MS. Neurology 1999; 53(8):1698–704.

40. Freeborough PA, Fox NC. Modeling brain deformations in Alzheimer disease by fluid registration of serial 3D MR images. J Comput Assist Tomogr 1998;22(5):838–43.

41. Fox NC, Jenkins R, Leary SM, et al. Progressive cerebral atrophy in MS—a serial study using registered, volumetric MRI. Neurology 2000;54(4): 807–12.

42. Smith SM. Fast robust automated brain extraction. Hum Brain Mapp 2002;17(3):143–55.

43. Lin X, Tench CR, Turner B, et al. Spinal cord atrophy and disability in multiple sclerosis over four years: application of a reproducible automated technique in monitoring disease progression in a cohort of the interferon beta-1a (Rebif) treatment trial. J Neurol Neurosurg Psychiatry 2003;74(8):1090–4.

44. Losseff NA, Webb SL, O'Riordan JI. Spinal cord atrophy and disability in multiple sclerosis. A new reproducible and sensitive MRI method with potential to monitor disease progression. Brain 1996; 19(3):701–8.

45. Horsfield MA. Magnetization transfer imaging in multiple sclerosis. J Neuroimaging 2005;15(4):58S–67S.

46. Barker GJ, Tofts PS, Gass A. An interleaved sequence for accurate and reproducible clinical measurement of magnetization transfer ratio. Magn Reson Imaging 1996;14(4):403–11.

47. Inglese M, Horsfield MA, Filippi M. Scan-rescan variation of measures derived from brain magnetization transfer ratio histograms obtained in healthy volunteers by use of a semi-interleaved magnetization transfer sequence. AJNR Am J Neuroradiol 2001; 22(4):681–4.

48. Barbosa S, Blumhardt LD, Roberts N, et al. Magnetic resonance relaxation time mapping in multiple sclerosis—normal-appearing white matter and the invisible lesion load. Magn Reson Imaging 1994; 12:33–42.

49. Neema M, Stankiewicz J, Arora A, et al. T1-and T2-based MRI measures of diffuse gray matter and white matter damage in patients with multiple sclerosis. J Neuroimaging 2007;17(Suppl 1):16S–21S.

50. Kidd D, Barker GJ, Tofts PS, et al. The transverse magnetization decay characteristics of longstanding lesions and normal-appearing white matter in multiple sclerosis. J Neurol 1997;244(2):125–30.

51. Butler JP, Reeds JA, Dawson SV. Estimating solutions of first kind integral equations with nonnegative constraints and optimal smoothing. Society for Industrial and Applied Mathematics Journal on Numerical Analysis 1981;18(3):381–97.

52. Whittall KP, MacKay AL, Graeb DA, et al. In vivo measurement of T2 distributions and water contents in normal human brain. Magn Reson Med 1997; 37(1):34–43.

53. Laule C, Kozlowski P, Leung E, et al. Myelin water imaging of multiple sclerosis at 7 T: correlations with histopathology. Neuroimage 2008;40(4):1575–80.

54. Rovaris M, Gass A, Bammer R, et al. Diffusion MRI in multiple sclerosis. Neurology 2005;65(10):1526–32.

55. Horsfield MA, Larsson HBW, Jones DK, et al. Diffusion magnetic resonance imaging in multiple sclerosis. J Neurol Neurosurg Psychiatry 1998;64(1):S80–84.

56. Basser PJ, Mattiello J, LeBihan D. MR diffusion tensor spectroscopy and imaging. Biophys J 1994; 66(1):259–67.

57. Turner R, LeBihan D, Maier J, et al. Echo-planar imaging of intravoxel incoherent motion. Radiology 1990;177(2):407–14.

58. Horsfield MA. Mapping eddy current induced fields for the correction of diffusion weighted echo planar images. Magn Reson Imaging 1999;17(9):1335–45.

59. Zhuang JC, Hrabe J, Kangarlu A, et al. Correction of eddy-current distortions in diffusion tensor images using the known directions and strengths of diffusion gradients. J Magn Reson Imaging 2006;24(5):1188–93.

60. Andersson JLR, Skare S. A model-based method for retrospective correction of geometric distortions in diffusion-weighted EPI. Neuroimage 2002;16(1): 177–99.

61. Mori S, Crain BJ, Chacko VP, et al. Three-dimensional tracking of axonal projections in the brain by magnetic resonance imaging. Ann Neurol 1999; 45(2):265–9.

62. Jones DK, Travis AR, Eden G, et al. PASTA: point-wise assessment of streamline tractography attributes. Magn Reson Med 2005;53(6):1462–7.

63. Smith SM, Jenkinson M, Johansen-Berg H, et al. Tract-based spatial statistics: voxelwise analysis of multi-subject diffusion data. Neuroimage 2006; 31(4):1487–505.

64. Jones DK. Determining and visualizing uncertainty in estimates of fiber orientation from diffusion tensor MRI. Magn Reson Med 2003;49(1):7–12.

65. Pagani E, Filippi M, Rocca MA, et al. A method for obtaining tract specific diffusion tensor MRI measurements in the presence of disease: application to patients with clinically isolated syndromes suggestive of multiple sclerosis. Neuroimage 2005; 26(1):258–65.

66. Tuch DS. Q-Ball imaging. Magn Reson Med 2004; 52(6):1358–72.

67. Tournier JD. Direct estimation of the fiber orientation density function from diffusion-weighted MRI data using spherical deconvolution. Neuroimage 2004; 23(3):1176–85.

68. Ostergaard L, Weisskoff RM, Chesler DA, et al. High resolution measurement of cerebral blood flow using intravascular tracer bolus passages. 1. Mathematical approach and statistical analysis. Magn Reson Med 1996;36(5):715–25.

69. Boxerman JL, Schmainda KM, Weisskoff RM. Relative cerebral blood volume maps corrected for contrast agent extravasation significantly correlate with glioma tumor grade, whereas uncorrected maps do not. AJNR Am J Neuroradiol 2006;27(4):859–67.

70. Gunther M, Bock M, Schad LR. Arterial spin labeling in combination with a look-locker sampling strategy: inflow turbo-sampling EPI-FAIR (ITS-FAIR). Magn Reson Med 2001;46(5):974–84.

71. Petersen ET, Zimine I, Ho YC, et al. Non-invasive measurement of perfusion: a critical review of arterial spin labelling techniques. Br J Radiol 2006; 79(944):688–701.

72. Adhya S, Johnson G, Herbert J, et al. Pattern of hemodynamic impairment in multiple sclerosis: dynamic susceptibility contrast perfusion MR imaging at 3.0 T. Neuroimage 2006;33(4): 1029–35.

73. Rashid W, Parkes LM, Ingle GT, et al. Abnormalities of cerebral perfusion in multiple sclerosis. J Neurol Neurosurg Psychiatry 2004;75(9):1288–93.

74. Inglese M, Adhya S, Johnson G, et al. Perfusion magnetic resonance imaging correlates of neuropsychological impairment in multiple sclerosis. J Cereb Blood Flow Metab 2008;28(1):164–71.

75. Zijdenbos AP, Forghani R, Evans AC. Automatic "pipeline" analysis of 3-D MRI data for clinical trials: application to multiple sclerosis. IEEE Trans Med Imaging 2002;21(10):1280–91.

76. Xinapse Systems Limited. Jim image analysis software page. Available at: http://www.xinapse.com. Accessed March 10, 2008.

77. 3D Slicer. Available at: http://www.slicer.org. Accessed March 10, 2008.

78. Gering DT, Nabavi A, Kikinis R, et al. An integrated visualization system for surgical planning and guidance using image fusion and an open MR. J Magn Reson Imaging 2001;13(6):967–97.

79. U.S. Food and Drug Administration. Good clinical practice in FDA-related clinical trials page. Available at: http://www.fda.gov/oc/gcp/. Accessed March 10, 2008.

80. The Association of Electrical and Medical Equipment Manufacturers. Digital imaging and communications in medicine page. Available at: http://dicom.nema.org. Accessed March 10, 2008.

81. Liu LF, Meier D, Polgar-Turcsanyi M, et al. Multiple sclerosis medical image analysis and information management. J Neuroimaging 2005;15(4):103S–17S.

Conventional MR Imaging

Anthony Traboulsee, MD[a],*, David K.B. Li, MD[b]

KEYWORDS

- Conventional MRI • Multiple sclerosis
- Guidelines • Diagnosis

Multiple sclerosis (MS) is a common disease and is the leading cause of nontraumatic disability in young adults. Most patients have a relapsing and remitting disease course (RRMS) characterized by acute exacerbations of inflammatory demyelination (attacks or relapses), including optic neuritis, transverse myelitis, and brainstem syndromes. A small proportion will present with a slowly evolving neurologic syndrome, typically a progressive myelopathy or cerebellar syndrome (primary progressive MS [PPMS]). Establishing an early and accurate diagnosis of MS allows for the initiation of therapies that can prevent future attacks of central nervous system (CNS) inflammation and potentially impact long-term disability. No single test is diagnostic for MS, including MR imaging of the brain, which, although extremely sensitive for detecting lesions typical of MS, lacks pathologic specificity. Where MR imaging technology is available, it would be rare for an individual with MS or suspected MS not to undergo brain and possibly spinal MR imaging as part of their diagnostic work-up or routine follow-up.

Conventional MR imaging refers to techniques routinely used in clinical practice, including T1 (T1W) and T2 (or similar) weighted (T2W) sequences and the use of contrast agents. The goals of conventional imaging in MS can be summarized as follows:

1. Routine investigation in patients with symptoms suspicious for MS
2. To establish an early diagnosis of MS in high-risk patients who have had a single clinically isolated syndrome (CIS) of definite demyelination such as optic neuritis, transverse myelitis, or brainstem/cerebellum inflammation
3. To rule out alternative diagnoses that are clinical or radiologic mimics of MS
4. To predict the short- and long-term clinical prognosis
5. To monitor the response to disease-modifying therapy
6. To monitor for complications of therapy

Conventional MR imaging techniques also serve an important role as robust, quantitative outcome measures in clinical trials of new therapies. This topic is covered in further detail elsewhere in this issue. This review includes a standardized imaging protocol for the diagnosis and monitoring of MS patients, a description of typical and unusual features of MR imaging in MS, imaging features for unique MS populations including pediatric MS, and the role of MR imaging in the diagnosis and routine follow-up of MS patients.

STANDARDIZED MR IMAGING PROTOCOL

MR imaging is the most important paraclinical test for the diagnosis of MS; however, inconsistent protocols can undermine its usefulness. An expert panel of radiologists and neurologists with experience in the clinical diagnosis and management of MS has established a basic minimum set of imaging sequences that are recommended in the investigation of suspected MS.[1] Furthermore, the Consortium of MS Centers standardized MR imaging guidelines provide a consistent protocol that allows for comparison of imaging studies over time for an individual patient on the same

[a] Department of Medicine, Division of Neurology, University of British Columbia, 2211 Wesbrook Mall, Room s199, Vancouver, British Columbia V6T 2B5, Canada
[b] Department of Radiology, University of British Columbia, 2211 Wesbrook Mall, Vancouver, British Columbia V6T 2B5, Canada
* Corresponding author.
E-mail address: trabouls@interchange.ubc.ca (A. Traboulsee).

Neuroimag Clin N Am 18 (2008) 651–673
doi:10.1016/j.nic.2008.07.001
1052-5149/08/$ – see front matter © 2008 Elsevier Inc. All rights reserved.

neuroimaging.theclinics.com

scanner or across scanners (**Table 1**). This protocol improves the accuracy and reliability for detecting new disease activity that many clinicians rely on for early diagnosis and for ongoing treatment decisions.

The minimum sequences that should be included for an MR imaging study of the brain are as follows: axial T2 (echo time [TE], 80–120 ms) and PD (TE, 15–40 ms) weighted, axial fluid-attenuated inversion recovery (FLAIR), axial pre- and postcontrast T1W, and sagittal FLAIR (covering the corpus callosum). Lesion intensity increases with longer TE. Posterior fossa lesions are best seen on T2W images, and FLAIR or PD is preferred for periventricular and juxtacortical lesion detection. A slice thickness of 3 mm or less with no gap (contiguous) provides for improved lesion detection[2,3] and may compensate for smaller lesions being missed by edge blurring associated with fast acquisition techniques.[4] Standardized acquisition of axial images parallel to the subcallosal line that joins the genu and splenium of the corpus callosum is important for comparison across serial studies.

Contrast can be helpful in establishing an early diagnosis by detecting new lesion activity and ruling out alternative diagnoses. A standard dose of gadolinium (Gd) (0.1 mmol/kg) with a minimum 5-minute delay after injection is given before acquiring the postcontrast T1W sequences. There

---

Table 1
The Consortium of MS Centers standardized brain and spinal cord MR imaging protocol

Brain MR Imaging Sequence	Diagnostic Scan for Clinically Isolated Syndrome	New Baseline or follow-up Scan in Definite MS	Comment
Three-plane scout	Recommended	Recommended	Axial sections through the subcallosal line (joins the undersurface of the rostrum and splenium of the corpus callosum)
Sagittal FLAIR	Recommended	Recommended	Useful for corpus callosum lesions
Axial fast spin or turbo spin-echo PD/T2	Recommended	Recommended	TE_1 <30 ms TE_2 >80 ms Useful for infratentorial lesions missed by FLAIR
Axial FLAIR	Recommended	Recommended	Useful for most white matter lesions including juxtacortical
Axial precontrast T1	Optional	Optional	Useful for T1 black hole assessment
Three-dimensional T1	Optional	Optional	Useful for brain volume measures
Axial postcontrast T1	Recommended	Optional	Minimum 5-min delay using a standard dose
Spinal cord MR imaging sequence			Spinal cord MR imaging following contrast-enhanced brain MR imaging (no further contrast is needed) sequence
Three-plane localizer			Three-plane localizer
Precontrast sagittal T1			Postcontrast sagittal T1
Sagittal fast spin-echo PD/T2			Sagittal fast spin-echo PD/T2
Axial fast spin-echo PD/T2 through lesions			Postcontrast axial T1 through lesions
Three-dimensional T1 (optional)			Axial fast spin-echo PD/T2 through lesions
Postcontrast sagittal T1			Three-dimensional T1 (optional)
Postcontrast axial T1 through lesions			

Slice thickness should be ≤3 mm with no interslice gap (contiguous) on a ≥1.0 T closed MR imaging scanner.
Adapted from Simon JH, Li D, Traboulsee A, et al. Standardized MRI protocol for multiple sclerosis: Consortium of MS Centers (CMSC) Consensus Guidelines. AJNR Am J Neuroradiol 2006;27:455; with permission.

can be potential advantages of higher (double or triple) doses of contrast, using a longer (15-minute) delay before collecting the postcontrast T1W images and incorporating a magnetization transfer sequence to increase the number and intensity of contrast-enhancing lesions;[5,6] however, these modifications are not essential for routine clinical imaging. In general, because newly diagnosed MS patients tend to be young (between the ages of 20 and 40 years), and because MS is not usually associated with renal disease, the use of Gd would not be contraindicated owing to concern regarding nephrogenic systemic fibrosis and Gd contrast administration in patients with decreased renal function.

Spinal cord imaging can be extremely helpful in the diagnostic work-up of suspected MS. A phase array coil is recommended, and, depending on the symptoms, coverage may include both cervical and thoracic cord. Sagittal sequences include pre- and postcontrast T1W and fast spin-echo PD/T2 with a slice thickness of 3 mm or less (contiguous). Axial PD/T2 and postcontrast T1W are acquired through suspicious lesions. If spinal cord imaging is to be performed at the same time as brain MR imaging, no additional contrast is required.

Most centers use a field strength of 1.5 T or greater. More lesions can be detected at higher field strengths[7] which, in some situations, may allow for an earlier diagnosis of MS.[8] The minimum recommended field strength is 1.0 T; however, lesion detection in some older 0.5 T systems has been similar to that seen at 1.5 T.[9] It is recommended that the patient keep a copy of their study on portable media should they move to an area with a different center. A comparison of studies over time allows for a better understanding of individual lesion evolution, resolution, and the behavior of contrast enhancement that may aid in diagnostic interpretation or therapeutic strategies.

IMAGING FEATURES OF TYPICAL LESIONS IN MULTIPLE SCLEROSIS

T2 lesions on brain MR imaging are characteristic of well-established, definite MS (Fig. 1A–H),[10,11] and the absence of these lesions should lead to careful reevaluation of the diagnosis.[12] Early in the disease course at the time of the first clinical symptoms (CIS), approximately 20% of patients in whom MS will develop within the next 5 to 20 years will have a normal brain on MR imaging initially.[13] Even patients who have definite MS after sustaining two clinical attacks may have a paucity of lesions that do not meet current radiologic criteria for MS. This finding is more common in MS

subgroups, including Asian opticospinal MS (OSMS)[14] and variants such as neuromyelitis optica (NMO) or Devic's disease;[15] therefore, an MR image of the brain with minimal abnormalities does not rule out the diagnosis of MS but may necessitate further supportive investigations including evoked potentials, cerebral spinal fluid (CSF) analysis, spinal cord imaging, anti–aquaporin-4 antibody testing, and follow-up brain MR imaging as symptoms evolve over time.

Postmortem studies in MS subjects have validated that MS plaques correspond to the hyperintense lesions seen on T2/PD and FLAIR images.[16] They appear higher in signal intensity (or bright) because of longer T2 relaxation times (see Fig. 1A–C). T2 lesions are not specific for plaque age, the degree of myelin and axon loss, or the amount of edema and inflammation.[17] Loss of myelin creates a more hydrophilic environment, and the increased water gives a brighter T2/PD signal and a darker T1W appearance. Infections, ischemia, tumors, and other causes of inflammation also affect lesion water content and can cause similar MR imaging signal changes, limiting the specificity for any individual lesion.

MS lesions vary in size and location and have a periventricular predominance. It would be unusual to have sparing of this region in MS. The lesions typically develop in a perivenular pattern as immune cells migrate across the blood-brain barrier and induce a cascade of inflammation and demyelination. These areas may appear as Dawson fingers or elongated flame-shaped lesions best seen on sagittal FLAIR images oriented along subependymal veins in the corona radiata and centrum semiovale, perpendicular to the walls of the ventricle (Fig. 1D).[18] Lesions can occur in any structure containing myelin, including the cortex. Cortical plaques occur commonly in MS[19] but are difficult to see on MR studies, even with special sequences,[20–23] owing to similarities in signal intensities of MS lesions and grey matter and the partial volume effects of CSF within the adjacent sulci.[24] Lesions are often seen in the temporal lobes, grey-white matter junction (juxtacortical) (Fig. 1G), brainstem, cerebellum (Fig. 1F), optic nerves, and spinal cord. Corpus callosum lesions occur frequently in all stages of MS, ranging from 51% of CIS patients[25] to 93% of MS patients compared to only 2% of patients with white matter disease due to other causes.[26] Some non-MS disorders in which involvement of the corpus callosum has been reported include stroke,[27] cerebral autosomal dominant arteriopathy with subcortical infarctions,[28] lymphoma,[29] Sjogren's disease,[30] and progressive multifocal leukoencephalopathy (Fig. 2).[31]

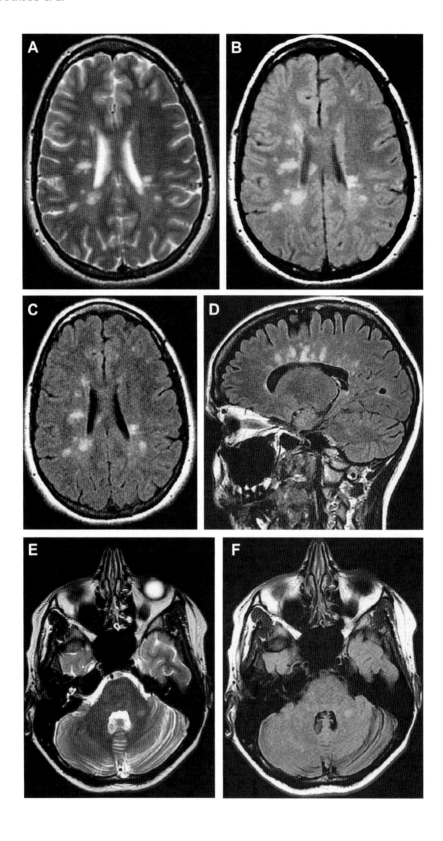

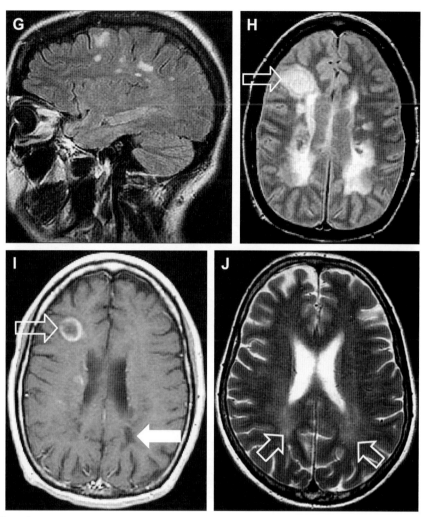

Fig. 1. (*continued*)

Four percent of healthy individuals of all ages can have periventricular changes that cannot be distinguished from MS.[32] With increasing age, nonspecific MR imaging abnormalities (unidentified bright objects [UBOs]) become increasingly common.[33] These objects are more frequent in women, and a few small UBOs are common by the early to mid-forties.[34] UBOs are usually isointense on T1W sequences, whereas approximately 30% of MS lesions appear hypointense (dark or

---

Fig. 1. Typical MS lesions are ovoid and ≥3 mm in diameter and are easily identified on T2W (*A*), proton density weighted (*B*), and FLAIR (*C*) images. They can occur anywhere in the brain, spinal cord, or optic nerves, and a periventricular distribution is common (*A–C*). Lesions in the corpus callosum (*D*) as well as flame-shaped perivenular lesions (*D*) are characteristic of MS. In general, T2/PD sequences are optimal for posterior fossa lesion detection (*E*) when compared with FLAIR (*F*); however, FLAIR is better for periventricular (*C*) and juxtacortical lesions that are in contact with the cortex (*G*). T2/PD and FLAIR will detect the majority of MS plaques but are not specific to lesion age or severity (*H*). The corresponding Gd-enhanced T1 images will detect newly active lesions due to transient breakdown of the blood-brain barrier (*I, open arrow*). T1 hypointense lesions that do not enhance and persist for 6 or more months are permanent or chronic black holes and represent lesions with the greatest tissue damage (*I, closed arrow*). Diffusely abnormal white matter (DAWM) is present in 17% of RRMS patients visible on T2W images as large, diffuse lesions with poorly defined boundaries, usually located around the ventricles (*J, open arrow*). DAWM corresponds with extensive loss of myelin phospholipids and variable degrees of axonal loss. DAWM spares the subcortical U fibers.

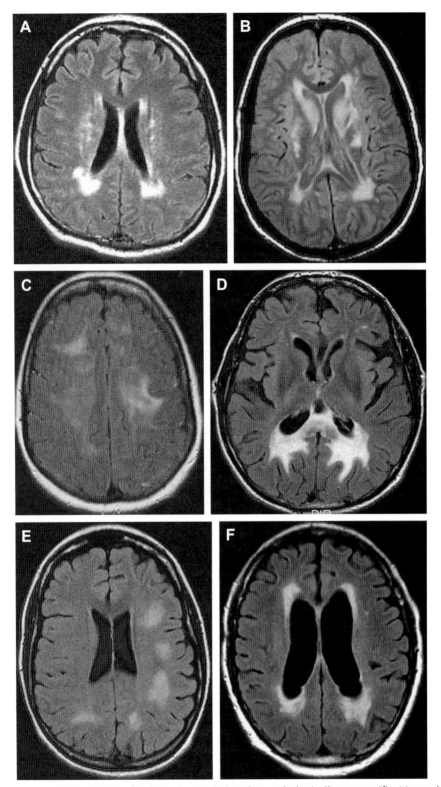

Fig. 2. MR imaging is highly sensitive for detecting MS lesions but pathologically nonspecific. Many white matter diseases can mimic the appearance of MS. Examples included here are primary vasculitis of the central nervous system (*A*), cerebral autosomal dominant angiopathy with subcortical infarcts and leukoencephalopathy (*B*), lymphoma (*C, D*), acute disseminated encephalomyelitis (*E*), chronic hypertension (*F*), nonspecific unidentified bright objects (*G*), and enlarged perivascular spaces (*H*).

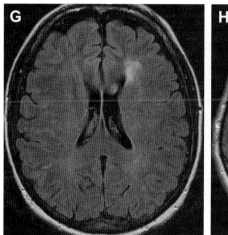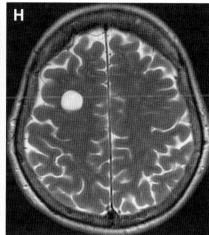

Fig. 2. (*continued*)

so-called "black holes") on T1W sequences. Patients with chronic hypertension can have confluent white matter lesions indistinguishable from those seen in patients with long-standing MS.[35] Normal structures can also be misinterpreted as false-positive lesions, including flow artifacts, volume averaging between slices, and enlarged perivascular Virchow-Robin spaces. Virchow-Robin spaces usually appear as punctate white matter lesions and commonly occur in the lower third of the corpus striatum, the midbrain, and caudal to the lenticular nucleus[36–38] Cases of giant perivascular spaces have also been reported (see **Fig. 2H**).[39,40]

The addition of T2W gradient echo images to detect hemosiderin-related susceptibility changes from occult hemorrhage may be helpful when CNS vasculitis is also under consideration.[41] The diagnosis of primary CNS vasculitis, also known as primary angiitis of the CNS (PACNS), is one of the most challenging problems in clinical neurology. The pathology of PACNS is a segmental necrotizing vasculitis. Leptomeningeal and cortical vessels are predominantly involved, especially small vessels 200 to 500 μm in diameter and precapillary arterioles less than 200 μm in diameter. T2 hyperintense lesions consistent with ischemia or infarction may be seen, particularly involving the subcortical white matter, deep white matter, or deep grey matter in the territory of small- to medium-sized vessels.[42] The cerebral hemispheres are affected more often than the posterior fossa; however, these findings are nonspecific, and the differential diagnosis of multiple T2 hyperintense lesions is a lengthy one. Occult hemorrhage can be seen in approximately 10% of patients with PACNS on T2W gradient echo images. This hemorrhage usually consists of single or multiple punctate areas

of signal void in the subcortical or deep white matter, representing hemosiderin.

An MS relapse refers to an episode of neurologic disturbance of the type seen in MS when clinico-pathologic studies have established that the causative lesions are inflammatory and demyelinating in nature.[12] T2W imaging techniques (ie, T2W, PD, or FLAIR) are the most sensitive conventional technique for detecting MS plaques but do not distinguish between acute and chronic lesions. The MR imaging correlate of new disease activity is the appearance of Gd enhancement on the post-contrast T1W image and new or enlarging T2 lesions (**Fig. 3**). Gd does not normally cross the intact blood-brain barrier. New MS lesions pathologically coincide with disruption of the blood-brain barrier and inflammation and appear on T1W imaging as Gd-enhancing lesions. Weekly MR imaging studies demonstrate that Gd enhancement always occurs before or during the development of all new T2 lesions[43] and represents breakdown of the blood-brain barrier as proinflammatory T cells infiltrate into the brain parenchyma.[44] Nevertheless, the enhancement is transient, with most lesions disappearing within 4 weeks (range, 1 to 16 weeks),[45,46] while a permanent T2 lesion remains as the only evidence of new disease activity relative to the previous MR imaging study. The enhancement pattern can change with evolution and resolution of inflammation from diffuse to nodular and ringlike. The enhancement is more often solid and homogeneous with fresh lesions, particularly when they are small, and may appear as ringlike with lesions that are larger and several weeks old. In rare cases where extremely large MS lesions appear tumefactive, the "open ring" sign favors demyelination over

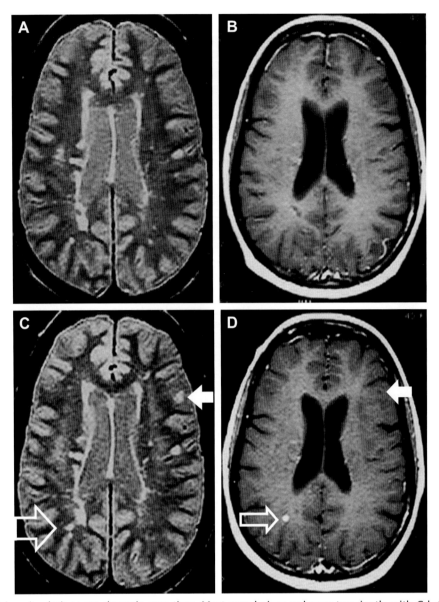

Fig. 3. MR imaging lesions are dynamic over time. Most new lesions enhance transiently with Gd. Often, this enhancement is accompanied by the formation of a new T2 lesion. Although the Gd enhancement will disappear as the inflammation resolves, a new permanent T2 lesion remains. Gd enhancement may also occur in pre-existing T2 lesions and is a sign of reactivation. Persistent Gd enhancement for more than 3 months would be extremely unusual for MS lesions. In many cases, the only evidence of recent disease activity is the detection of a new T2 lesion, especially when MR imaging studies are preformed infrequently. (A) Baseline PD image showing multiple T2 lesions, none of which enhance on the corresponding T1 postcontrast image (B). One month later, a new enhancing lesion is detected (D, open arrow) along with a corresponding new T2 lesion (C, open arrow). There is an additional new T2 lesion (arrow) that did not enhance (closed arrow).

tumor or abscess.[47] Gd enhancement is sensitive to steroids and other anti-inflammatory treatments used in MS. In clinical practice, less than 30% of untreated MS patients have evidence of Gd-enhancing lesions during a routine MR imaging study because of the transient enhancement that is characteristic of active MS lesions and the seemingly random occurrence of new disease activity. The most common evidence of previous MS lesion activity is the accumulation of new T2 and enlarging T2 lesions since the last clinical scan.

The use of Gd can help detect new MS lesion activity or rule out confounding diagnoses that could be missed by PD/T2W imaging alone. Some diagnoses include meningiomas, small neoplasms, vascular malformations, and leptomeningeal disease such as sarcoidosis. Leptomeningeal enhancement is rare in MS.[48] In contrast, enhancement of the optic sheath is common at the time of optic neuritis when specialized MR imaging sequences are used to view the optic nerves.[49] A potential false-positive MR imaging finding is Gd within a vessel situated in a deep sulcus. Verifying the presence of a lesion on the corresponding T2W, PD, or FLAIR image or a follow-up scan can help clarify this finding.

New or enlarging T2 lesions also represent new inflammation and provide complimentary information on disease activity that is given by the detection of contrast-enhancing lesions. On average, MS patients develop four to five new MR imaging lesions per year, with great variability among individuals,[50] with some having no new activity and others having dozens of new lesions. T2 lesions increase in size during the acute phase mostly due to edema associated with inflammatory infiltrates, reaching their maximum size within 4 weeks.[51] The inflammatory process is self-limiting, and the lesions slowly decrease in size over the next 6 to 8 weeks as edema resolves and possibly remyelination occurs. Unlike Gd enhancement, which is transient and disappears, most new lesions leave a residual T2 lesion. Preexisting T2 lesions can reactivate with re-enhancement only, enlarge on T2W images, or both. Eventually, after many reactivations, lesions may fuse with adjacent lesions, and what may have started out as several small lesions may end up forming large confluent lesions.[52] Annually, there is commonly net accumulation of new and enlarging lesions that increases the total T2 volume or burden of disease (T2 BOD) by 5% to 10% per year.[53] The absence of Gd-enhancing lesions or ongoing stability of T2 BOD does not necessarily indicate that the disease is quiescent. Low-grade migration of immune cells across the blood-brain barrier occurs in the absence of a detectable Gd enhancement, and the regions of the grey and white matter that appear normal on conventional MR imaging are often damaged with pathologic evidence of ongoing inflammation, demyelination, and axonal loss.[54,55] Much of current imaging research has been focused on developing advanced techniques to directly or indirectly monitor this subtle or occult disease activity in MS patients.

Three additional MR imaging features that are common in MS include T1W black holes (see Fig. 1I), diffusely abnormal white matter (Fig. 1J), and cerebral atrophy (Fig. 4). T1W black holes are a subset of MS lesions that have a stronger correlation with disability than seen with T2 BOD.[56] On the precontrast T1W images, the majority of MS lesions are isointense to surrounding white matter; approximately 30% are hypointense with a signal intensity less than or equal to grey matter. A small proportion of these lesions may enhance on the postcontrast T1W images, representing new inflammation with edema (acute black holes). Approximately half of acute black holes will resolve within 3 months of their appearance. The remaining black holes that are chronic (persistent for a minimum of 6 months after their first appearance) represent a subset of lesions with greater axonal loss and more extracellular fluid[57] when compared with chronic T2 lesions that are isointense on T1W images. T1W black holes are more prevalent in MS than in vascular disease.[58] Although the presence of black holes has limited diagnostic value, an increase in their number over time may be an indication of clinically significant disease progression and could lead to a change in patient management.[59,60]

Not all lesions are discrete on MR imaging. Large diffuse lesions may be visible on T2W MR imaging with poorly defined boundaries. These areas of diffusely abnormal or "dirty" appearing white matter (DAWM) have similar intensity to gray matter on T2W scans and are most commonly found around the ventricles, adjacent to the trigone and occipital horn, the body of the lateral ventricles, and the centrum semiovale. DAWM can extend over several contiguous slices and were present in 17% of RRMS patients in one study.[61] Pathologic examination of DAWM lesions in several MS patients has demonstrated consistent and extensive loss of myelin phospholipids within all of the lesions with variable degrees of axonal loss.[62] The degree of these changes is intermediate to those found in normal appearing white matter and MS plaques. DAWM spares the subcortical U fibers, a frequent location of MS plaques. The specificity and utility of DAWM in the diagnosis of MS is unknown.

MR imaging studies can readily detect brain atrophy, occurring in 47% to 100% of MS patients,[63,64] and is an important feature that underscores the chronic, irreversible tissue loss that most likely is a major contributing factor to permanent clinical disability.[65] It is more severe and evident in patients with secondary progressive MS than RRMS.[66] With quantitative measures, atrophy can sometimes be detected after a single attack of demyelination (CIS) before the diagnosis of MS is established and in the presence of a small

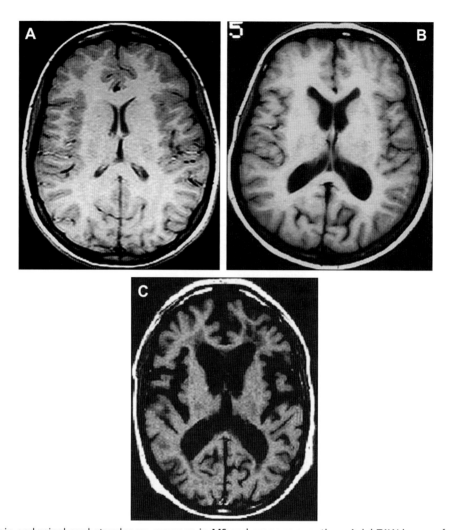

Fig. 4. Brain and spinal cord atrophy are common in MS and progress over time. Axial T1W image of a healthy volunteer (A), RRMS patient with moderate cerebral atrophy (B), and RRMS patient with severe atrophy (C) with enlargement of ventricles and widening of sulci due to loss of brain parenchyma.

T2 BOD.[67] Atrophy is progressive during the course of MS. The video available at http://www.neuroimaging.theclinics.com demonstrates progressive cerebral atrophy in a patient with RRMS imaged over 8 years. Initially, there appears to be a subtle widening of the sulci and some mild ventricular enlargement. The changes are more dramatic after month 48, when there is also an accompanying increase in T2 lesion burden around the ventricles. Annually, MS patients lose 0.6% to 0.8% of brain volume compared with 0.3% for healthy controls.[68–70] There is an associated increase in ventricle size of 1.6 mL/year in MS compared with 0.3 mL/year in healthy age-matched control subjects. In one study, this increase was equivalent to 17 to 24 mL of tissue loss per year.[71] Detecting progressive brain volume loss is of potential clinical importance when assessing treatment response or failure, because increasing evidence suggests that more potent MS therapies can delay this process.[72] The benefit of treatment on preventing brain atrophy can be masked by the effects of "pseudoatrophy" that occurs shortly after starting therapy and is presumed to be due to shifts in brain water and edema.

CONVENTIONAL MR IMAGING OF THE SPINAL CORD: COMMON FINDINGS AND ROLE IN MULTIPLE SCLEROSIS

Spinal cord lesions can be found in 50% to 90% of patients who have clinically definite MS (CDMS).[73] Spinal cord lesions are more commonly visible in the cervical cord than the thoracic cord (Fig. 5).[74]

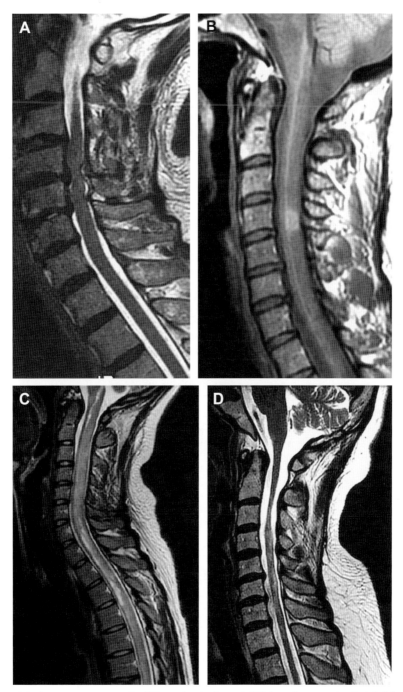

Fig. 5. Spinal cord lesions are common in MS, and spinal cord MR imaging can be helpful in diagnostically challenging cases to rule out alternative diagnoses including cervical spinal canal stenosis (*A*). Unlike in brain MR imaging, age-related lesions do not occur in the spinal cord. MS lesions in the spinal cord tend to be discrete and rarely have any mass effect (*B*). A long extensive spinal cord lesion (LESCL) (*C, D*) spanning at least three vertebral segments coinciding with an acute transverse myelitis would be suspicious for neuromyelitis optica rather than MS. LESCLs often improve; however, severe focal cord atrophy is common (*D* shows an acute LESCL below an area of severe cord atrophy).

These lesions tend to involve the posterior and lateral regions, are asymmetric, and occupy less than half the area of the cord on axial images.[75] The lesions rarely extend beyond two vertebral segments. Early in MS, brain MR imaging is more likely to be positive than spinal MR imaging, even if the initial symptoms involve the cord. In patients presenting with spinal cord symptoms, 55% have lesions that can be detected on MR imaging of the spinal cord, whereas 91% have an abnormal brain on MR imaging.[76]

For patients who have presenting symptoms involving the spinal cord, a brain and spinal cord MR imaging scan are recommended, especially if the symptoms have not resolved, to exclude structural diseases that can mimic MS such as spinal canal stenosis, vascular malformations, and neoplasms. Spinal MR imaging may be useful when brain MR imaging is normal or equivocal and MS is still under consideration.[77] In 115 CIS patients with optic neuritis, 27% had lesions on spinal cord MR imaging compared with 70% who had brain lesions.[78] CIS patients with nine or more T2 lesions on brain MR imaging are more likely to have a spinal cord lesion when compared with CIS patients with normal brain MR imaging (45% versus 12%). Using the revised McDonald diagnostic criteria,[79] spinal cord MR imaging improved the evidence for dissemination in space (DIS) for 3 of 44 patients. When followed prospectively, 11 of 63 CIS patients developed new spinal cord lesions at 1 year. When compared with using brain MR imaging alone, the detection of spinal cord lesions had little impact on the number of patients being diagnosed with CDMS, changing the diagnosis for one additional patient within 1 year and two additional patients within 3 years of follow-up.[78] Nevertheless, the combination of spinal cord lesions with an abnormal brain MR image can improve the diagnostic confidence of MS when other diseases are under consideration, especially in diagnostically uncertain cases. In contrast to brain MR imaging studies, T2W spinal cord lesions do not develop with normal aging or chronic hypertension and diabetes.[80] Spinal cord lesions were found in 6% of patients with other neurologic diseases, including vasculitis and other inflammatory conditions.[74] Spinal cord lesions are often asymptomatic in MS patients, in contrast to those caused by vasculitis or other inflammatory, infectious, and metabolic disorders. A partial list of conditions that sometimes mimic the appearance of a spinal cord presentation of MS clinically and radiologically includes tumors (primary, metastatic, lymphoma), inflammatory disorders (systemic lupus, Sjogren's disease, sarcoidosis),

infection, and nutritional (vitamin B_{12}) deficiencies. Occasionally, a solitary MS lesion in the cord can mimic the appearance of a spinal cord tumor. A brain MR image along with CSF studies can prevent unnecessary surgical removal or biopsy.

UNUSUAL VARIANTS OF MULTIPLE SCLEROSIS

Clinically, MS is heterogeneous, and the findings of MR imaging can be equally variable. Within the broad spectrum of idiopathic or autoimmune demyelinating disorders, several variants may occasionally be seen. A long extensive spinal cord lesion (LESCL) spanning at least three vertebral segments coinciding with an acute transverse myelitis would be extremely rare in MS (see **Fig. 5**), whereas these findings occur frequently in NMO. The acute NMO lesion tends to be central and is often associated with cord swelling. The LESCL is a transient finding, with improvement often leaving a residual T2 lesion or patchy T2 lesions indistinguishable from MS. Depending on the severity of the attack and the degree of recovery, there can be severe spinal cord atrophy. The relative absence of brain lesions helps to distinguish NMO from MS.[81] Other unusual lesion types seen in NMO include tumefactive demyelinating lesions, optic chiasm enhancement,[82] lesions involving the periaquaductal grey matter, and hypothalamic lesions.[83]

Tumefactive demyelinating lesions are an uncommon presentation occurring in both children and adults and can be confused with high-grade tumors, especially if the lesion is solitary, which is common (**Fig. 6**). Patients who present with a tumefactive demyelinating lesion as their first clinical attack may be at a lower risk for developing MS.[84] Mass effect can be minimal or sometimes moderate, and an open ring enhancement pattern is common. Over time, these lesions tend to decrease in size. Large lesions in the centrum semiovale and disseminated lesions throughout the brainstem can be seen with the Marburg variant of MS.[85] Balo's concentric sclerosis is another rare, acute, and sometimes fatal variant of MS that is also associated with large lesions. The lesions have concentric layers of normal or remyelinated white matter alternating with regions of acute demyelination. These types of lesions are increasingly seen in other MS patients, suggesting that this radiologic finding is not necessarily a hallmark of a malignant disease course.[86] Over time, the lesions can become diffusely homogenous.

ROLE OF CONVENTIONAL MR IMAGING IN CLINICALLY ISOLATED SYNDROME AND IN ESTABLISHING THE DIAGNOSIS OF MULTIPLE SCLEROSIS

MR imaging aids in the clinical assessment of patients with possible MS by providing further evidence for a CNS disease with lesion DIS and in time. Patients with MS often present in one of five ways:

1. A single attack typical of demyelination (CIS)
2. Multiple attacks of demyelination
3. Progressive neurologic syndrome suspicious for PPMS
4. Symptoms suspicious for demyelination but unclear
5. Incidental finding on an MR image performed for non-MS symptoms

The interpretation of the findings on MR imaging and the criteria that can be applied depend in part on which of these groups is being considered. MR imaging is not required for the diagnosis of MS when patients present with clinical evidence of lesion DIS and in time. Nonetheless, it enables one to establish an early diagnosis after a single clinical attack (CIS) and aids in ruling out alternative disorders.

CIS refers to a classic syndrome of demyelination typically seen in MS populations. The syndrome includes optic neuritis, transverse myelitis, or a brainstem syndrome. Symptoms need to last for at least 24 hours, and neurologic abnormalities must be documented by an experienced clinician. Occasionally, CIS is preceded by a flulike syndrome, but, more commonly, it is unprovoked, occurring spontaneously. Approximately half of CIS patients sustain another event within the next 5 years and therefore have CDMS. Abnormal brain MR imaging (two or more lesions >3 mm in diameter and typical of MS) is seen in 50% to 65% of CIS patients and is the best single predictor of future MS.[87,88] Approximately 80% of CIS patients with abnormal MR imaging compared with 20% of those with a normal initial brain MR image will subsequently develop CDMS. In many countries, CIS individuals with abnormal brain MR imaging (at high risk of CIS conversion to definite MS) qualify for treatment with MS therapies even before their final diagnosis is established.

The main principle of diagnosis in MS is to demonstrate evidence of multiple lesions in the CNS consistent with inflammation affecting different locations (DIS) and the development of new lesions over months or years (dissemination in time [DIT]). In 2001, the Poser diagnostic criteria[89] were replaced by the International Panel or McDonald criteria.[12] An important achievement of the McDonald criteria was to formally incorporate MR imaging findings typical of MS into the diagnostic scheme. This inclusion allows for an earlier diagnosis when clinical evidence is lacking for DIS or DIT. By demonstrating additional lesions as well as new clinically silent disease activity (new T2 lesions or new Gd-enhancing lesions) on a follow-up brain (or spinal) MR image, CIS patients can proceed from a possible diagnosis of MS to definite MS. In one recent study of high-risk CIS patients enrolled in a treatment trial of interferon beta-1b, all patients had abnormal brain MR imaging (at least two lesions) required for enrollment. Forty percent of CIS patients had a Gd-enhancing lesion, 72% had nine or more T2 lesions, and 12% had a low number of T2 lesions (between two and four).[90] Within 3 months, 10% of the 176 patients on placebo had a second clinical attack compared with 40% who met McDonald criteria (either had a clinical or MR imaging relapse). At 2 years, the numbers increased to 44% having had a second clinical attack and 85% having either a clinical or MR imaging relapse (McDonald definite MS).[91] Patients with multiple abnormalities on the initial brain MR imaging (Gd enhancement, >9 T2 lesions, or meeting DIS criteria) were at the greatest risk for converting to definite MS over the 2-year period.[92]

In 2005, two important revisions were added to the diagnostic criteria.[79] The first revision allows the presence of a spinal cord lesion to have a similar significance as a brainstem (infratentorial) lesion. The second revision allows the identification of new T2 lesions as evidence for DIT, having a greater sensitivity than using new Gd lesions only.[93]

The McDonald criteria incorporated a modification of the Barkhof criteria of MR imaging abnormalities for evidence of DIS (**Table 2**). Several studies have demonstrated that these criteria have greater specificity (73%–78%) for diagnosing MS after a single attack while maintaining good sensitivity (73%–82%) when compared with the earlier Paty[94] and Fazekas[95] criteria (sensitivity of 88%, specificity of 54%).[25] In addition to the number of lesions seen, it is important to recognize that the type and strategic location of the lesions are also critical. In patients with an appropriate clinical syndrome (ie, consistent with demyelination), the MR imaging criteria that provide evidence for DIS (modified Barkhof criteria) must include three of the four MR imaging features as follows:

1. One or more enhancing lesions (brain or spinal cord) or nine or more T2 lesions (brain or spinal cord)

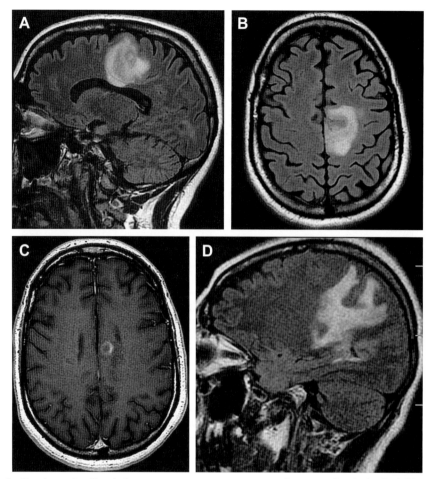

Fig. 6. Tumefactive demyelinating lesions are an uncommon presentation occurring in both children and adults and can be confused with high-grade tumors or abscess, especially if the lesion is solitary. Mass effect can be minimal or sometimes moderate (*A*, sagittal FLAIR), and an open ring enhancement pattern is common and favors demyelination (*B*, axial FLAIR; *C*, axial postcontrast T1). These unusual lesion types can also be seen in neuromyelitis optica (*D–G*). Over time, the lesions tend to decrease in size consistent with demyelination (*E*, baseline FLAIR; *F*, 1 month; and *G*, 6 month follow-up MR image).

2. Three or more periventricular lesions
3. One or more juxtacortical lesions
4. One or more infratentorial lesions or spinal cord lesions

In general, T2 lesions should be 3 mm or more in diameter. FLAIR sequences, especially in the sagittal plane, are optimal for detecting juxtacortical lesions, whereas T2W sequences are generally superior for infratentorial lesion detection. Juxtacortical lesions must be in contact with the cortex to be distinguished from subcortical lesions. For centers that routinely use Gd for diagnostic MR imaging, the minimum number of lesions necessary to fulfill the criteria for DIS is two (eg, one juxtacortical lesion and one infratentorial lesion) as long as one of the two lesions enhances with Gd.

For centers that do not use Gd, or if no Gd lesions are present, the minimum number of lesions required is five (depending on lesion location). There are two situations in which meeting the MR imaging criteria is optional: (1) in patients with evidence of two clinical or other paraclinical (visual evoked potential) signs, or (2) when CSF analysis demonstrates the presence of oligoclonal banding or an elevated IgG index. In the latter situation, only two brain lesions are required for DIS. In one study, approximately 20% of CIS patients with normal brain MR imaging at the time of their first symptoms subsequently developed CDMS within the 20 years of follow-up;[87] however, it would be unusual in chronic MS for brain MR imaging to remain normal (notable exceptions include many cases of Asian OSMS and NMO).

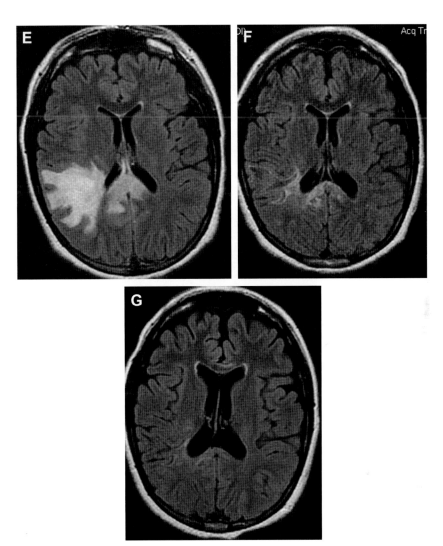

Fig. 6. *(continued)*

Table 2
Prevalence of common MR imaging abnormalities in clinically isolated syndromes (CIS) consistent
with demyelination and early relapsing-remitting MS (RRMS) patients

MR Imaging Feature	Prevalence in CIS (%)	Prevalence in Early RRMS (%)
Normal cranial MR imaging	18	3
Periventricular lesions (three or more)	47	73
Juxtacortical lesions	51	73
Gd-enhancing lesions	38	61
Infratentorial lesions	38	58
Nine or more cranial lesions	41	73
Corpus callosum lesions	51	79
Oval lesions	53	76

Data from Barkhof F, Filippi M, Miller DH, et al. Comparison of MRI criteria at first presentation to predict conversion to clinically definite multiple sclerosis. Brain 1997;120:2059.

Although other lesions types and locations are commonly seen in MS (eg, corpus callosum lesions and flame-shaped Dawson fingers), these do not improve the predictive value of the original Barkhof criteria for determining which CIS patients will develop CDMS; therefore, they are not included in the current criteria. These features, when present, provide additional confidence to the diagnosis.

For the diagnosis of MS, all patients require clinical or subclinical (ie, MR imaging) evidence of new disease activity (DIT) occurring no earlier than 1 month after the onset of the first clinical episode. This cut-off was chosen to avoid including subjects with evolving demyelinating syndromes, such as acute disseminated encephalomyelitis (ADEM), who generally are at a low risk for subsequently developing MS. The original MR imaging criterion for DIT is the presence of new Gd-enhancing lesions at least 3 months after the first MR imaging in an anatomic location separate from the original clinical syndrome.[12] This cut-off is based on natural history studies in which MS lesions rarely continue to enhance 3 months after their initial appearance. The 2005 revision allows for the development of new T2 lesions 1 month or more after the last MR image to also satisfy DIT criteria (**Box 1**). The yield of detecting new lesions increases with time; however, this relies on using standardized MR imaging protocols with similar coverage, slice orientation, slice thickness, and, ideally, no interslice gap to reliably distinguish new lesions from lesions that were previously missed due to incomplete coverage. These criteria have been validated when applied to patients with a documented clinically isolated episode of demyelination of the CNS and allow for an earlier diagnosis of MS before the second clinical attack occurs.

The role of MR imaging in detecting new clinically silent disease activity as evidence supporting the diagnosis of MS was also recommended by the Therapeutics and Technology Assessment Subcommittee of the American Academy of Neurology after an extensive review of the relevant literature concerning the utility of MR imaging in suspected MS, including studies published that had validated the earlier McDonald diagnostic criteria.[96] The committee recommended less stringent MR imaging criteria for DIS of three or more white matter lesions larger than 3 mm, or two Gd-enhancing lesions that would be highly predictive of MS. This recommendation reflects current clinical practice, particularly in North America, because patients with a well-documented CIS who also have two characteristic T2 lesions 3 mm or more in diameter, one of which is ovoid

---

Box 1
MR imaging criteria for evidence of disease disseminated in space and in time

For dissemination of lesions in space (DIS) in relapse onset MS, three of four of the following (modified Barkhof criteria):

1. One Gd-enhancing brain or spinal cord lesion OR nine or more brain and/or spinal cord T2 lesions
2. One or more infratentorial OR spinal cord lesions
3. One or more juxtacortical lesions (must be in contact with cortex)
4. Three or more periventricular lesions

For dissemination of lesions in space (DIS) in PPMS, two of three of the following:

1. Nine or more brain T2 lesions OR four or more brain T2 lesions in addition to abnormal visual evoked potentials
2. Two or more spinal cord lesions
3. Positive CSF for oligoclonal banding

For dissemination of lesions in time (DIT) using a standardized MR imaging protocol, one of two of the following:

1. Gd-enhancing lesion 3 months or more after the first MR imaging or onset of symptoms
2. New T2 lesion 1 month or more after the initial MR imaging

---

or periventricular, are started on disease-modifying therapy. The CHAMPS pivotal CIS clinical trial with interferon beta-1a given intramuscularly once weekly was the first study that showed a clear benefit in delaying the onset of MS when compared with patients treated with placebo only.[97]

Other studies have shown that, even in the presence of a few T2 lesions, as many as 42% of patients who have optic neuritis still do not develop CDMS within 10 years of follow-up.[98] An important ongoing follow-up study of CIS patients demonstrated that 18% of those with abnormal brain MR imaging initially (ie, high risk) did not develop further clinical attacks over the 20 years of prospective observation.[87] Some early MR imaging features that are predictive of an earlier conversion to definite MS include the number of DIS criteria that are met.[99] The McDonald diagnostic criteria were based on natural history studies using older MR imaging technology with field strengths ranging from 0.5 to 1.5 T, slice thicknesses of 5 to 10 mm, and variable interslice gaps. Current MR imaging protocols with 3-mm contiguous slices and high field strengths of

3.0 T or greater can increase the number of asymptomatic lesions that are detected, increasing the number of patients who meet MR imaging criteria for both DIS and DIT;[7,8] therefore, some clinicians may wait until evidence of new disease activity is present on MR imaging or clinically before initiating chronic immune-modulating therapy.

The high sensitivity and specificity of the revised McDonald criteria apply to carefully selected patients with classic symptoms of MS. Ten patients with symptoms similar to demyelination but who were eventually proven to have another disease such as vasculitis were excluded from the studies used to develop the diagnostic MR imaging criteria.[100] Because the sensitivity and specificity of these criteria do not necessarily apply to patients who have unusual or unclear presentations, and because the necessary clinical information may not be available at the time of the request for the MR imaging, there is a potential for overdiagnosis when the diagnosis is based on imaging findings alone. A 1993 study of 99 suspected MS patients found that 3% of patients had a false-positive diagnosis of MS when only MR imaging criteria were used without any clinical information.[101] Since then, both the availability and sensitivity of MR imaging for detecting lesions have improved. In a more recent study, 103 patients were referred to an MS center for possible MS because of one or more T2 lesions found on brain MR imaging. Only 11% of these patients were determined to have clinically definite or possible MS.[102] In another small retrospective study of 28 patients initially suspected of having MS but proven to have another disorder, 11% met McDonald MR imaging criteria for DIS compared with 71% who met the criteria of the Therapeutics and Technology Assessment Subcommittee of the American Academy of Neurology.[103] MR imaging lesions lack pathologic specificity, and when only MR imaging criteria are used, there is an increased risk of a false-positive diagnosis. More research is needed to improve the specificity of MR imaging criteria when the clinical syndrome is less clear. The report that accompanies a diagnostic MR imaging study should comment on whether the lesions are typical of demyelination in addition to whether there are sufficient lesions to meet DIS or DIT criteria. MS should never be diagnosed on the basis of MR imaging findings alone in the absence of appropriate clinical history.

ROLE OF MR IMAGING IN THE DIAGNOSIS OF PRIMARY PROGRESSIVE MULTIPLE SCLEROSIS

A minority of MS patients (10% to 15%) have a progressive neurologic syndrome of an evolving myelopathy or ataxia and never have clinical relapses. Although PPMS patients may have features on MR imaging that are classic for MS, this form of MS tends to be less inflammatory. In one large study of 943 patients who had PPMS, only 14% had Gd-enhancing lesions at the beginning of the 2-year treatment trial with glatiramer acetate (PROMISE trial).[104] Furthermore, new T2 lesion development is also much less frequent, with only 48% of PPMS patients showing a new lesion within 2 years of follow-up. A retrospective study of 261 PPMS patients (clinically defined with at least 1 year of progression) found that, although 64% had nine or more T2 lesions on brain MR imaging and 61% had one or more spinal cord lesions, 20% of patients had less than four T2 lesions;[105] therefore, the MR imaging requirements for PPMS are less stringent than for relapsing-onset MS (see **Box 1**). In addition to evidence of disease progression for at least 1 year, the revised McDonald diagnostic criteria for DIS in PPMS require two of the three following criteria: (1) nine or more brain lesions OR four or more brain lesions and abnormal visual evoked potential; (2) more than two spinal cord lesions; or (3) positive CSF for oligoclonal banding or an elevated IgG index.

Approximately 80% of PPMS patients have positive CSF, and the DIS criteria can be met by brain or spinal cord MR imaging alone. In most cases, both studies should be performed. It would be unusual not to have some brain abnormalities on MR imaging in established PPMS. Even in the presence of an abnormal brain on MR imaging, spinal cord MR imaging is helpful to rule out comorbidity with cervical spinal canal stenosis in patients with a progressive spinal cord syndrome or an alternative diagnosis including low-grade tumors (eg, ependymoma).

SPECIAL POPULATIONS: PEDIATRIC AND OPTICOSPINAL MULTIPLE SCLEROSIS

Four percent of all MS patients present before the age of 16 years.[106] Ninety-eight percent of pediatric MS patients will present with a relapsing-remitting course.[107] MR imaging features are similar to that in adults; however, pediatric CIS patients have more infratentorial lesions than adult RRMS patients.[108] Less than one quarter of patients had Gd-enhancing lesions at the time of their first presentation in a large French study of 116 subjects (KIDMUS);[109] however, another study showed that 9 of 20 RRMS pediatric patients (44%) had enhancing lesions.[110] Both of these studies showed a similar proportion (approximately 50%) of pediatric CIS and early MS patients meeting McDonald MR imaging criteria for DIS. These findings are not that different from recent validation studies of the McDonald criteria reported in adult CIS.[99]

Younger patients (less than 10 years old) may differ more evidently from adults, presenting with diffuse, bilateral white matter changes with ill-defined borders that subsequently improve; however, the similarity of imaging features in ADEM may make it difficult to distinguish early cases of ADEM from those of MS. The literature on ADEM lacks consistency in the diagnostic criteria used, and the imaging features of ADEM may overlap with those of CIS and MS.[111] The imaging features of ADEM are variable. Characteristic lesions include large, bilateral, multifocal, subcortical white matter lesions.[112] Involvement of the corpus callosum and the presence of Dawson's fingers favor MS. Grey matter structures can be affected in MS; however, in ADEM, bilateral thalamic or basal ganglia lesions can be prominent. ADEM lesions tend to be stable or improve within 6 months, and the development of new lesions over time or of clinical attacks will often favor a diagnosis of MS. The prognostic role of the first MR imaging study at the time of pediatric CIS is under study. It is expected that an abnormal MR imaging study in pediatric patients will have similar importance for representing a high risk for the development of MS as it does in adults. Tumefactive lesions can also occur in pediatric CIS and MS and may be misdiagnosed as tumor or abscess.[113]

Much of our knowledge about the natural history of MS comes from studies conducted in North America and Europe; however, MS is a global disease. Although the differential diagnosis may vary among regions (eg, human T-cell lymphotrophic virus, tuberculosis, sarcoidosis, Behçet's and Lyme disease), the clinical and MR imaging features are usually indistinguishable from those of "Western" MS.[114] In South-East Asia (including Japan, Korea, China, Taiwan, Singapore, Malaysia, Philippines, Thailand, and Vietnam), most patients will have classic or Western MS with the typical MR imaging features described earlier. One third of patients will have OSMS that is clinically restricted to the optic nerves and spinal cord with relatively sparing of disease on brain MR imaging.[14] Many patients with OSMS will have attacks with LESCL and a high positive rate of anti–aquaporin-4 antibodies.[115]

MR IMAGING FOR FOLLOW-UP

The first clear role for follow-up MR imaging using a standardized protocol is to monitor high-risk CIS patients to establish an early diagnosis by demonstrating new disease activity. It is certainly worthwhile to use this approach if there is any ambiguity concerning the diagnosis, especially when spinal cord MR imaging, CSF, and evoked potentials are all normal.

Once patients have an established diagnosis of MS, the required frequency of routine imaging is less clear. There is often a desire to monitor treatment response by the presence or absence of new lesion development over time, especially in patients early in the disease course or in those having frequent or disabling clinical relapses. Some evidence suggests that the number of lesions early in the disease course and some of the early changes are predictive of future disability 20 years later.[87] The main criticisms of performing routine imaging to monitor individual patients are as follows: (1) lesions only correlate partially with current disability (the clinical-radiologic paradox);[116] (2) new lesions do not necessarily predict future relapses[117] or disability; and (3) diffuse evolving damage cannot be easily monitored by conventional MR imaging[118] and contributes independently to disability.[119] A "stable" MR image may give a false sense of global disease stability.

Several clinical guidelines have been published based on expert opinion on how to incorporate MR imaging changes into individualized patient management.[59,120] New lesion development and progressive atrophy occur at all stages of MS, including the earliest stages (CIS and RRMS) and progressive forms (secondary and primary). MR imaging changes may influence clinical practice in RRMS patients for whom a variety of disease-modifying therapies exists. Once patients are in the slow progressive phase, routine MR imaging is less likely to impact on clinical decisions until effective therapies are established. Nevertheless, utilization of a standardized MR imaging protocol and reporting are essential if accurate and quantitative assessment of new or worsening disease status over time is required. The evolving MR imaging features that are considered worrisome include new Gd-enhancing lesions, new T2 lesions, an increased T2 BOD, an increased number and volume of chronic black holes, and progressive cerebral atrophy. Rapid and easy to use segmentation tools for quantitatively reporting these latter outcomes are not readily available.

The third important role of conventional MR imaging is in the assessment of patients who have unexpected symptoms or sudden deterioration. Whenever a secondary diagnosis is suspected or the original diagnosis is under review, in addition to CSF studies, visual evoked potentials, or other neurophysiologic testing, additional brain and spinal cord MR imaging can provide valuable diagnostic information. The three main areas of concern include (1) unexpected deterioration due to a new independent condition (tumor, abscess, stroke, spinal canal stenosis); (2) complication of disease-modifying therapy (eg, progressive multifocal leukoencephalopathy); and (3) reassessing the original diagnosis. The aging MS population is at risk for ischemic stroke as a secondary diagnosis. It would be particularly challenging to assess MR imaging for lacunar strokes within a field of chronic MS lesions. Diffusion-weighted MR imaging may help in assessing acute from chronic lesions.

MS lesions that present as a tumor-like mass may resemble a glioblastoma multiforme, abscess, or lymphoma. The open ring sign of Gd enhancement is more common in large tumor-like MS lesions, and demyelinating lesions tend to have less mass effect and surrounding edema when compared with similar sized tumors and should decrease in size over time. Unexpected complications that have developed include progressive multifocal leukoencephalopathy, which does not normally occur in MS patients. With the introduction of more potent immunomodulatory therapies for MS, a few cases have developed in patients treated with a combination of natalizumab and interferon beta-1a intramuscularly once weekly.[121] Clinical and MR imaging guidelines have been proposed for monitoring patients on this therapy;[122] however, early progressive multifocal leukoencephalopathy can have a similar appearance on MR imaging as MS lesions, making it challenging to sort out clinically as well as radiologically.

Misdiagnosis at the time of clinical presentation is less likely with the routine use of brain and spinal cord MR imaging to exclude common structural diseases that can clinically mimic MS such as spinal canal stenosis (see **Fig. 5**), vascular malformations, and most neoplasia. Patients diagnosed with MS based on nonspecific symptoms and minimal abnormalities on initial MR imaging of the brain warrant reinvestigation and careful follow-up. Diagnosing other inflammatory diseases such as Sjogren's syndrome, systemic lupus erythematosus, and sarcoidosis can be more challenging due to the nonspecific nature of their lesions on MR imaging. It is not uncommon to come across case series, such as those with CNS involvement with Sjogren's syndrome, in which the MR imaging appearance and the clinical evolution resemble MS.[30] Cervical spondylitic myelopathy can coexist with or mimic the symptoms of progressive MS. This situation is less likely to occur with the routine use of spinal cord MR imaging in the initial diagnostic work-up of patients.

SUMMARY

Conventional MR imaging techniques that are readily available on all clinical scanners include T1W (pre- and postcontrast enhancement) and T2W (or variations) sequences. MR imaging is exquisitely sensitive for detecting clinically asymptomatic lesions; however, these lesions are pathologically nonspecific. A variety of features favor MS, including ovoid lesions, corpus callosum involvement, a lack of mass effect, Dawson's fingers, a transient Gd enhancement pattern, and spinal cord lesions. The spectrum of MR imaging abnormalities among individuals with MS is variable, with extremes ranging from relatively bland, minimally abnormal MR imaging to large tumor-like lesions. The first important step in assessing MR imaging in the diagnostic work-up is to determine whether the abnormalities are usual for MS or atypical. The second step is to determine whether the pattern of lesions provides additional evidence for DIS and DIT, giving additional support to the clinical suspicion in patients who have had a single neurologic episode consistent with demyelination. To monitor changes over time, to establish the diagnosis, or to determine the treatment response, a standardized MR imaging protocol should be used. This practice will allow reliable and confident determination of changes between studies performed at the same or different MR imaging unit.

REFERENCES

1. Simon JH, Li D, Traboulsee A, et al. Standardized MRI protocol for multiple sclerosis: Consortium of MS Centers (CMSC) consensus guidelines. AJNR Am J Neuroradiol 2006;27:455–61.
2. Filippi M, Marciano N, Capra R, et al. The effect of imprecise repositioning on lesion volume measurements in patients with multiple sclerosis. Neurology 1997;49:274–6.
3. Rovaris M, Rocca MA, Capra R, et al. A comparison between the sensitivities of 3-mm and 5-mm thick serial brain MRI for detecting lesion volume changes in patients with multiple sclerosis. J Neuroimaging 1998;8:144–7.
4. Rydberg JN, Riederer SJ, Rydberg CH, et al. Contrast optimization of fluid-attenuated inversion recovery (FLAIR) imaging. Magn Reson Med 1995;34:868–77.
5. Filippi M, Yousry T, Campi A, et al. Comparison of triple dose versus standard dose gadolinium-DTPA for detection of MRI enhancing lesions in patients with MS. Neurology 1996;46:379–84.
6. Silver NC, Good CD, Barker GJ, et al. Sensitivity of contrast enhanced MRI in multiple sclerosis: effects of gadolinium dose, magnetization transfer contrast

and delayed imaging. Brain 1997;120(Pt 7): 1149–61.

7. Keiper MD, Grossman RI, Hirsch JA, et al. MR identification of white matter abnormalities in multiple sclerosis: a comparison between 1.5 T and 4 T. AJNR Am J Neuroradiol 1998;19:1489–93.

8. Wattjes MP, Harzheim M, Kuhl CK, et al. Does high-field MR imaging have an influence on the classification of patients with clinically isolated syndromes according to current diagnostic MR imaging criteria for multiple sclerosis? AJNR Am J Neuroradiol 2006;27:1794–8.

9. Lee DH, Vellet AD, Eliasziw M, et al. MR imaging field strength: prospective evaluation of the diagnostic accuracy of MR for diagnosis of multiple sclerosis at 0.5 and 1.5 T. Radiology 1995;194:257–62.

10. Young IR, Hall AS, Pallis CA, et al. Nuclear magnetic resonance imaging of the brain in multiple sclerosis. Lancet 1981;2:1063–6.

11. Robertson WD, Li DK, Mayo JR, et al. Assessment of multiple sclerosis lesions by magnetic resonance imaging. Can Assoc Radiol J 1987;38:177–82.

12. McDonald WI, Compston A, Edan G, et al. Recommended diagnostic criteria for multiple sclerosis: guidelines from the International Panel on the diagnosis of multiple sclerosis. Ann Neurol 2001;50: 121–7.

13. Brex PA, Ciccarelli O, O'Riordan JI, et al. A longitudinal study of abnormalities on MRI and disability from multiple sclerosis. N Engl J Med 2002;346:158–64.

14. Kira J. Multiple sclerosis in the Japanese population. Lancet Neurol 2003;2:117–27.

15. Wingerchuk DM, Weinshenker BG. Neuromyelitis optica. Curr Treat Options Neurol 2005;7:173–82.

16. Stewart WA, Hall LD, Berry K, et al. Magnetic resonance imaging (MRI) in multiple sclerosis (MS): pathological correlation studies in eight cases. Neurology 1986;36:320.

17. Barnes D, Munro PM, Youl BD, et al. The longstanding MS lesion: a quantitative MRI and electron microscopic study. Brain 1991;114:1271–80.

18. Horowitz AL, Kaplan RD, Grewe G, et al. The ovoid lesion: a new MR observation in patients with multiple sclerosis. AJNR Am J Neuroradiol 1989;10:303–5.

19. Pirko I, Lucchinetti CF, Sriram S, et al. Gray matter involvement in multiple sclerosis. Neurology 2007; 68:634–42.

20. Geurts JJ, Pouwels PJ, Uitdehaag BM, et al. Intracortical lesions in multiple sclerosis: improved detection with 3D double inversion-recovery MR imaging. Radiology 2005;236(1):254–60.

21. Wattjes MP, Lutterbey GG, Gieseke J, et al. Double inversion recovery brain imaging at 3 T: diagnostic value in the detection of multiple sclerosis lesions. AJNR Am J Neuroradiol 2007;28:54–9.

22. Nelson F, Poonawalla AH, Hou P, et al. Improved identification of intracortical lesions in multiple sclerosis with phase-sensitive inversion recovery in combination with fast double inversion recovery MR imaging. AJNR Am J Neuroradiol 2007;28: 1645–9.

23. Geurts JJ, Bo L, Pouwels PJ, et al. Cortical lesions in multiple sclerosis: combined postmortem MR imaging and histopathology. AJNR Am J Neuroradiol 2005;26:572–7.

24. Kidd D, Barkhof F, McConnell R, et al. Cortical lesions in multiple sclerosis. Brain 1999;122:17–26.

25. Barkhof F, Filippi M, Miller DH, et al. Comparison of MRI criteria at first presentation to predict conversion to clinically definite multiple sclerosis. Brain 1997;120:2059–69.

26. Gean-Marton AD, Vezina LG, Marton KI, et al. Abnormal corpus callosum: a sensitive and specific indicator of multiple sclerosis. Radiology 1991;180: 215–21.

27. Giroud M, Dumas R. Clinical and topographical range of callosal infarction: a clinical and radiological correlation study. J Neurol Neurosurg Psychiatry 1995;59:238–42.

28. Abe K, Murakami T, Matsubara E, et al. Clinical features of CADASIL. Ann N Y Acad Sci 2002; 977:266–72.

29. Buhring U, Herrlinger U, Krings T, et al. MRI features of primary central nervous system lymphomas at presentation. Neurology 2001;57:393–6.

30. Morgen K, McFarland HF, Pillemer SR. Central nervous system disease in primary Sjogren's syndrome: the role of magnetic resonance imaging. Semin Arthritis Rheum 2004;34:623–30.

31. Whiteman ML, Post MJ, Berger JR, et al. Progressive multifocal leukoencephalopathy in 47 HIV-seropositive patients: neuroimaging with clinical and pathologic correlation. Radiology 1993;187:233–40.

32. Yetkin FZ, Haughton VM, Papke RA, et al. Multiple sclerosis: specificity of MR for diagnosis. Radiology 1991;178:447–51.

33. Hunt AL, Orrison WW, Yeo RA, et al. Clinical significance of MRI white matter lesions in the elderly. Neurology 1989;39:1470–4.

34. de Leeuw FE, de Groot JC, Achten E, et al. Prevalence of cerebral white matter lesions in elderly people: a population based magnetic resonance imaging study. The Rotterdam Scan Study. J Neurol Neurosurg Psychiatry 2001;70:9–14.

35. van Swieten JC, Geyskes GG, Derix MM, et al. Hypertension in the elderly is associated with white matter lesions and cognitive decline. Ann Neurol 1991;30:825–30.

36. Takao M, Koto A, Tanahashi N, et al. Pathologic findings of silent hyperintense white matter lesions on MRI. J Neurol Sci 1999;167:127–31.

37. Jungreis CA, Kanal E, Hirsch WL, et al. Normal perivascular spaces mimicking lacunar infarction: MR imaging. Radiology 1988;169:101–4.

38. Williams DW III, Elster AD, Kramer SI. Neurosarcoidosis: gadolinium-enhanced MR imaging. J Comput Assist Tomogr 1990;14:704–7.

39. Salzman KL, Osborn AG, House P, et al. Giant tumefactive perivascular spaces. AJNR Am J Neuroradiol 2005;26:298–305.

40. Fanous R, Midia M. Perivascular spaces: normal and giant. Can J Neurol Sci 2007;34:5–10.

41. Pomper MG, Miller TJ, Stone JH, et al. CNS vasculitis in autoimmune disease: MR imaging findings and correlation with angiography. AJNR Am J Neuroradiol 1999;20:75–85.

42. Harris KG, Yuh WT. Intracranial vasculitis. Neuroimaging Clin N Am 1994;4:773–97.

43. Lai M, Hodgson T, Gawne-Cain M, et al. A preliminary study into the sensitivity of disease activity detection by serial weekly magnetic resonance imaging in multiple sclerosis. J Neurol Neurosurg Psychiatry 1996;60:339–41.

44. Nesbit GM, Forbes GS, Scheithauer BW, et al. Multiple sclerosis: histopathologic and MR and/or CT correlation in 37 cases at biopsy and three cases at autopsy. Radiology 1991;180:467–74.

45. Kermode AG, Tofts PS, Thompson AJ, et al. Heterogeneity of blood-brain barrier changes in multiple sclerosis: an MRI study with gadolinium-DTPA enhancement. Neurology 1990;40:229–35.

46. Cotton F, Weiner HL, Jolesz FA, et al. MRI contrast uptake in new lesions in relapsing-remitting MS followed at weekly intervals. Neurology 2003;60:640–6.

47. Masdeu JC, Drayer BP, Anderson RE, et al. Multiple sclerosis–when and how to image. American College of Radiology (ACR) Appropriateness Criteria. Radiology 2000;215(Suppl):547–62.

48. Barkhof F, Valk J, Hommes OR, et al. Meningeal Gd-DTPA enhancement in multiple sclerosis. AJNR Am J Neuroradiol 1992;13:397–400.

49. Demaerel P, Robberecht W, Casteels I, et al. Focal leptomeningeal MR enhancement along the chiasm as a presenting sign of multiple sclerosis. J Comput Assist Tomogr 1995;19:297–8.

50. Paty DW. Magnetic resonance imaging in the assessment of disease activity in multiple sclerosis. Can J Neurol Sci 1988;15:266–72.

51. Willoughby EW, Grochowski E, Li DKB, et al. Serial magnetic resonance scanning in multiple sclerosis: a second prospective study in relapsing patients. Ann Neurol 1989;25:43–9.

52. Koopmans RA, Li DK, Grochowski E, et al. Benign versus chronic progressive multiple sclerosis: magnetic resonance imaging features. Ann Neurol 1989;25:74–81.

53. Paty DW, Li DK, Oger JJ, et al. Magnetic resonance imaging in the evaluation of clinical trials in multiple sclerosis. Ann Neurol 1994;36(Suppl):S95–6.

54. Trapp BD, Peterson J, Ransohoff RM, et al. Axonal transection in the lesions of multiple sclerosis. N Engl J Med 1998;338:278–85.

55. Kutzelnigg A, Lucchinetti CF, Stadelmann C, et al. Cortical demyelination and diffuse white matter injury in multiple sclerosis. Brain 2005;128(Pt 11):2705–12.

56. Truyen L, van Waesberghe JH, van Waldorvoon MA, et al. Accumulation of hypointense lesions ("black holes") on T1 spin-echo MRI correlates with disease progression in multiple sclerosis. Neurology 1996;47(6):1469–76.

57. van Walderveen MA, Barkhof F, Pouwels PJ, et al. Neuronal damage in T1-hypointense multiple sclerosis lesions demonstrated in vivo using proton magnetic resonance spectroscopy. Ann Neurol 1999;46:79–87.

58. Uhlenbrock D, Sehlen S. The value of T1-weighted images in the differentiation between MS, white matter lesions, and subcortical arteriosclerotic encephalopathy (SAE). Neuroradiology 1989;31:203–12.

59. Freedman MS, Patry DG, Grand'Maison F, et al. Treatment optimization in multiple sclerosis. Can J Neurol Sci 2004;31:157–68.

60. Karussis D, Biermann LD, Bohlega S, et al. A recommended treatment algorithm in relapsing multiple sclerosis: report of an international consensus meeting. Eur J Neurol 2006;13:61–71.

61. Zhao GJ, Li DK, Wang XY, et al. MRI of dirty-appearing white matter in MS. Neurology 2000;54:A121.

62. Moore GR, Laule C, MacKay A, et al. Dirty-appearing white matter in multiple sclerosis: preliminary observations of myelin phospholipid and axonal loss. J Neurol, in press.

63. Liu C, Edwards S, Gong Q, et al. Three dimensional MRI estimates of brain and spinal cord atrophy in multiple sclerosis. J Neurol Neurosurg Psychiatry 1999;66:323–30.

64. Filippi M, Mastronardo G, Rocca MA, et al. Quantitative volumetric analysis of brain magnetic resonance imaging from patients with multiple sclerosis. J Neurol Sci 1998;158:148–53.

65. Miller DH, Barkhof F, Frank JA, et al. Measurement of atrophy in multiple sclerosis: pathological basis, methodological aspects and clinical relevance. Brain 2002;125:1676–95.

66. van Walderveen MA, Barkhof F, Tas MW, et al. Patterns of brain magnetic resonance abnormalities on T2-weighted spin echo images in clinical subgroups of multiple sclerosis: a large cross-sectional study. Eur Neurol 1998;40(2):91–8.

67. Brex PA, Jenkins R, Fox NC, et al. Detection of ventricular enlargement in patients at the earliest clinical stage of MS. Neurology 2000;54:1689–91.

68. Fox NC, Jenkins R, Leary SM, et al. Progressive cerebral atrophy in MS: a serial study using registered, volumetric MRI. Neurology 2000;54:807–12.

69. Rudick RA, Fisher E, Lee JC, et al. Use of the brain parenchymal fraction to measure whole brain atrophy in relapsing-remitting MS: Multiple Sclerosis Collaborative Research Group. Neurology 1999; 53:1698–704.

70. Rovaris M, Comi G, Rocca MA, et al. Short-term brain volume change in relapsing-remitting multiple sclerosis: effect of glatiramer acetate and implications. Brain 2001;124:1803–12.

71. Ge Y, Grossman RI, Udupa JK, et al. Brain atrophy in relapsing-remitting multiple sclerosis and secondary progressive multiple sclerosis: longitudinal quantitative analysis. Radiology 2000;214:665–70.

72. Miller DH, Soon D, Fernando KT, et al. MRI outcomes in a placebo-controlled trial of natalizumab in relapsing MS. Neurology 2007;68:1390–401.

73. Tartaglino LM, Friedman DP, Flanders AE, et al. Multiple sclerosis in the spinal cord: MR appearance and correlation with clinical parameters. Radiology 1995;195(3):725–32.

74. Bot JC, Barkhof F, Lycklama G, et al. Differentiation of multiple sclerosis from other inflammatory disorders and cerebrovascular disease: value of spinal MR imaging. Radiology 2002;223:46–56.

75. Thielen KR, Miller GM. Multiple sclerosis of the spinal cord: magnetic resonance appearance. J Comput Assist Tomogr 1996;20:434–8.

76. Lee KH, Hashimoto SA, Hooge JP, et al. Magnetic resonance imaging of the head in the diagnosis of multiple sclerosis: a prospective 2-year follow-up with comparison of clinical evaluation, evoked potentials, oligoclonal banding, and CT. Neurology 1991;41:657–60.

77. Thorpe JW, Kidd D, Moseley IF, et al. Spinal MRI in patients with suspected multiple sclerosis and negative brain MRI. Brain 1996;119(Pt 3):709–14.

78. Dalton CM, Brex PA, Miszkiel KA, et al. Spinal cord MRI in clinically isolated optic neuritis. J Neurol Neurosurg Psychiatry 2003;74:1577–80.

79. Polman CH, Reingold SC, Edan G, et al. Diagnostic criteria for multiple sclerosis: 2005 revisions to the McDonald criteria. Ann Neurol 2005;58(6):840–6.

80. Lycklama G, Thompson A, Filippi M, et al. Spinal-cord MRI in multiple sclerosis. Lancet Neurol 2003;2:555–62.

81. Wingerchuk DM, Lennon VA, Pittock SJ, et al. Revised diagnostic criteria for neuromyelitis optica. Neurology 2006;66:1485–9.

82. Costa RM, Santos AC, Costa LS. An unusual chiasmal visual defect in a patient with neuromyelitis optica: case report. Arq Bras Oftalmol 2007;70:153–5.

83. Pittock SJ, Weinshenker BG, Lucchinetti CF, et al. Neuromyelitis optica brain lesions localized at sites of high aquaporin 4 expression. Arch Neurol 2006; 63:964–8.

84. Kepes JJ. Large focal tumor-like demyelinating lesions of the brain: intermediate entity between multiple sclerosis and acute disseminated encephalomyelitis? A study of 31 patients. Ann Neurol 1993;33:18–27.

85. Capello E, Mancardi GL. Marburg type and Balo's concentric sclerosis: rare and acute variants of multiple sclerosis. Neurol Sci 2004;25(Suppl 4): S361–3.

86. Canellas AR, Gols AR, Izquierdo JR, et al. Idiopathic inflammatory-demyelinating diseases of the central nervous system. Neuroradiology 2007;49: 393–409.

87. Fisniku LK, Brex PA, Altmann DR, et al. Disability and T2 MRI lesions: a 20-year follow-up of patients with relapse onset of multiple sclerosis. Brain 2008; 131:808–17.

88. Cole SR, Beck RW, Moke PS, et al. The National Eye Institute visual function questionnaire: experience of the ONTT. Optic Neuritis Treatment Trial. Invest Ophthalmol Vis Sci 2000;41:1017–21.

89. Poser CM, Paty DW, Scheinberg L, et al. New diagnostic criteria for multiple sclerosis: guidelines for research protocols. Ann Neurol 1983;13: 227–31.

90. Barkhof F, Polman CH, Radue EW, et al. Magnetic resonance imaging effects of interferon beta-1b in the BENEFIT study: integrated 2-year results. Arch Neurol 2007;64:1292–8.

91. Kappos L, Freedman MS, Polman CH, et al. Effect of early versus delayed interferon beta-1b treatment on disability after a first clinical event suggestive of multiple sclerosis: a 3-year follow-up analysis of the BENEFIT study. Lancet 2007;370:389–97.

92. Polman C, Kappos L, Freedman MS, et al. Subgroups of the BENEFIT study: risk of developing MS and treatment effect of interferon beta-1b. J Neurol 2008;255:480–7.

93. Dalton CM, Brex PA, Miszkiel KA, et al. New T2 lesions enable an earlier diagnosis of multiple sclerosis in clinically isolated syndromes. Ann Neurol 2003;53:673–6.

94. Paty DW, Oger JJ, Kastrukoff LF. Magnetic resonance imaging (MRI) in the diagnosis of multiple sclerosis: a prospective study with comparison of clinical evaluation, evoked potentials, oligoclonal banding and computerized tomography. Neurology 1988;38:180–5.

95. Fazekas F, Offenbacher H, Fuchs S, et al. Criteria for an increased specificity of MRI interpretation in elderly subjects with suspected multiple sclerosis. Neurology 1988;38:1822–5.

96. Frohman EM, Goodin DS, Calabresi PA, et al. The utility of MRI in suspected MS: report of the Therapeutics and Technology Assessment Subcommittee of the American Academy of Neurology. Neurology 2003;61:602–11.

97. Jacobs LD, Beck RW, Simon JH, et al. Intramuscular interferon beta-1a therapy initiated during a first

demyelinating event in multiple sclerosis. CHAMPS Study Group. N Engl J Med 2000;343:898–904.

98. Beck RW, Trobe JD, Moke PS, et al. High- and low-risk profiles for the development of multiple sclerosis within 10 years after optic neuritis: experience of the optic neuritis treatment trial. Arch Ophthalmol 2003;121:944–9.

99. Korteweg T, Tintore M, Uitdehaag B, et al. MRI criteria for dissemination in space in patients with clinically isolated syndromes: a multicentre follow-up study. Lancet Neurol 2006;5(3):221–7.

100. Uitdehaag BM, Geurts JJ, Barkhof F, et al. The utility of MRI in suspected MS: report of the Therapeutics and Technology Assessment Subcommittee. Neurology 2004;63:1140.

101. Schiffer R, Giang D, Mushlin A, et al. Perils and pitfalls of magnetic resonance imaging in the diagnosis of multiple sclerosis. J Neuroimaging 1993;3:81–8.

102. Carmosino MJ, Brousseau KM, Arciniegas DB, et al. Initial evaluations for multiple sclerosis in a university multiple sclerosis center: outcomes and role of magnetic resonance imaging in referral. Arch Neurol 2005;62:585–90.

103. Nielsen JM, Korteweg T, Barkhof F, et al. Overdiagnosis of multiple sclerosis and magnetic resonance imaging criteria. Ann Neurol 2005;58:781–3.

104. Wolinsky JS. The PROMiSe trial: baseline data review and progress report. Mult Scler 2004; 10(Suppl 1):S65–71.

105. de Seze J, Debouverie M, Waucquier N, et al. Primary progressive multiple sclerosis: a comparative study of the diagnostic criteria. Mult Scler 2007;13:622–5.

106. Sadovnick AD, Ebers GC. Epidemiology of multiple sclerosis: a critical overview. Can J Neurol Sci 1993;20:17–29.

107. Banwell B, Shroff M, Ness JM, et al. MRI features of pediatric multiple sclerosis. Neurology 2007;68: S46–53.

108. Ghassemi R, Antel SB, Narayanan S, et al. Lesion distribution in children with clinically isolated syndromes. Ann Neurol 2008;63:401–5.

109. Mikaeloff Y, Adamsbaum C, Husson B, et al. MRI prognostic factors for relapse after acute CNS inflammatory demyelination in childhood. Brain 2004;127:1942–7.

110. Hahn CD, Shroff MM, Blaser SI, et al. MRI criteria for multiple sclerosis: evaluation in a pediatric cohort. Neurology 2004;62:806–8.

111. Menge T, Hemmer B, Nessler S, et al. Acute disseminated encephalomyelitis: an update. Arch Neurol 2005;62:1673–80.

112. Hynson JL, Kornberg AJ, Coleman LT, et al. Clinical and neuroradiologic features of acute disseminated encephalomyelitis in children. Neurology 2001;56:1308–12.

113. McAdam LC, Blaser SI, Banwell BL. Pediatric tumefactive demyelination: case series and review of the literature. Pediatr Neurol 2002;26:18–25.

114. Chong HT, Ramli N, Lee KH, et al. Magnetic resonance imaging of Asians with multiple sclerosis was similar to that of the West. Can J Neurol Sci 2006;33(1):95–100.

115. Nakashima I, Fujihara K, Miyazawa I, et al. Clinical and MRI features of Japanese patients with multiple sclerosis positive for NMO-IgG. J Neurol Neurosurg Psychiatry 2006;77:1073–5.

116. Barkhof F. The clinico-radiological paradox in multiple sclerosis revisited. Curr Opin Neurol 2002; 15:239–45.

117. Petkau J, Reingold SC, Held U, et al. Magnetic resonance imaging as a surrogate outcome for multiple sclerosis relapses. Mult Scler 2008;14: 70–8.

118. Filippi M. Non-conventional MR techniques to monitor the evolution of multiple sclerosis. Neurol Sci 2001;22:195–200.

119. Traboulsee A, Dehmeshki J, Peters KR, et al. Disability in multiple sclerosis is related to normal appearing brain tissue MTR histogram abnormalities. Mult Scler 2003;9:566–73.

120. Rieckmann P. [Escalating immunomodulatory therapy of multiple sclerosis. Update (September 2006)]. Nervenarzt 2006;77:1506–18 [in German].

121. Langer-Gould A, Atlas SW, Green AJ, et al. Progressive multifocal leukoencephalopathy in a patient treated with natalizumab. N Engl J Med 2005;353(4):375–81.

122. Yousry TA, Major EO, Ryschkewitsch C, et al. Evaluation of patients treated with natalizumab for progressive multifocal leukoencephalopathy. N Engl J Med 2006;354:924–33.

Brain Atrophy Assessment in Multiple Sclerosis: Importance and Limitations

Antonio Giorgio, MD[a,b], Marco Battaglini, MSc[a],
Stephen M. Smith, DPhil[b], Nicola De Stefano, MD[a],*

KEYWORDS

- Brain atrophy • Multiple sclerosis • Tissue damage

The recent development of computational methods that, using conventional magnetic resonance (MR) images, are able to provide sensitive and reproducible measures of brain volumes has allowed an indirect quantification of cerebral tissue loss in many neurologic disorders. These methods can be easily implemented at any MR center and have been extensively used in the study of multiple sclerosis (MS), increasing the interest in cerebral tissue loss (brain atrophy) as a marker to accurately assess and monitor the pathologic evolution of the disease.[1–4] Brain volume loss has been recognized as an important feature of MS from the earliest disease stages and, in this complex disease, is the expression of a generalized process involving various tissue components of the brain.

This article reviews the most recent literature on the use of brain atrophy as a measure of disease progression in MS. Particular attention is paid to the methods used for these assessments, the clinical relevance of global and regional volume loss, and the potential limitations of these measurements.

MEASURING BRAIN VOLUMES

There are many valid approaches to obtaining MR imaging–based measures of brain volume changes. On the basis of the amount of operator intervention, they can be grouped into manual, semi-manual, and fully automated. Clearly, when compared with manual ones, automated analysis methods provide better reproducibility and reduce reliance on time-consuming user intervention. More generally, methods for measuring brain volumes can be broadly divided into two categories depending on whether brain volumes are measured cross-sectionally or longitudinally **(Table 1)**.

Cross-Sectional Methods

These methods need a single image as input and measure the current atrophy state. They are generally based on segmentation of the brain tissues.

The first of these approaches to assess global brain atrophy is based on the measurement of the brain parenchymal fraction (BPF).[5] The brain volume is calculated by measuring the difference in volumes inside a mesh over the exterior surface of the brain and inside the ventricles. A partial volume correction is employed to limit the impact of cerebrospinal fluid (CSF) within the cerebral sulci. Differences in the field of interest and segmentation partially cancel out because only one segmentation is performed to obtain the ratio of volume of parenchymal brain tissue to the total volume within the outer surface of the brain. This method is highly

The study was supported in part by a grant of the Associazione Italiana Sclerosi Multipla.
[a] Neurology and Neurometabolic Unit, Department of Neurological and Behavioural Sciences, University of Siena, Viale Bracci 2, 53100 Siena, Italy
[b] Oxford University Centre for Functional MRI of the Brain (FMRIB), Department of Clinical Neurology, University of Oxford, Headington, Oxford OX3 9DU, UK
* Corresponding author.
E-mail address: destefano@unisi.it (N. De Stefano).

Neuroimag Clin N Am 18 (2008) 675–686
doi:10.1016/j.nic.2008.06.007

Table 1
Methods used for measuring brain atrophy

Type of Method	Features
Cross-sectional	
BPF[5]	Calculation of the ratio of brain parenchyma volume to the total volume within the outer surface of the brain
BICCR[6]	Brain tissue volume measured with respect to the volume of the inner table of the skull
Fuzzy connectedness algorithm[7]	Each brain compartment considered a fuzzy connected set
Alfano's method[8]	Brain volumes obtained automatically with a multispectral relaxometry approach
TDS[9]	Brain volumes segmented by using a digital brain atlas
SABRE[10]	Individualized Talairach brain maps used for different brain regions in each hemisphere
Free Surfer[11,12]	Calculation of cortical thickness after inflation of the folded cortical surface
SIENAX[14]	Global and regional brain volume measurements normalized for subject head size
VBM[16,18,19]	Assessment of voxelwise brain tissue "concentrations"
Longitudinal	
BBSI[20]	Volume changes measured by subtracting baseline and follow-up scans
SIENA and SIENAr[21,23]	Volume changes assessed by estimating the local shift in brain edges across the brain and its voxelwise extension for regional assessments

Abbreviations: BBSI, brain boundary shift integral; BICCR, brain to intracranial capacity ratio; BPF, brain parenchymal fraction; SABRE, semiautomatic brain region extraction; SIENAX, structural image evaluation, using normalization, of atrophy; TDS, template-driven segmentation; VBM, voxel-based morphometry.

accurate, and the results are highly reproducible across different images from the same brain acquired over a short period of time (1 week), with a coefficient of variation less than 0.2%.[5]

A similar method has been proposed by Collins and colleagues.[6] With the brain to intracranial capacity ratio (BICCR), brain tissue is segmented as a primary step. The volume of brain tissue (or of any compartment) is measured with respect to the volume of the inner table of the skull.

Another method uses the fuzzy connectedness algorithm[7] on dual-echo, fast spin-echo MR images for segmenting and estimating the volume of the white matter (WM), grey matter (GM), and CSF, each one detected as a fuzzy connected set.

Additional methods for measuring brain volumes in different brain compartments are the one described by Alfano and colleagues[8] and the template-driven segmentation method (TDS).[9] In the first method, WM, GM, and CSF volumes are obtained with an unsupervised, automated segmentation of the brain using a multispectral relaxometric MR approach. In TDS, the initial signal

intensity–based statistical tissue classification is subsequently refined using a digital brain atlas as an anatomic template. This template, which is subdivided into over 120 anatomic labels, is matched to a given subject's image using a combination of automated linear and nonlinear registration algorithms. Similarly, a more recent technique[10] (SABRE) provides a semiautomatic brain region extraction and uses individualized Talairach brain maps for each subject to delineate and quantify different brain regions in each hemisphere. In this context, certainly interesting is an image analysis technique (Free Surfer) that segments out the cortex from the brain, avoiding the confound coming from gyral folding by inflating the folded cortical surface.[11,12] This approach has allowed highly accurate measurements not only of overall cortical thickness but also of local cortical thickness in different regions.[13]

The cross-sectional version of the structural image evaluation using the normalization of atrophy (SIENA) method (SIENAX)[14] (part of the FMRIB Software Library [FSL]; www.fmrib.ox.ac.uk) is an increasingly used method that estimates global and regional brain tissue volumes normalized for subject head size. It starts by extracting brain and skull images from the single whole-head input data.[15] The brain image is then affine-registered to a canonical image (MNI152 image) in a standardized space (using the skull image to provide the scaling cue), a procedure that provides a spatial normalization (scaling) factor for each subject. Next, tissue-type segmentation with partial volume estimation is performed[15] to calculate the total volume of brain tissue, including separate estimates of volumes of GM, WM and ventricular CSF. As is true for other methods, this calculation can be extended to include selective measures of multiple brain regions by using standard-space masks. This cross-sectional version of the SIENA longitudinal method gives a test-retest reproducibility of brain volume measures of about 0.5%.

Specific regional measures of volume changes can also be obtained more indirectly by using the voxel-based morphometry (VBM) approach.[16] This method is widely used for characterizing regional volume and tissue "concentration" differences in conventional MR images. Mainly, it is used to make voxelwise comparisons of the local concentration of GM regions between two groups of subjects. The procedure is relatively straightforward and involves a spatial normalization of high-resolution images from all subjects in a study into the same stereotactic space. This normalization is followed by a segmentation of the GM from the spatially normalized images and then a smoothing of the GM segments. Voxelwise parametric statistical tests which compare the smoothed GM images from the two groups are performed. Corrections for multiple comparisons are most frequently made using the theory of Gaussian random fields. VBM is most commonly performed using the statistical parametric mapping (SPM) software package. A VBM-style

analysis is also straightforward to carry out with FSL tools.[16,17] In this situation, a voxelwise general linear model is applied using permutation-based nonparametric testing.[18] The comparison of the classical VBM approach and the FSL-VBM approach on the same data set shows similar changes in cortical GM areas (**Fig. 1**).[19]

Longitudinal Methods

Longitudinal methods need two sets of MR images acquired at different times as input. They measure the atrophy rate. Each of the previously described cross-sectional methods can give a measure of the atrophy rate by assessing the differences of measurement results at different time points; however, a more precise measurement is obtained when serial scans from an individual are accurately registered and the cerebral volume changes are derived directly.[2] Explicit examples of registration-based methods that can be used for this purpose are brain boundary shift integral (BBSI)[20] and SIENA.[21]

In BBSI,[20] volume changes over time are measured by subtracting baseline and follow-up scans. The method defines a region that lies near the borders of the baseline and registered follow-up brains. The BBSI technique is based on integrating the differences in intensities over this region. Scan intensities are normalized by dividing each scan by its respective mean, calculated over the interior region. The intensities are bounded by a clipping function based on a predefined upper and lower intensity for each scan. Dividing the integrated differences by the span of the clipping function provides a measure of the global brain volume loss.

Another increasingly popular approach to measuring total brain volume change directly is the SIENA method,[21] also part of FSL. This method assesses brain volume changes by estimating

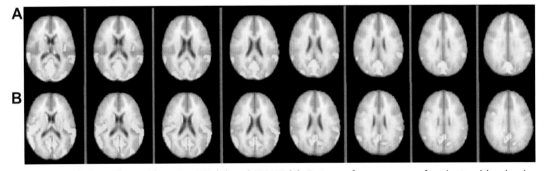

Fig. 1. VBM analysis performed by using FSL (*A*) and SPM05 (*B*). Data are from a group of patients with relapsing-remitting MS compared with a group of normal controls. The color overlay is created on top of the MNI152 standard brain. Brain voxels with significant GM loss in MS patients are shown in yellow ($P < .05$, corrected). Note how the two methods show similar local GM atrophy.

directly the local shifts in brain edges across the entire brain. SIENA starts by extracting brain and skull images from the two time point whole-head input data.[15] The two brain images are then aligned to each other[15] (using the skull images to constrain the registration scaling). Both brain images are re-sampled into the space halfway between the two, avoiding bias in atrophy estimation due to asymmetric interpolation blurring. Next, tissue-type segmentation is performed[15] to find brain/nonbrain edge points, and then perpendicular edge displacement (between the two time points) is estimated at these edge points. The displacement is estimated by aligning the peaks of the spatial derivatives of the intensity profiles of the two images to subvoxel accuracy. The mean edge displacement is converted into a global estimate of percentage brain volume change (PBVC) between the two time points. SIENA has been extended to allow the voxelwise statistical analysis of atrophy across subjects.[22,23] This approach takes a SIENA-derived edge "flow image" (edge displacement between the time points) for each subject and warps this to align with a standard space edge image. The resulting images from all subjects are fed into voxelwise statistical analysis to find statistically significant localized difference in atrophy between the two groups of subjects.

In a recent study,[24] the BBSI and SIENA methods were compared using the same data set. The two methods were in excellent agreement with each other. There was close correlation between the two measures ($r = 0.87$, $P < .0001$, median absolute difference = 0.25%), and even the absolute scaling of the two measures was close. With both methods, the measurements had an error of less than 0.2%, in agreement with previously published estimations of the overall error rate. Furthermore, another recent study[25] has shown that registration-based techniques appear to be more precise and sensitive than segmentation-based methods in measuring brain atrophy, with BBSI and SIENA providing comparable results. Despite this finding, measures made with different techniques usually cannot be compared directly (although their measurements of change may be correlated), and sensitivities to change may be different.

GLOBAL BRAIN ATROPHY

Since the earliest MR imaging studies in MS, marked atrophy of the brain has been recognized as an important feature of the late disease stages. Today, the availability of high-quality MR images and cutting-edge signal post-processing methods has allowed us to measure even small changes in brain volume occurring over relatively short periods of time (months). Serial MR imaging studies have demonstrated that brain volume loss occurs at a rate of around 0.5% to 1% per year in MS patients[4,26] compared with a rate of about 0.1% to 0.3% per year in healthy subjects.[27,28]

Brain atrophy appears to proceed relentlessly throughout the course of MS even at the earliest stages.[2-4] In subjects at presentation with clinically isolated syndrome (CIS) suggestive of MS, it has been demonstrated that significantly greater ventricular enlargement occurs in persons in whom MS develops when compared with persons who remain stable.[29,30] Several cross-sectional studies have shown that brain volume also is significantly reduced in relapsing-remitting (RR) MS subjects when compared with age-matched controls.[5,20,31,32] Similarly, significant and diffuse brain atrophy is reported in patients with the secondary progressive (SP) and primary progressive (PP) forms of the disease.[20,33-39] In a mixed population of MS patients (benign MS, RRMS, SPMS, and PPMS), a significant brain volume loss in each patient group was found, as well as a greater ventricle enlargement in patients than in normal controls[20]; however, in general, the rate of brain atrophy progression seems to be substantially independent of the MS subtype.[40]

BRAIN ATROPHY IN GREY AND WHITE MATTER

Several MR[41-44] and histologic[45-49] studies have suggested that, even though MS is a demyelinating disorder, cortical GM pathology is also present. Many of the previously mentioned computational methods for measurement of brain volumes have been used successfully to selectively measure GM volumes in MS patients.

Several studies have demonstrated that GM volume loss is consistently present in MS patients from the earliest disease stages. For example, a decrease of GM fractional volume has been detected in CIS patients in whom clinically definite MS developed 3 years later,[50] and cortical GM loss has been found in early RRMS patients.[31,51-53] Other studies have tried to gain insights into the temporal evolution of GM atrophy in the early course of the disease. In particular, it has been demonstrated that GM volume loss may evolve over time periods as short as 1.5 to 2 years[54,55] or less than 1 year[56] in RRMS patients.

One of the most intriguing observations of MR studies assessing brain atrophy in MS has been that the pathology underlying cerebral volume loss seems to have a different impact in different GM regions. Overall, the studies have agreed in finding the frontal, temporal, and parietal lobes as the most involved (atrophic) cortical GM regions in MS patients.[2,57–62] Although global measures have generically found a diffuse reduction of brain volumes in MS patients without major differences between clinical phenotypes and disease stages, selective regional measures have demonstrated differences in brain regional involvement in the progressive and relapsing forms of MS,[63] or a progressive involvement of the cortical regions in patients with long disease duration or increasing disability.[13,61,62,64] Atrophy seems to start in frontotemporal areas, specifically involving the superior temporal gyrus and superior and middle frontal gyri, and to extend to other clinically relevant areas (eg, the motor cortex) in more advanced disease phases.[13]

Atrophy of the deep GM also occurs in MS. Normalized bicaudate volume has been found to be lower in MS patients than in normal controls,[65] with no correlation with whole-brain atrophy or lesion volume. Thalamic volume reduction up to 25% in RRMS patients and up to 35% in SPMS patients has been observed in several recent cross-sectional and longitudinal studies.[58,66–69] A longitudinal study of early PPMS patients[59] found bilateral atrophy of the thalamus at baseline, which also extended to the putamen, caudate, and other cortical and infratentorial areas after 1 year. The thalamus seemed to be the only GM compartment involved in pediatric MS.[70] All of these studies, demonstrating that there are specific deep GM regions (eg, thalamus and caudate nuclei) that can be involved earlier and more strongly than other regions in the pathologic process, provide additional evidence of the high relevance of GM pathology from the earliest stages of MS. Two of these studies bring the most relevant support to this hypothesis. By combining histopathologic methods and quantitative MR measures, they have elegantly shown that both RRMS[66] and SPMS[69] patients have comparable ex vivo loss of thalamic neurons and in vivo thalamic volume decrease.

Interestingly, when compared with GM volumes, decreases of WM volumes in MS are much less frequently reported. No WM atrophy has been found in CIS patients in whom clinically definite MS developed 3 years later[50] and in early RRMS over an 18-month[55] or 2-year[54] follow-up. Nevertheless, decreases of WM volume have been reported in other studies of relapsing[31,52,71] and progressive[59,71] MS patients. Moreover, in a 9-year longitudinal study of a group of MS patients with a wide range of disease duration, the midsagittal corpus callosum size decreased independently of the disease course at the rate of about 1.8% per year.[72] This decrease adds to the significant atrophy of central brain regions (ie, lateral ventricles) that also largely progresses over time in all MS stages and subtypes.[2,29,30,62,73,74]

CLINICAL RELEVANCE OF BRAIN ATROPHY

In the last decade or so, many studies have investigated whether robust MR correlates of clinical change do exist in MS. The results have often been disappointing, probably explained by the fact that attention has been mostly focused on focal pathologic damage (ie, lesions) in WM. Focal WM lesions do not lead to disability progression in a simple way, and focal demyelination alone cannot explain entirely the pathologic process leading to clinical disability.[75–78] Brain atrophy measures, by reflecting tissue loss (mostly myelin and axonal damage or loss) in both abnormal and normal appearing brain, may correlate with disability better than measures of focal demyelination or inflammation.

Both global brain[71,79–81] and selective GM[51,61,63,82] measures of volume loss have been closely associated with disability. Greater brain atrophy is generally found in CIS subjects in whom MS develops when compared with those in whom it does not[29,30] and, in established MS, brain atrophy is greater in patients who show sustained progression of disability than in those who are clinically stable.[32,38,83] In longitudinal studies of relapsing and progressive MS patients, brain volume at early stages seems to be a good predictor of disability status at follow-up, suggesting that atrophy is a relevant marker of disease progression and may even precede the development of measurable disability.[36,84]

Interestingly, specific aspects of clinical dysfunction have been linked to regional brain atrophy. For example, longitudinal studies have shown a persisting association between segmental callosal atrophy and disability status, even at early disease stages.[72,85] Also, the decline in ambulatory function (ie, Timed Walk Test) has been related to atrophy of periventricular and brainstem regions,[62] whereas a focal thinning of the precentral gyrus and primary visual cortex has been related to the motor and visual scores of the Expanded Disability Status Scale, respectively.[60]

Several MR studies have linked cognitive impairment to brain atrophy in MS. This impairment is an increasingly recognized clinical aspect of the disease observed in about 40% to 60% of patients, even including a proportion of those with early disease stage.[86,87] Although increasing cognitive impairment may sometimes proceed in parallel with increasing T2 MR imaging lesion load, the magnitude of the correlation between neuropsychologic scores and T2 lesion volume has been found to be weak or moderate.[88,89] By contrast, cognitive impairment has been found to be associated with measures of cerebral atrophy, and the importance of decreasing brain volumes (rather than increasing lesion load) to MS-related cognitive impairment has been suggested in several studies.[68,90–92] In particular, cortical atrophy has been found to be significantly higher in cognitively impaired than in cognitively preserved RRMS patients[91] and, in both RRMS and SPMS patients, has been the best predictor of verbal memory impairment and neurobehavioral symptoms.[93] In other studies, the atrophy of the frontal cortex has been found to be related to reduced cognitive functions,[94] and right and left frontal atrophy has been associated with auditory/verbal memory and episodic and working memory deficits, respectively.[95]

The results of the previously mentioned studies strongly suggest the notion that brain atrophy (in particular, selective GM atrophy) is a good marker of unfavorable disease outcome in MS; however, its correlation with clinical disability is far from perfect. In a complex disease such as MS, several other factors (eg, spinal cord damage, cortical adaptation to injury, genetic predisposition to injury repair) can all contribute to weaken this relationship and should be considered when interpreting the clinical relevance of this and other MR imaging measures.[96,97]

USE OF BRAIN ATROPHY AS AN ENDPOINT IN CLINICAL TRIALS

After MR-derived measures of brain volume changes were established as a sensitive, reproducible, and accurate index of brain tissue damage, they were used in several clinical trials to assess treatment efficacy.[5,33,83,98–102] Nevertheless, only rarely has a treatment effect on brain atrophy been demonstrated.

Common characteristics of the studies using brain volume change as an endpoint are the relatively short follow-up period (mostly 2 to 3 years) and the increase of the atrophy rate occurring during the first period of treatment with anti-inflammatory agents. The latter finding is an important point that needs to be discussed.

Several lines of evidence suggest that the large brain atrophy rates found at the beginning of an anti-inflammatory therapy may be more a reflection of the resolution of inflammatory edema than a consequence of the irreversible loss of axons and myelin. In agreement with this, in many cases, the atrophy rate reduces after the first treatment period (ie, after the inflammatory edema is resolved), and, often, this lower rate is maintained over the remaining treatment period.[99,103] In patients who had severe and rapidly evolving MS who underwent autologous hematopoietic stem cell transplantation,[104] this procedure was associated (in addition to an immediate and longstanding suppression of focal demyelination and inflammatory activity) with a large and progressive atrophy (about 1.4% per year) over the first 2 years after treatment and to a significant and sustained reduction of volume loss in the subsequent 3 years (about 0.4% per year).[105] Indeed, in CIS patients, in whom a minor resolution of inflammatory edema is expected, treatment with interferon beta-1a was shown to be effective in slowing progressive brain tissue loss.[101]

Against this background, it is evident that measures of brain volume changes are sensitive and accurate enough to provide a robust index of efficacy in clinical trials; however, it is also clear that in a complex disease such as MS in which inflammation, demyelination, and neurodegeneration contribute to chronic disease progression, brain atrophy can be considered a good index of clinical outcome only when the study design entails relatively long follow-up periods.

UNDERSTANDING AND INTERPRETING BRAIN ATROPHY

The pathologic correlates of brain atrophy are arguably more complex in MS than in many other neurodegenerative disorders. In the brain of a patient who has MS, demyelination and inflammation add to neurodegeneration, and, as a consequence, loss of brain components such as myelin and glial cells contributes with that of neurons and axons to the total loss of tissue volume. Nevertheless, the mechanisms leading to atrophy in MS are still inadequately understood.

Axonal damage may lead to retrograde neurodegeneration and cause brain atrophy.[106,107] Because the corticospinal tracts and frontal periventricular WM are preferential sites for MS lesions,[89] WM pathology in MS may lead to a selective retrograde injury to frontal, temporal, and motor areas of the cortex. This injury could explain, for example, the characteristic pattern of cortical atrophy found in the studies mentioned previously.[2,57–62]

Interestingly, although a significant proportion of neuroaxonal damage is dependent on focal WM changes,[108] other studies[13,51,107] have shown that widespread neocortical loss and thinning can be found even in patients with minimal cerebral lesion load. This observation suggests that retrograde changes from focal WM lesions cannot explain the full range of findings. Pathologic studies have shown that neuroaxonal damage and loss may occur via mechanisms that are independent of those causing demyelination and are likely related to the presence of an abnormal glia-axonal interaction even with low or absent inflammation.[49,109] In agreement with this, apoptotic neuronal death unrelated to axonal transection has been found in the cortex of MS patients.[49] It is possible that factors that are not directly connected with lesion formation may also have a significant role in determining brain atrophy in MS.

Although the interpretation of brain atrophy measures can reasonably be framed in terms of a mutual contribution of demyelination, inflammation, and neurodegeneration, brain tissue also includes a significant extracellular compartment. MR studies have shown indirectly that, in the MS brain, water content is increased in inflammatory lesions[110] and normal-appearing tissue.[111] Direct histopathologic measures confirm the expansion of the extracellular space over the course of the disease.[112] In this context, dramatic changes in water content that can affect interpretation of brain volume measurements might also include dialysis (with volume increases up to 3%)[113] and acute dehydration or rehydration.[114] Similarly, as discussed previously, the short-term decreases in brain volume reported (eg, in anti-inflammatory treatments[83,99,103,115,116]) should be accounted for a decrease in water content (ie, "pseudoatrophy") rather than for a real "atrophy" arising from myelin loss and neuroaxonal degeneration.

Generic factors such as life habits, genetic load, and concomitant paraphysiologic conditions may affect brain volume measurements and need to be taken into account when interpreting brain atrophy in MS patients. For example, alcohol abuse is associated with changes in water content and structural brain damage leading to brain volume changes that can partially recover after therapeutic sobriety.[22] Also, there is some evidence that the ApoE genotype, by influencing the ability to respond to injury, may have a significant role in tissue damage leading to atrophy.[117,118] Similarly, although it is known that brain atrophy progresses with age, this seems to be more pronounced when aging is complicated by the presence of smoking, diabetes, and other cardiovascular risk factors.[119]

PITFALLS AND LIMITATIONS OF MR IMAGING–DERIVED MEASURES OF BRAIN ATROPHY

Despite the accuracy of MR imaging–derived measures of brain atrophy, various sources of error can affect the estimation of brain volume changes. Clearly, the quality of image acquisition (ie, image resolution, signal-to-noise ratio) has a crucial role. For example, poor contrast in images may cause suboptimal tissue classification when intensity-based tissue segmentation is used. Also, artifacts due to head motion and inhomogeneities in radio frequency can cause intensity variations in the image and problems in threshold-based segmentation, particularly in methods that rely on high-resolution data to perform accurate regional analysis.[11,12] Additional problems may arise in the presence of partial head acquisition. In this situation, the differences in the amount of brain image acquired at two time points might be erroneously confounded with brain volume changes. This issue can be overcome in registration-based methods by using standard-space–based limits for the bottom and top slices of the brain.[15]

In interpreting the brain atrophy occurring in MS, the decrease in cortical GM volumes might be overestimated owing to the fact that cerebral cortical lesions, which appear to be common in MS,[49,120] are virtually invisible with conventional MR sequences. Such lesions, which have been detected recently by using specific MR imaging sequences,[44,121,122] may affect segmentation between the cortex and the CSF, such that the former may be erroneously decreased in volume.

Although image segmentation is usually aided by multiple-contrast acquisitions, most segmentation methods produce the best results on T1-weighted acquisitions.[123] In this context, less reliable results are usually obtained when post-gadolinium, T1-weighted images are used to estimate brain volume changes. This characteristic is particularly important for data derived from multicenter trials, because, in these studies, post-gadolinium images (used to assess brain MR imaging lesion activity) are often the only T1-weighted data available. Practically, the presence of the contrast agent in the central nervous system causes both poor contrast MR images and suboptimal brain extraction. For example, in a data set on 55 RRMS patients who underwent identical pre- and post-gadolinium T1-weighted MR imaging at baseline and 1 year later, the correlation between the two sets of T1-weighted images was limited (Pearson correlation = 0.71; M. Battaglini and N. De Stefano, personal observation, 2008). The measurements of global brain volume changes could be improved by using a more accurate approach for brain extraction[124] (the Pearson correlation on the previous set of data was 0.86; **Fig. 2**); however, with post-gadolinium, T1-weighted images, an accurate classification of GM and WM is not possible.

Although most of the methods for assessing brain volume changes tend to be largely automated, they hide several complexities that should be appreciated to understand the possible sources of measurement errors. For example, the removal of non-brain tissue may be imperfect

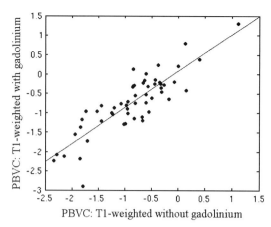

Fig. 2. The correlation between percentage brain volume changes (PBVC) obtained by using T1-weighted MR images with and without injection of gadolinium (Pearson's correlation = 0.86, *P* < .001). Data are from a group of 55 patients with RRMS who underwent the acquisition of both T1-weighted sequences at baseline and after 1 year.

(eg, incorrect inclusion of eyes, periorbital fat, and other non-brain structures). In this case, manual editing[125] or a more accurate brain extraction procedure[124] may decrease volume overestimation and reduce variability. Also, all registration-based methods suffer from the well-known issue of ambiguity of interpretation (eg, apparent changes due to tissue loss or systematic alignment changes), which easily can occur with poor imaging resolution or large anatomic variation across subjects.[126] When serial changes in brain volume are measured using technically demanding approaches, such as voxel-based assessments or model-based parcellation techniques, high-quality MR image acquisition is mandatory. In this context, measures of brain atrophy should take advantage of the continuous development of image acquisition (eg, high MR fields, new sequences) and post-processing procedures (eg, intensity normalization, segmentation, and coregistration) that can significantly improve the final output.

SUMMARY

Despite the important issues that still need to be solved, the meaning of brain atrophy in MS has a great potential and represents one of the most interesting and promising in vivo measures of unfavorable disease outcome. Future studies are warranted to answer important questions such as when and at what rate atrophy starts to develop in MS, how exactly atrophy relates to the complex MS pathology, how it relates to prognosis, whether atrophy distribution is clinically important, and

whether an "atrophy threshold" exists. Long follow-up studies and combined histologic and MR imaging studies can provide an answer to at least some of these questions.

REFERENCES

1. Zivadinov R. Can imaging techniques measure neuroprotection and remyelination in multiple sclerosis? Neurology 2007;68:S72–82 [discussion: S91–76].
2. De Stefano N, Battaglini M, Smith SM. Measuring brain atrophy in multiple sclerosis. J Neuroimaging 2007;17(Suppl 1):10S–5S.
3. Simon JH. Brain atrophy in multiple sclerosis: what we know and would like to know. Mult Scler 2006; 12:679–87.
4. Bermel RA, Bakshi R. The measurement and clinical relevance of brain atrophy in multiple sclerosis. Lancet Neurol 2006;5:158–70.
5. Rudick RA, Fisher E, Lee JC, et al. Use of the brain parenchymal fraction to measure whole brain atrophy in relapsing-remitting MS. Multiple Sclerosis Collaborative Research Group. Neurology 1999; 53:1698–704.
6. Collins DL, Montagnat J, Zijdenbos AP, et al. Automated estimation of brain volume in multiple sclerosis with BICCR. Lect Notes Comput Sci 2001;2082: 141–7.
7. Udupa JK, Wei L, Samarasekera S, et al. Multiple sclerosis lesion quantification using fuzzy-connectedness principles. IEEE Trans Med Imaging 1997; 16:598–609.
8. Alfano B, Brunetti A, Covelli EM, et al. Unsupervised, automated segmentation of the normal brain using a multispectral relaxometric magnetic resonance approach. Magn Reson Med 1997;37: 84–93.
9. Guttmann CR, Benson R, Warfield SK, et al. White matter abnormalities in mobility-impaired older persons. Neurology 2000;54:1277–83.
10. Dade LA, Gao FQ, Kovacevic N, et al. Semiautomatic brain region extraction: a method of parcellating brain regions from structural magnetic resonance images. Neuroimage 2004;22: 1492–502.
11. Fischl B, Sereno MI, Dale AM. Cortical surface-based analysis. II. Inflation, flattening, and a surface-based coordinate system. Neuroimage 1999; 9:195–207.
12. Dale AM, Fischl B, Sereno MI. Cortical surface-based analysis. I. Segmentation and surface reconstruction. Neuroimage 1999;9:179–94.
13. Sailer M, Fischl B, Salat D, et al. Focal thinning of the cerebral cortex in multiple sclerosis. Brain 2003;126:1734–44.

14. Smith SM, Zhang Y, Jenkinson M, et al. Accurate, robust, and automated longitudinal and cross-sectional brain change analysis. Neuroimage 2002;17:479–89.

15. Smith SM, Jenkinson M, Woolrich MW, et al. Advances in functional and structural MR image analysis and implementation as FSL. Neuroimage 2004;23(Suppl 1):S208–219.

16. Ashburner J, Friston KJ. Voxel-based morphometry–the methods. Neuroimage 2000;11:805–21.

17. Good CD, Johnsrude IS, Ashburner J, et al. A voxel-based morphometric study of ageing in 465 normal adult human brains. Neuroimage 2001;14: 21–36.

18. Nichols TE, Holmes AP. Nonparametric permutation tests for functional neuroimaging: a primer with examples. Hum Brain Mapp 2002;15:1–25.

19. Battaglini M, Smith SM, Douad G, et al. Voxel-based analysis of global and neocortical progression of brain atrophy in RRMS [abstract]. ISMRM 2007.

20. Fox NC, Jenkins R, Leary SM, et al. Progressive cerebral atrophy in MS: a serial study using registered, volumetric MRI. Neurology 2000;54:807–12.

21. Smith SM, De Stefano N, Jenkinson M, et al. Normalized accurate measurement of longitudinal brain change. J Comput Assist Tomogr 2001;25: 466–75.

22. Bartsch AJ, Homola G, Biller A, et al. Manifestations of early brain recovery associated with abstinence from alcoholism. Brain 2007;130:36–47.

23. De Stefano N, Jenkinson M, Guidi L, et al. Voxel-level cross-subject statistical analysis of brain atrophy in early relapsing remitting MS patients. Int Soc Magn Reson Med [book of abstracts]. 2003;2:2625.

24. Smith SM, Rao A, De Stefano N, et al. Longitudinal and cross-sectional analysis of atrophy in Alzheimer's disease: cross-validation of BSI, SIENA and SIENAX. Neuroimage 2007;36:1200–6.

25. Anderson VM, Fernando KT, Davies GR, et al. Cerebral atrophy measurement in clinically isolated syndromes and relapsing remitting multiple sclerosis: a comparison of registration-based methods. J Neuroimaging 2007;17:61–8.

26. Anderson VM, Fox NC, Miller DH. Magnetic resonance imaging measures of brain atrophy in multiple sclerosis. J Magn Reson Imaging 2006;23: 605–18.

27. Coffey CE, Wilkinson WE, Parashos IA, et al. Quantitative cerebral anatomy of the aging human brain: a cross-sectional study using magnetic resonance imaging. Neurology 1992;42:527–36.

28. Pfefferbaum A, Mathalon DH, Sullivan EV, et al. A quantitative magnetic resonance imaging study of changes in brain morphology from infancy to late adulthood. Arch Neurol 1994;51:874–87.

29. Brex PA, Jenkins R, Fox NC, et al. Detection of ventricular enlargement in patients at the earliest clinical stage of MS. Neurology 2000;54:1689–91.

30. Dalton CM, Brex PA, Jenkins R, et al. Progressive ventricular enlargement in patients with clinically isolated syndromes is associated with the early development of multiple sclerosis. J Neurol Neurosurg Psychiatry 2002;73:141–7.

31. Chard DT, Griffin CM, Parker GJ, et al. Brain atrophy in clinically early relapsing-remitting multiple sclerosis. Brain 2002;125:327–37.

32. Rudick RA, Fisher E, Lee JC, et al. Brain atrophy in relapsing multiple sclerosis: relationship to relapses, EDSS, and treatment with interferon beta-1a. Mult Scler 2000;6:365–72.

33. Turner B, Lin X, Calmon G, et al. Cerebral atrophy and disability in relapsing-remitting and secondary progressive multiple sclerosis over four years. Mult Scler 2003;9:21–7.

34. Stevenson VL, Miller DH, Leary SM, et al. One year follow up study of primary and transitional progressive multiple sclerosis. J Neurol Neurosurg Psychiatry 2000;68:713–8.

35. Rovaris M, Judica E, Gallo A, et al. Grey matter damage predicts the evolution of primary progressive multiple sclerosis at 5 years. Brain 2006;129:2628–34.

36. Sastre-Garriga J, Ingle GT, Chard DT, et al. Grey and white matter volume changes in early primary progressive multiple sclerosis: a longitudinal study. Brain 2005;128:1454–60.

37. Leary SM, Miller DH, Stevenson VL, et al. Interferon beta-1a in primary progressive MS: an exploratory, randomized, controlled trial. Neurology 2003;60: 44–51.

38. Ingle GT, Stevenson VL, Miller DH, et al. Two-year follow-up study of primary and transitional progressive multiple sclerosis. Mult Scler 2002;8: 108–14.

39. Filippi M, Rovaris M, Iannucci G, et al. Whole brain volume changes in patients with progressive MS treated with cladribine. Neurology 2000;55:1714–8.

40. Kalkers NF, Ameziane N, Bot JC, et al. Longitudinal brain volume measurement in multiple sclerosis: rate of brain atrophy is independent of the disease subtype. Arch Neurol 2002;59:1572–6.

41. Matthews PM, De Stefano N, Narayanan S, et al. Putting magnetic resonance spectroscopy studies in context: axonal damage and disability in multiple sclerosis. Semin Neurol 1998;18:327–36.

42. Filippi M, Inglese M. Overview of diffusion-weighted magnetic resonance studies in multiple sclerosis. J Neurol Sci 2001;186(Suppl 1):S37–43.

43. Chard DT, Griffin CM, McLean MA, et al. Brain metabolite changes in cortical grey and normal-appearing white matter in clinically early relapsing-remitting multiple sclerosis. Brain 2002;125: 2342–52.

44. Calabrese M, De Stefano N, Atzori M, et al. Detection of cortical inflammatory lesions by double inversion recovery magnetic resonance imaging in patients with multiple sclerosis. Arch Neurol 2007; 64:1416–22.

45. Bjartmar C, Trapp BD. Axonal and neuronal degeneration in multiple sclerosis: mechanisms and functional consequences. Curr Opin Neurol 2001;14: 271–8.

46. Lucchinetti CF, Bruck W, Lassmann H. Evidence for pathogenic heterogeneity in multiple sclerosis. Ann Neurol 2004;56:308.

47. Bruck W. Inflammatory demyelination is not central to the pathogenesis of multiple sclerosis. J Neurol 2005;252(Suppl 5):v10–15.

48. Wegner C, Esiri MM, Chance SA, et al. Neocortical neuronal, synaptic, and glial loss in multiple sclerosis. Neurology 2006;67:960–7.

49. Peterson JW, Bo L, Mork S, et al. Transected neurites, apoptotic neurons, and reduced inflammation in cortical multiple sclerosis lesions. Ann Neurol 2001;50:389–400.

50. Dalton CM, Chard DT, Davies GR, et al. Early development of multiple sclerosis is associated with progressive grey matter atrophy in patients presenting with clinically isolated syndromes. Brain 2004;127: 1101–7.

51. De Stefano N, Matthews PM, Filippi M, et al. Evidence of early cortical atrophy in MS: relevance to white matter changes and disability. Neurology 2003;60:1157–62.

52. Ge Y, Grossman RI, Udupa JK, et al. Brain atrophy in relapsing-remitting multiple sclerosis: fractional volumetric analysis of gray matter and white matter. Radiology 2001;220:606–10.

53. Quarantelli M, Ciarmiello A, Morra VB, et al. Brain tissue volume changes in relapsing-remitting multiple sclerosis: correlation with lesion load. Neuroimage 2003;18:360–6.

54. Tiberio M, Chard DT, Altmann DR, et al. Gray and white matter volume changes in early RRMS: a 2-year longitudinal study. Neurology 2005;64: 1001–7.

55. Chard DT, Griffin CM, Rashid W, et al. Progressive grey matter atrophy in clinically early relapsing-remitting multiple sclerosis. Mult Scler 2004;10: 387–91.

56. Valsasina P, Benedetti B, Rovaris M, et al. Evidence for progressive gray matter loss in patients with relapsing-remitting MS. Neurology 2005;65:1126–8.

57. Prinster A, Quarantelli M, Orefice G, et al. Grey matter loss in relapsing-remitting multiple sclerosis: a voxel-based morphometry study. Neuroimage 2006;29:859–67.

58. Carone DA, Benedict RH, Dwyer MG, et al. Semi-automatic brain region extraction (SABRE) reveals superior cortical and deep gray matter atrophy in MS. Neuroimage 2006;29:505–14.

59. Sepulcre J, Sastre-Garriga J, Cercignani M, et al. Regional gray matter atrophy in early primary progressive multiple sclerosis: a voxel-based morphometry study. Arch Neurol 2006;63:1175–80.

60. Calabrese M, Atzori M, Bernardi V, et al. Cortical atrophy is relevant in multiple sclerosis at clinical onset. J Neurol 2007;254:1212–20.

61. Charil A, Dagher A, Lerch JP, et al. Focal cortical atrophy in multiple sclerosis: relation to lesion load and disability. Neuroimage 2007;34:509–17.

62. Jasperse B, Vrenken H, Sanz-Arigita E, et al. Regional brain atrophy development is related to specific aspects of clinical dysfunction in multiple sclerosis. Neuroimage 2007;38:529–37.

63. Pagani E, Rocca MA, Gallo A, et al. Regional brain atrophy evolves differently in patients with multiple sclerosis according to clinical phenotype. AJNR Am J Neuroradiol 2005;26:341–6.

64. Chen JT, Narayanan S, Collins DL, et al. Relating neocortical pathology to disability progression in multiple sclerosis using MRI. Neuroimage 2004; 23:1168–75.

65. Bermel RA, Innus MD, Tjoa CW, et al. Selective caudate atrophy in multiple sclerosis: a 3D MRI parcellation study. Neuroreport 2003;14:335–9.

66. Wylezinska M, Cifelli A, Jezzard P, et al. Thalamic neurodegeneration in relapsing-remitting multiple sclerosis. Neurology 2003;60:1949–54.

67. Audoin B, Davies GR, Finisku L, et al. Localization of grey matter atrophy in early RRMS: a longitudinal study. J Neurol 2006;253:1495–501.

68. Houtchens MK, Benedict RH, Killiany R, et al. Thalamic atrophy and cognition in multiple sclerosis. Neurology 2007;69:1213–23.

69. Cifelli A, Arridge M, Jezzard P, et al. Thalamic neurodegeneration in multiple sclerosis. Ann Neurol 2002;52:650–3.

70. Mesaros S, Rocca MA, Absinta M, et al. Evidence of thalamic gray matter loss in pediatric multiple sclerosis. Neurology 2008;70:1107–12.

71. Tedeschi G, Lavorgna L, Russo P, et al. Brain atrophy and lesion load in a large population of patients with multiple sclerosis. Neurology 2005; 65:280–5.

72. Martola J, Stawiarz L, Fredrikson S, et al. Progression of non–age-related callosal brain atrophy in multiple sclerosis: a 9-year longitudinal MRI study representing four decades of disease development. J Neurol Neurosurg Psychiatry 2007;78: 375–80.

73. Luks TL, Goodkin DE, Nelson SJ, et al. A longitudinal study of ventricular volume in early relapsing-remitting multiple sclerosis. Mult Scler 2000;6: 332–7.

74. Dalton CM, Miszkiel KA, O'Connor PW, et al. Ventricular enlargement in MS: one-year change at various stages of disease. Neurology 2006;66:693–8.

75. McDonald WI, Miller DH, Thompson AJ. Are magnetic resonance findings predictive of clinical outcome in therapeutic trials in multiple sclerosis? The dilemma of interferon-beta. Ann Neurol 1994; 36:14–8.

76. McDonald WI. Rachelle Fishman-Matthew Moore Lecture. The pathological and clinical dynamics of multiple sclerosis. J Neuropathol Exp Neurol 1994;53:338–43.

77. Trapp BD, Ransohoff R, Rudick R. Axonal pathology in multiple sclerosis: relationship to neurologic disability. Curr Opin Neurol 1999;12:295–302.

78. Trapp BD, Bo L, Mork S, et al. Pathogenesis of tissue injury in MS lesions. J Neuroimmunol 1999;98: 49–56.

79. Sanfilipo MP, Benedict RH, Sharma J, et al. The relationship between whole brain volume and disability in multiple sclerosis: a comparison of normalized gray vs. white matter with misclassification correction. Neuroimage 2005;26:1068–77.

80. Losseff NA, Wang L, Lai HM, et al. Progressive cerebral atrophy in multiple sclerosis: a serial MRI study. Brain 1996;119(Pt 6):2009–19.

81. Ge Y, Grossman RI, Udupa JK, et al. Brain atrophy in relapsing-remitting multiple sclerosis and secondary progressive multiple sclerosis: longitudinal quantitative analysis. Radiology 2000;214:665–70.

82. Bakshi R, Benedict RH, Bermel RA, et al. Regional brain atrophy is associated with physical disability in multiple sclerosis: semiquantitative magnetic resonance imaging and relationship to clinical findings. J Neuroimaging 2001;11:129–36.

83. Molyneux PD, Kappos L, Polman C, et al. The effect of interferon beta-1b treatment on MRI measures of cerebral atrophy in secondary progressive multiple sclerosis. European Study Group on interferon beta-1b in secondary progressive multiple sclerosis. Brain 2000;123(Pt 11):2256–63.

84. Fisher E, Rudick RA, Simon JH, et al. Eight-year follow-up study of brain atrophy in patients with MS. Neurology 2002;59:1412–20.

85. Pelletier J, Suchet L, Witjas T, et al. A longitudinal study of callosal atrophy and interhemispheric dysfunction in relapsing-remitting multiple sclerosis. Arch Neurol 2001;58:105–11.

86. Feinstein A, Kartsounis LD, Miller DH, et al. Clinically isolated lesions of the type seen in multiple sclerosis: a cognitive, psychiatric, and MRI follow up study. J Neurol Neurosurg Psychiatry 1992;55:869–76.

87. Amato MP, Ponziani G, Pracucci G, et al. Cognitive impairment in early-onset multiple sclerosis: pattern, predictors, and impact on everyday life in a 4-year follow-up. Arch Neurol 1995;52:168–72.

88. Rovaris M, Filippi M, Falautano M, et al. Relation between MR abnormalities and patterns of cognitive impairment in multiple sclerosis. Neurology 1998;50:1601–8.

89. Filippi M, Tortorella C, Rovaris M, et al. Changes in the normal appearing brain tissue and cognitive impairment in multiple sclerosis. J Neurol Neurosurg Psychiatry 2000;68:157–61.

90. Zivadinov R, De Masi R, Nasuelli D, et al. MRI techniques and cognitive impairment in the early phase of relapsing-remitting multiple sclerosis. Neuroradiology 2001;43:272–8.

91. Amato MP, Bartolozzi ML, Zipoli V, et al. Neocortical volume decrease in relapsing-remitting MS patients with mild cognitive impairment. Neurology 2004;63:89–93.

92. Benedict RH, Zivadinov R. Predicting neuropsychological abnormalities in multiple sclerosis. J Neurol Sci 2006;245:67–72.

93. Sanfilipo MP, Benedict RH, Weinstock-Guttman B, et al. Gray and white matter brain atrophy and neuropsychological impairment in multiple sclerosis. Neurology 2006;66:685–92.

94. Locatelli L, Zivadinov R, Grop A, et al. Frontal parenchymal atrophy measures in multiple sclerosis. Mult Scler 2004;10:562–8.

95. Tekok-Kilic A, Benedict RH, Weinstock-Guttman B, et al. Independent contributions of cortical gray matter atrophy and ventricle enlargement for predicting neuropsychological impairment in multiple sclerosis. Neuroimage 2007;36:1294–300.

96. Matthews PM, Arnold DL. Magnetic resonance imaging of multiple sclerosis: new insights linking pathology to clinical evolution. Curr Opin Neurol 2001;14:279–87.

97. Mainero C, De Stefano N, Iannucci G, et al. Correlates of MS disability assessed in vivo using aggregates of MR quantities. Neurology 2001;56:1331–4.

98. Frank JA, Richert N, Bash C, et al. Interferon-beta-1b slows progression of atrophy in RRMS: three-year follow-up in NAb− and NAb+ patients. Neurology 2004;62:719–25.

99. Hardmeier M, Wagenpfeil S, Freitag P, et al. Rate of brain atrophy in relapsing MS decreases during treatment with IFNbeta-1a. Neurology 2005;64:236–40.

100. Gasperini C, Paolillo A, Giugni E, et al. MRI brain volume changes in relapsing-remitting multiple sclerosis patients treated with interferon beta-1a. Mult Scler 2002;8:119–23.

101. Filippi M, Rovaris M, Inglese M, et al. Interferon beta-1a for brain tissue loss in patients at presentation with syndromes suggestive of multiple sclerosis: a randomised, double-blind, placebo-controlled trial. Lancet 2004;364:1489–96.

102. Rovaris M, Comi G, Rocca MA, et al. Short-term brain volume change in relapsing-remitting

multiple sclerosis: effect of glatiramer acetate and implications. Brain 2001;124:1803–12.

103. Miller DH, Soon D, Fernando KT, et al. MRI outcomes in a placebo-controlled trial of natalizumab in relapsing MS. Neurology 2007;68:1390–401.

104. Mancardi GL, Saccardi R, Filippi M, et al. Autologous hematopoietic stem cell transplantation suppresses Gd-enhanced MRI activity in MS. Neurology 2001;57:62–8.

105. Roccatagliata L, Rocca M, Valsasina P, et al. The long-term effect of AHSCT on MRI measures of MS evolution: a five-year follow-up study. Mult Scler 2007;13:1068–70.

106. Trapp BD, Peterson J, Ransohoff RM, et al. Axonal transection in the lesions of multiple sclerosis. N Engl J Med 1998;338:278–85.

107. Evangelou N, Konz D, Esiri MM, et al. Size-selective neuronal changes in the anterior optic pathways suggest a differential susceptibility to injury in multiple sclerosis. Brain 2001;124:1813–20.

108. Arnold DL. Changes observed in multiple sclerosis using magnetic resonance imaging reflect a focal pathology distributed along axonal pathways. J Neurol 2005;252(Suppl 5):v25–29.

109. Garbern JY, Yool DA, Moore GJ, et al. Patients lacking the major CNS myelin protein, proteolipid protein 1, develop length-dependent axonal degeneration in the absence of demyelination and inflammation. Brain 2002;125:551–61.

110. Helms G. T2-based segmentation of periventricular paragraph sign volumes for quantification of proton magnetic paragraph sign resonance spectra of multiple sclerosis lesions. MAGMA 2003;16:10–6.

111. Whittall KP, MacKay AL, Li DK, et al. Normal-appearing white matter in multiple sclerosis has heterogeneous, diffusely prolonged T(2). Magn Reson Med 2002;47:403–8.

112. Evangelou N, Esiri MM, Smith S, et al. Quantitative pathological evidence for axonal loss in normal appearing white matter in multiple sclerosis. Ann Neurol 2000;47:391–5.

113. Walters RJ, Fox NC, Crum WR, et al. Haemodialysis and cerebral oedema. Nephron 2001;87:143–7.

114. Mellanby AR, Reveley MA. Effects of acute dehydration on computerized tomographic assessment of cerebral density and ventricular volume. Lancet 1982;2:874.

115. Rao AB, Richert N, Howard T, et al. Methylprednisolone effect on brain volume and enhancing lesions in MS before and during IFNbeta-1b. Neurology 2002;59:688–94.

116. Zivadinov R, Rudick RA, De Masi R, et al. Effects of IV methylprednisolone on brain atrophy in relapsing-remitting MS. Neurology 2001;57:1239–47.

117. De Stefano N, Bartolozzi ML, Nacmias B, et al. Influence of apolipoprotein E epsilon4 genotype on brain tissue integrity in relapsing-remitting multiple sclerosis. Arch Neurol 2004;61:536–40.

118. Enzinger C, Ropele S, Smith S, et al. Accelerated evolution of brain atrophy and "black holes" in MS patients with APOE-epsilon 4. Ann Neurol 2004;55:563–9.

119. Enzinger C, Fazekas F, Matthews PM, et al. Risk factors for progression of brain atrophy in aging: six-year follow-up of normal subjects. Neurology 2005;64:1704–11.

120. Kidd D, Barkhof F, McConnell R, et al. Cortical lesions in multiple sclerosis. Brain 1999;122(Pt 1):17–26.

121. Geurts JJ, Pouwels PJ, Uitdehaag BM, et al. Intracortical lesions in multiple sclerosis: improved detection with 3D double inversion-recovery MR imaging. Radiology 2005;236:254–60.

122. Kangarlu A, Bourekas EC, Ray-Chaudhury A, et al. Cerebral cortical lesions in multiple sclerosis detected by MR imaging at 8 Tesla. AJNR Am J Neuroradiol 2007;28:262–6.

123. Miller DH, Barkhof F, Frank JA, et al. Measurement of atrophy in multiple sclerosis: pathological basis, methodological aspects and clinical relevance. Brain 2002;125:1676–95.

124. Battaglini M, Smith SM, Brogi S, et al. Enhanced brain extraction improves the accuracy of brain atrophy estimation. Neuroimage 2008;40:583–9.

125. Jasperse B, Valsasina P, Neacsu V, et al. Intercenter agreement of brain atrophy measurement in multiple sclerosis patients using manually-edited SIENA and SIENAX. J Magn Reson Imaging 2007;26:881–5.

126. Bookstein FL. "Voxel-based morphometry" should not be used with imperfectly registered images. Neuroimage 2001;14:1454–62.

The Use of MR Imaging as an Outcome Measure in Multiple Sclerosis Clinical Trials

Robert A. Bermel, MD[a], Elizabeth Fisher, PhD[b],
Jeffrey A. Cohen, MD[a],*

KEYWORDS

- Magnetic resonance imaging • Multiple sclerosis
- Clinical trials • Outcomes

RATIONALE FOR MR IMAGING AS AN OUTCOME MEASURE IN MULTIPLE SCLEROSIS CLINICAL TRIALS

Multiple sclerosis (MS) is characterized pathologically by multifocal central nervous system (CNS) lesions with a combination of inflammatory demyelination and axon loss. These processes are likely tempered by innate mechanisms of remyelination and neural plasticity, the rates of which are insufficient to compensate for the ongoing pathologic changes in most patients. Even without complete knowledge of MS pathogenesis, promising new therapies are actively being evaluated. Clinical trials of any new therapeutic agent depend on sensitive indices of disease activity to detect benefit. These measures ideally should be directly linked to the mechanism of disease.

The principal impetus for use of MR imaging as an outcome measure in MS clinical trials is potentially greater sensitivity to change and treatment effects compared with clinical measures. The ultimate goal of MS disease therapy is to prevent relapses and accumulation of neurologic disability. Demonstration of benefit on these aspects is required for regulatory approval of new treatments. The direct relevance to patient outcome is at the expense of efficiency, however. Even

when tested in patients preselected for a high risk for relapse or disability progression, required sample sizes are large and follow-up relatively prolonged, rendering phase III trials resource-intensive. In addition, in several neurologic diseases, including MS, clinical manifestations often develop late, sometimes after substantial irreversible tissue damage has accumulated. Likewise, in phase II trials, insensitive outcomes are undesirable, because the potential for treatment-related adverse events and placebo-related disease activity necessitates small sample sizes. The inefficiency of clinical outcomes is of even greater concern, because the availability of effective therapies for MS increasingly necessitates inclusion of an active treatment comparator for practical and ethical reasons in the testing of new therapies,[1] which substantially increases the sample size, complexity, and cost of clinical trials. Thus, there is great impetus to develop more sensitive outcome measures.[2,3]

Lesion activity on MR imaging exceeds clinically apparent relapses 5- to 10-fold, providing a much more sensitive measure of the disease process.[4] Statistical power is further enhanced by the continuous nature of some MR imaging variables. When analyzed by a blinded "central reading center" within a clinical trial, MR imaging data provide

[a] Mellen Center for MS Treatment and Research, Neurological Institute, Cleveland Clinic Foundation, 9500 Euclid Avenue, Cleveland, OH 44195, USA
[b] Biomedical Engineering, Lerner Research Institute, Cleveland Clinic Foundation, 9500 Euclid Avenue, Cleveland, OH 44195, USA
* Corresponding author.
E-mail address: cohenj@ccf.org (J. A. Cohen).

Neuroimag Clin N Am 18 (2008) 687–701
doi:10.1016/j.nic.2008.06.008

an independent quantitative means to supplement potentially subjective clinical ratings.[5] MR imaging raw data can be archived and reanalyzed to assess for reproducibility or even extract new variables that were unrecognized at the initial time of the study.

Therefore, MR imaging has received substantial consideration as a potential surrogate measure for MS clinical trials. Prentice[6] defined stringent formal criteria for a surrogate measure. At this time, despite the promise of MR imaging, it does not fulfill the requirements of a surrogate measure. Nevertheless, there are many advantages to using MR imaging–based outcome measures in MS clinical trials (Box 1). MR imaging is useful as the primary end point in early trials providing preliminary evidence of efficacy and as secondary and exploratory end points in pivotal trials providing supporting evidence of efficacy corroborating clinical measures. At all stages of drug development, MR imaging provides data on safety and mechanism of action.

Standard MR imaging measures in MS clinical trials include measures of lesion activity (gadolinium-enhancing [GdE] lesions and new or enlarged T2-hyperintense lesions) and measures of disease severity or burden (total T2-hyperintense lesion volume, total T1-hypointense lesion volume, and whole-brain atrophy). The field has substantial experience in implementing these measures in multicenter clinical trials, estimating the required sample size, statistical analysis of the data generated, and assessing the results of these analyses. A variety of new MR imaging measures potentially provide additional pathologic specificity, or sensitivity to change and treatment effects (magnetization transfer imaging [MTI], diffusion tensor imaging [DTI], proton magnetic resonance spectroscopy [^{1}HMRS], regional atrophy, and functional MR imaging [fMR imaging]) (see Table 1).

STANDARD MR IMAGING MEASURES OF DISEASE ACTIVITY
Gadolinium-Enhancing Lesions

Lesions that are hyperintense on T1 images after administration of gadolinium (Gd) represent focal areas of blood-brain barrier (BBB) disruption, which are presumed to represent areas of active inflammation in MS. After the acute inflammatory stage, MS lesions typically cease to enhance over 2 to 4 weeks. Therefore, GdE activity on a single scan provides information on disease activity over a relatively narrow time window. When scans are performed at frequent (eg, monthly) intervals, the total number or volume of GdE lesions provides a cumulative measure of disease activity over the entire interval. Periods of clinical worsening correlate with increased GdE lesion burden.[7] The relation between GdE lesion activity and neurologic disability is weak over short intervals but stronger over longer intervals. Two factors account for the poor correlation: (1) lesions frequently occur in noneloquent regions of brain and (2) studies have not been sufficiently long to capture the cumulative disability that results only after years of lesion accrual.

Several technical factors must be addressed to ensure valid analysis of GdE lesions in clinical trials. The dose of Gd, time from injection to scanning, and acquisition parameters must be standardized. Higher contrast doses (eg, triple dose) and a planned delay to imaging increase the sensitivity of enhancing lesion detection.[8,9] It remains uncertain whether the GdE lesions detected with different doses of contrast represent comparable pathologic processes, however. Scan acquisition and pulse sequence should be designed to minimize the intrusion of T2 effects into the postcontrast scans, which could lead to false-positive results. Image processing software must allow review by the operator to "veto" pixels incorrectly identified as GdE lesions (eg, blood vessels). In general, total GdE lesion number and volume vary in parallel. A therapeutic agent conceivably could alter lesion evolution but not lesion initiation; as a result, it could decrease GdE volume but not the number of GdE lesions, dissociating the two measures. Therefore, in general, both parameters should be measured in a clinical trial.

Box 1
Advantages of adding MR imaging–derived outcome measures to MS clinical trials

1. Higher sensitivity to disease activity

2. Easy blinding of MR imaging raters to treatment and clinical status (independent analysis and greater objectivity)

3. Greater precision and reproducibility over clinical measures

4. Can provide continuous variables on linear scales

5. Potential retrieval of raw data for post-hoc analyses

6. More closely represents the underlying pathologic findings, potentially yielding drug mechanism–specific information

The degree of the relative advantages varies, based on the specific measure chosen (Table 1).

Table 1
Relative strengths of different MR imaging–based outcome measures

Modality	Pathologic Finding Assessed	Specificity	Multicenter Feasibility
Measures of inflammatory activity			
T2 lesions	Combined	+	++++
GdE lesions	Acute inflammation	++	++++
Measures of axonal/neuronal integrity			
T1 "black holes"	Axons/myelin	++	++++
Whole-brain atrophy	Combined	+	++++
GM atrophy	Combined	++	+++
MTR	Myelin	+++	++
Magnetic resonance spectroscopy	Axons	++++	++
DTI	Axons/myelin	+++	++
fMRI	Function	++	+

New or Enlarged T2-Hyperintense Lesion Number

Because of their transient nature, GdE lesions on a single scan indicate disease activity at that time point only. Because GdE lesions are virtually always associated with T2-hyperintensity,[10] enumerating the number of T2 lesions that are new or enlarged on a follow-up scan compared with baseline provides a measure of lesion activity over that period. T2 lesions comprise a variety of tissue changes, including edema, inflammation, demyelination, remyelination, axon loss, and gliosis. Significant month-to-month fluctuation in T2 lesion volume is attributed to these biological factors as well as technical variability.[11] The criteria for lesion enlargement must take this into account and be defined in advance of data analysis. A typical definition is to classify a lesion as enlarged if it has a 50% increase in diameter (if smaller than 5 mm) or a 20% increase in diameter for a lesion larger than 5 mm.[12] To avoid double-counting T2 lesions that are also GdE, the parameter "combined unique active lesions" is useful.[13]

STANDARD MR IMAGING MEASURES OF DISEASE SEVERITY
T2-Hyperintense Lesion Volume

The most useful method of quantifying the overall "burden of disease" is total volume of abnormal T2-hyperintensity. Despite its lack of pathologic specificity, T2 lesion burden early in the disease strongly predicts long-term disability and brain atrophy.[14] When implementing T2 lesion burden

in a clinical trial, acquisition parameters must be standardized and optimized to maximize sensitivity and reproducibility. Reliable longitudinal detection of small T2 lesions requires protocols with thin tissue slices (generally 3 mm) without interslice gaps. Cerebrospinal fluid (CSF)–suppressed sequences, such as fluid-attenuated inversion recovery (FLAIR), increase sensitivity for periventricular and subcortical lesions compared with traditional T2-weighted or proton density–weighted sequences.[15] The same T2-weighted sequence (conventional spin-echo versus rapid acquisition with relaxation enhancement [RARE] versus a fluid-suppressed sequence) must be used across all sites.[16] Because lesion boundaries are indistinct, automated segmentation approaches are preferable to manual methods because of their greater precision. Conversely, with automated techniques, approaches to limit misclassification of lesions, which can have signal intensity similar to brain tissue or CSF depending on lesion stage and MR imaging pulse sequence, are necessary.[17]

T1-Hypointense Black Holes

A proportion of T2-hyperintense lesions (5%–20%) are hypointense on non-enhanced T1-weighted images, so-called "T1 black holes," representing areas with irreversible tissue loss and axonal destruction.[18] Approximately half of GdE lesions evolve into chronic T1 black holes, making baseline GdE lesion number a strong predictor of subsequent T1 black holes.[19] However, early GdE lesions themselves may appear transiently hypointense on T1-weighted images, due to edema. For this reason GdE lesions should be excluded from the total volume of T1 holes. Total T1 black hole volume correlates more strongly than T2 lesion volume with physical disability, although the absolute magnitude of the correlation remains modest. A stronger association between T1 black hole volume and whole-brain atrophy measures in most studies suggests that axonal disconnection from chronic lesions contributes at least in part to brain atrophy development.[20–22] Thus, total T1-hypointense lesion volume provides a measure of the burden of severe brain tissue destruction.

Whole-Brain Atrophy

Tissue loss can be viewed as the final common pathway for the wide variety of pathologic processes that occur in MS, which can be captured by measurement of whole-brain atrophy. This lack of specificity is an advantage and a shortcoming of brain atrophy as an outcome measure. Whole-brain atrophy becomes extremely apparent in the middle to late stages of the disease,[23,24] but it is detectable even in the earliest stages of the disease, suggesting substantial subclinical pathologic change.[25,26] Short-term whole-brain atrophy progression predicts long-term disability.[27]

Multiple techniques have been developed to measure brain atrophy,[28] including manual linear measurement of central or regional atrophy,[29] semiautomated or automated methods of measuring whole-brain atrophy using segmentation-based techniques,[20,22,30–32] and registration-based techniques to identify changes in brain volume over time.[33–35] Brain atrophy progression and treatment effects can be detected in a 2-year clinical trial when precise automated techniques that normalize brain volume are used.[22] Sample size estimates to demonstrate treatment benefit on whole-brain atrophy progression are similar to those required for lesion analyses. For example, to demonstrate a 50% effect size with 90% power, 44 subjects per arm are needed for a 2-year trial.[36]

An important issue with the use of brain atrophy in clinical trials is that the magnitude of change is small in short-term trials and different measures can produce conflicting results because of differences in reproducibility, susceptibility to artifacts, geometry as a function of anatomic site, and biologic factors determining the rate of atrophy in different structures.[37–39] In addition, brain volume fluctuates as a result of tissue water content related to hydration status and inflammatory activity. This issue is especially relevant to high-dose corticosteroids, which can induce "pseudoatrophy" depending on the timing of their use relative to scan acquisition.[40] Anti-inflammatory effects of MS disease-modifying agents can cause apparent acceleration of atrophy progression at the initiation of therapy.[22] Therefore, when using normalized brain atrophy as a key outcome measure in a clinical trial of an agent expected to have anti-inflammatory activity, it may be useful to use a scan obtained, for example, at month 3 as a revised baseline.

EXPLORATORY MR IMAGING MEASURES FOR CLINICAL TRIALS

MR imaging is useful to track the inflammatory components of MS. Inflammation alone, however, as currently measured by the lesions seen on conventional MR imaging, accounts incompletely for disability progression.[41,42] In studies of a variety of agents in secondary progressive MS, neurologic disability and brain atrophy continued to progress despite effective inhibition lesion activity on MR imaging.[43,44] Therefore, the MR imaging outcomes presented up to this point are unlikely to help in testing treatments targeting the progressive or degenerative component of MS, including potential neuroprotective or reparative strategies. Several imaging approaches have been proposed to provide additional pathologic specificity with greater ability to monitor tissue integrity within lesions visible on standard imaging, normal-appearing brain tissue (NABT), and gray matter (GM).

Magnetization Transfer Imaging

MTI quantifies the interaction between MR imaging–visible free water protons and MR imaging–invisible protons associated with macromolecules (proteins and lipids), providing a measure of tissue integrity, particularly myelin in the brain.[45] MT is quantified using the magnetization transfer ratio (MTR). Demyelination and decreased axonal density decrease MTR compared with normal tissue.[46] Whole-brain MTR correlates strongly with T2 lesion volume and with whole-brain atrophy,[47] raising some question of its added value in clinical trials. MTI provides information on preservation of tissue structure, however, distinguishing it from these other measures.

One approach is to measure MTR over the entire brain, generating a frequency distribution of MTR versus voxel count. Whereas normal controls have a narrow range of MTR values, patients who have MS have a higher proportion of voxels with low values, resulting in a lower mean and higher variance.[48–50] Whole-brain histogram analysis on a relatively large scale (82 patients from five centers) failed to show an effect on MTR for interferon β-1b in secondary progressive MS.[51] An alternative approach is to measure

MTR in defined regions, such as lesions, NABT, white matter, or GM. Following MTR in individual lesions over time, looking for stabilization (suggesting preservation of myelin and axons) or improvement (suggesting remyelination) is a potential way to test neuroprotective or repair strategies.[52] Benefit was demonstrated in small studies for intravenous methylprednisolone (IVMP)[53] and interferon-β[54] using this approach.

Inclusion of MTI in large-scale multicenter trials has been limited by technical issues and difficulty with standardization across sites. These impediments are not as great as with some other advanced imaging measures, however. Guidelines for incorporation of MTI into trials recently were published.[55]

Diffusion Tensor Imaging

With DTI, the diffusivity of water molecules is quantified in multiple spatial directions to determine the orientation and integrity of fiber tracts. As fiber tracts undergo axon loss, their spatial anisotropy is disrupted and molecules diffuse more equally in all directions. This is manifest as increased mean diffusivity and decreased fractional anisotropy. DTI seems to be sensitive to disease-related changes in NABT, even over short periods.[56–58] Analogous to MTI, DTI can be performed on the whole brain, yielding a frequency distribution of values, or in regions of interest. Both approaches can be applied longitudinally over time. A preliminary study suggested that DTI can be performed reproducibly at high field strength across multiple study sites.[59]

Proton Magnetic Resonance Spectroscopy

^{1}HMRS is a technique that derives a nuclear magnetic resonance spectrum from a volume of tissue, yielding relative concentrations of the major proton-yielding metabolites. The most prominent peak in the spectrum from the CNS is N-acetyl aspartate (NAA), almost exclusively contained within neurons and their processes. The concentration of NAA, measured most commonly as a ratio of NAA to creatine (Cr), decreases when there is neuronal dysfunction, damage, or axonal or neuronal loss.[60] Decreased NAA/Cr ratio was demonstrated within MS lesions[61] and in NABT.[62] Use of ^{1}HMRS in clinical trials has been limited, but studies of interferon-β[63–65] and glatiramer acetate[63] demonstrated treatment benefit.

Issues complicating the use of ^{1}HMRS in multicenter trials include the need for standardization of techniques across centers, and the limitations of single-voxel techniques (which are difficult to duplicate over time within patients). With the growing capability of whole-brain MRS techniques,[66,67] some of these issues may be overcome. New recommendations were published to facilitate the use of ^{1}HMRS in multicenter clinical trials.[68]

Spinal Cord Atrophy

A significant portion of the physical disability in MS results from spinal cord involvement and subsequent upper extremity and gait impairment. Patients who had MS were shown to have significant spinal cord atrophy compared with normal controls (up to 40% volume loss), particularly in primary progressive (PP) MS, which progresses over periods as short as 1 year.[69,70] Spinal cord atrophy has not yet been used as a supportive outcome in a major clinical trial, although this approach potentially is of interest, particularly in progressive disease. The principal impediment has been poor reproducibility.

Localized Brain Atrophy

It is possible to separate brain volumes into different compartments, using automated or manual parcellation software. One distinction of particular interest is GM versus white matter. Selective GM atrophy has been noted early in relapsing-remitting (RR) MS and PPMS and correlates with disease severity.[71–74] Measurement of lobar atrophy also is feasible and may correlate best with specific cognitive measures.[75,76] Localized measures of brain atrophy have not been applied prospectively in a major clinical trial. It may be possible to analyze preexisting data sets post hoc, however.

Functional MR Imaging

Focal damage in MS elicits not only attempted tissue repair but neural plasticity, with reassignment of function to other anatomic sites. fMR imaging can be used study the effects of MS on specific pathways and provides a way to interrogate these compensatory mechanisms. Most methods use the different magnetic properties of oxygenated and deoxygenated blood to identify regions of increased or decreased cerebral blood flow (called the blood oxygen level–dependent [BOLD] technique). There may be particular utility in using fMR imaging to study effects on fatigue, a consequence of the disease that has been difficult to quantify objectively thus far.[77] fMR imaging protocols highly dependent on a standardized methodology, as implemented by technicians and other study staff, rendering it challenging to implement longitudinally in multicenter trials.

PURPOSES SERVED BY MR IMAGING IN CLINICAL TRIALS

Some of the measures discussed here are now routinely incorporated into clinical trials at all stages of drug development, wherein they serve multiple purposes. Nevertheless, the emphasis is different in phase I, phase II, and phase III studies.

Subject Selection

MR imaging is commonly used to support the diagnosis of MS in clinical practice and, likewise, for enrollment in clinical trials. Increasingly, trials allow diagnosis of MS by criteria in which dissemination of pathologic change anatomically or over time is confirmed by MR imaging.[78] This effectively expands the pool of subjects eligible for clinical trials. MR imaging is also helpful in excluding subjects who have other neurologic diagnoses mimicking MS.

Requiring GdE lesions on a baseline MR imaging scan has been used as a way to enrich study populations with subjects more likely to experience ongoing disease activity during the trial, and thus able to demonstrate benefit from the intervention. The phenomenon of regression to the mean dictates that periods of activity may be followed by a quiescent period, however, even in the absence of therapy.[79] Therefore, the magnitude of benefit is difficult to quantify without a parallel placebo group.

If randomization is successful in large-scale trials, treatment groups should theoretically be well matched for MR imaging parameters at baseline. In smaller trials (those that are most likely to rely on MR imaging as an outcome measure), randomization may not be effective for all characteristics. Analysis of a screening MR imaging scan for a variable of interest (ie, the presence of GdE lesions) allows the investigators to balance the randomization of treatment allocation a priori, limiting potential confounders in small studies.[12] It is also possible to compensate for potential imbalances statistically; however, at times, results of this approach may be difficult to interpret.

Assessment of Efficacy

Given their increased sensitivity over clinical outcomes, MR imaging measures of MS disease activity are ideally suited to preliminary trials aimed at exploring efficacy of new immunomodulatory agents expected to have a rapid and prominent effect on lesion activity.[80] Use of MR imaging outcomes allows smaller sample size and shorter study duration, with less exposure of study populations to an agent with which there may be limited experience.

The effect of a novel treatment on cumulative disease severity can also be assessed by MR imaging. Quantifying the overall volume of T2 lesions is the most routinely performed measure of overall burden of disease, although whole-brain atrophy is becoming increasingly more common. Measures of cumulative tissue integrity can include T1 black hole volume and advanced MR imaging techniques.

Even in initial small-scale trials, a treatment's relative effect on different MR imaging measures can yield information about the kinetics and mechanism of action of the tested therapy. For instance, a potent suppression of GdE lesions would imply an anti-inflammatory mechanism of action, whereas an improvement on MTI or ^{1}HMRS-derived metrics would suggest tissue repair. The timing of an agent's biologic effect (influenced by its pharmacokinetics and pharmacodynamics) is often first identified in a phase I or phase II study using frequent MR imaging to monitor closely for the outcome of interest.

Monitoring Safety

In initial studies of novel therapies, scans obtained shortly after initiation of treatment can be used to monitor for unexpected increase in disease activity suggesting "reverse efficacy," as was seen in trials of interferon-γ, altered peptide ligand, and anti–tumor necrosis factor-α.[81–83] Increased tissue damage can occur despite a therapeutic decrease in inflammation, for example, the increased rate of brain atrophy seen after immunoablation with bone marrow transplantation rescue.[84] With emerging potent immunomodulatory therapies, neoplasia and opportunistic infection (eg, progressive multifocal leukoencephalopathy)[85] are concerns. Thus, MR imaging also functions as an important safety outcome measure. During development of the protocol, it must be decided whether MR imaging scans are to be monitored for safety issues at the central reading center or at the individual sites.

MR IMAGING IN PHASE I TRIALS

Phase I trials aim to expose a relatively small number of subjects to a new medication for a short period, monitoring primarily for safety concerns. In phase I trials, MR imaging is used primarily to determine eligibility and monitor adverse effects of therapy. MR imaging also can be incorporated to provide preliminary information on efficacy, but because of the typically short duration and small sample size of such trials, clear-cut evidence of efficacy is not expected.

MR IMAGING IN PHASE II TRIALS

At early stages of drug development, information about the magnitude and kinetics of benefit, side effects, and optimal dose needs to be generated to guide future definitive studies. In addition, exposure of subjects to a novel agent of unproved safety and efficacy needs to be minimized, as does exposure to placebo. Clinical outcomes (relapses and disability progression) are insufficiently sensitive to serve as the primary outcome for preliminary studies.

As a result, MR imaging-based studies have become standard for phase II (proof-of-concept) trials in MS. The most common approaches (**Fig. 1**) include frequent (most often monthly) scanning of subjects with active RRMS and enumeration of GdE lesions over periods ranging from 3 to 12 months. There now is substantial experience in the field with such designs, including trial conduct, subject selection, sample size estimation, and data analysis.[86–88] Natalizumab is one of several agents shown to be effective on MR imaging–based outcomes in a phase II proof-of-concept trial,[89] followed by successful phase III pivotal clinical trials.[90,91]

Data on which to base sample size estimates are available from a natural history cohort plus subjects involved in the placebo arms of clinical trials.[92] Assuming a 70% treatment effect on cumulative GdE lesion number (typical of the most recently tested therapies), a sample size of approximately 40 patients per arm provides 80% or greater statistical power in a parallel group design. Assuming rapid onset of therapeutic effect, follow-up for 3 months may be adequate to show efficacy. Nevertheless, longer follow-up often is desirable to avoid missing less prominent or more gradual benefit, confirm persistent efficacy, and provide additional safety data.

Several methods are used to increase the number of on-study events and improve power. One recruitment tactic selects for active subjects by requiring one or more GdE lesions on screening MR imaging. This approach usually is effective but can impede enrollment. In addition, some subjects may have decreased on-study activity after an active scan because of "regression to the mean." Other useful selection criteria (which probably are interrelated) are young age, short disease duration, and recent relapses. Another way potentially to augment on-study events is to increase Gd dose (eg, triple dose) and add a lag time between Gd administration and scanning.[9,93] The additional lesions detected by this approach have unclear pathogenic significance, however, and it is uncertain that this method actually improves the ability to detect differences across treatment groups.

The timing of MR imaging scans in the trial must be laid out to capture the expected effect

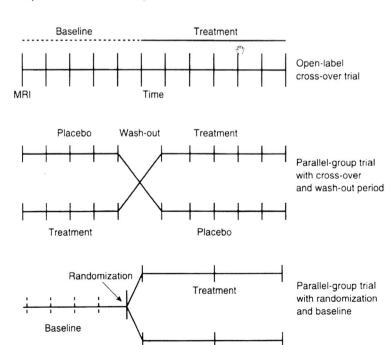

Fig. 1. Three-monthly MR imaging trial designs based on enhanced MR imaging. Vertical lines signify monthly scans. (*Top*) Crossover trial design. A typical design would include a 6-month baseline period followed by a 6-month treatment period. (*Middle*) Parallel-group design with crossover. (*Bottom*) Parallel-group trial with baseline run-in period. (*From* Frank JA, McFarland HF. How to participate in a multiple sclerosis clinical trial. Neuroimaging Clin North Am 2000;10:817–30; with permission.)

on GdE lesions, based on knowledge of the pharmacokinetics and pharmacodynamics of the tested agent. The ability to detect a difference across treatment groups also depends on patient population, specifically the degree to which patients are matched at baseline and their level of inflammatory activity. For an agent expected to have a delayed effect on GdE, early scans can be included to look for evidence of a deleterious increase in disease activity, but principal scans for analysis should be performed later, after a delay.

The intermittent use of IVMP to treat relapses can confound use of GdE as an outcome. IVMP suppresses GdE lesions for 4 to 8 weeks.[94] Delaying a protocol-dictated MR imaging scan to avoid this effect complicates visit scheduling and data analysis. If possible, the preferred approach is to obtain the scheduled scan before administration of IVMP.

A final decision involves whether to include a placebo-treated comparison group. A single-arm crossover design has the advantage that all subjects receive active therapy (after a prebaseline run-in period). Interpretation of the results assumes that GdE lesion activity would have remained constant in the absence of treatment, however, which is frequently invalid. A parallel-group placebo-controlled design is more robust, but there are practical and ethical issues with including a placebo arm. Such studies generally preselect patients who have active RRMS, for whom effective treatments are available. These concerns are partly addressed by keeping the duration of washout periods from prior therapies before study and potential placebo treatment on-study as short as possible and by explicit provisions for detection and treatment of unacceptable disease activity. Investigators and subjects need to be cognizant of this important issue, however.

Phase II designs based on enumeration of GdE lesions work well for agents with a rapid and prominent effect on GdE. If this is not the case, one runs the risk for erroneously discarding a potentially useful agent. There are several immunomodulatory agents expected to have modest or gradual on BBB integrity. From a practical perspective, this shortcoming also applies to testing agents with putative neuroprotective or reparative mechanisms of action. It remains uncertain how to conduct preliminary studies of such agents to obtain data supporting proof of concept before undertaking large-scale pivotal trials. Potential approaches include MTI, DTI, or ^{1}HMRS applied to lesions, specific pathways, or the whole brain.

MR IMAGING IN PHASE III TRIALS

Primary outcomes for phase III (pivotal) trials, which, when successful, lead to regulatory approval for new agents, remain relapses and disability progression. MR imaging metrics serve as important supportive measures, providing corroborating evidence of efficacy.[14,95,96] In all the most recent pivotal trials of new therapies, the effect size on imaging metrics has paralleled or exceeded clinical outcomes.[13,90,91] MR imaging also provides important information for interpreting the results of the study, including characteristics of the population, assessing whether the treatment groups were well matched at baseline, identifying factors predicting responders and nonresponders, and analyzing the effects of factors that can interfere with efficacy (eg, neutralizing antibodies).

Phase III trials in MS typically are large, based on the expected statistical power of clinical end points. In most trials, all subjects undergo standard MR imaging at entry and exit (or annually). Cost and logistics preclude frequent MR imaging of all subjects. Therefore, when included in phase III trials, more frequent or advanced MR imaging usually is performed as a substudy in a cohort of subjects at selected sites. If this approach is taken, separate power analyses are conducted to determine the size of the subset needed to show efficacy on MR imaging end points.[97] Similarly, substudies of advanced MR imaging techniques, which are important to advance the field, can be performed at selected sites with the necessary technical resources and expertise.

STATISTICAL CONSIDERATIONS WITH USE OF MR IMAGING IN TRIALS

A critical assumption in clinical trials is that the treatment groups are matched at baseline before study intervention, particularly on parameters serving as study outcomes or their correlates. In large studies, randomization generally is effective in balancing the characteristics of identified parameters and, it is assumed, unmeasured or unrecognized factors. In small studies, however, such as phase II MR imaging–based MS trials, it is common for treatment groups not to be matched on some MR imaging parameters. Ideally, to avoid this issue, some mechanism should be built into randomization to match the groups on the key MR imaging measures at baseline. One option is to evaluate scans locally at the sites or at the reading center before treatment allocation and to stratify randomization, although both approaches pose several practical hurdles.

Conceptually, it is helpful to distinguish the specific scanning technique performed at the study site (eg, a FLAIR scan) from the MR imaging measure determined at the reading center (eg, total T2-hyperintense lesion volume) from the outcome measure analyzed by the study statistician (eg, between-group difference in baseline to study end absolute change in T2-hyperintense lesion volume). Each step of this sequence must be tailored to the population being studied and biologic question being asked. The specific choice of outcome measure determines the statistical nature of the data. Numbers of GdE or new or enlarged T2 lesions are ordinal data, whereas lesion volume and brain atrophy data are continuous. In phase II studies, the primary outcome is cumulative number of GdE lesions, sometimes beginning after a lag period. A similar approach is used in frequent MR imaging substudies of phase III trials. The most common analytic approach (for lesion volumes and atrophy measurements) in phase III studies is between-group comparison of change from baseline to study end.

Although continuous measures are generally regarded as more robust, lesion volumes often show marked variability from subject to subject; thus, group aggregate change may be obscured. A frequent approach has been to analyze relative change in individual subjects. Subjects with small initial lesion volumes and resultant exaggerated relative (percent) change may inappropriately drive results in this method, however. Absolute within-subject change is therefore favored so as to avoid this effect.

Another issue is that the distribution of MR imaging lesion measurements is often highly skewed, with a few subjects exhibiting high lesion counts or volumes. These subjects can drive the results and, depending on treatment assignment, suggest treatment benefit when none exists or obscure true benefit. A variety of approaches can be used to analyze such data to de-emphasize the small number of highly active subjects, such as nonparametric statistical tests (including categoric data modeling and rank analyses), truncating the data, or transforming the data. This important issue must be considered not only when developing the statistical plan but also when estimating sample size and interpreting the results of the study.

PRACTICAL ASPECTS OF IMAGE ANALYSIS IN TRIALS

Ensuring the technical rigor of the MR imaging aspect of a clinical trial can be difficult. The expertise of a multidisciplinary team with members from neurology, radiology, MR imaging physics, biomedical engineering, computer science, and biostatistics is necessary to guarantee accurate acquisition and analysis of the data. **Fig. 2** depicts the work flow of MR imaging data in a multicenter clinical trial.

First, the acquisition protocol must generate images that can be quantified reliably and accurately yet be technically feasible at the participating study sites and tolerable to subjects. The MR imaging reading center must be able to receive, read, and analyze data reliably from the scanners

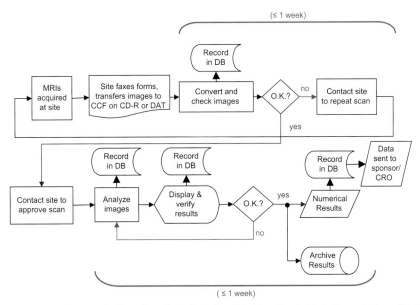

Fig. 2. Example MR imaging work flow for clinical trials. CCF, Cleveland Clinic Foundation; CD-R, recordable compact disc, CRO, clinical research organization, DAT, digital audio tape, DB, database. (*Courtesy of* Cleveland Clinic Foundation, Cleveland, OH; with permission.)

Table 2
Steps to ensure high-quality MR imaging data in a clinical trial

Study	MR Imaging Analysis Center Personnel	Participating Site Personnel
Before study		

Design MR imaging protocol with appropriate pulse sequences and consideration of:
    Ease of standardization across sites
    Reasonable acquisition time
    High tissue contrast/lesion conspicuity
    Resolution/slice thickness/coverage
	PI, RE	—

Select and evaluate MR imaging analysis software to ensure:
    High accuracy and reproducibility
    Functionality in multicenter studies
    Feasibility for a large number of scans (automation, user time required per scan)
	RE	—

Setup image analysis database, data handling, documentation, and standard operating procedures	RE, SC	—
Train MR imaging analysis center personnel	RE, Tech	—
Provide MR imaging manual to participating sites	SC	—
Train participating sites (investigators meeting)	RE, Tech	PI, SC, Tech
Evaluate site performance (MR imaging dummy scans)	RE, SC	SC, Tech
During study		

Communicate frequently with sites to ensure:
    Scans are sent to reading center in a timely manner
    Same scanner and protocol are used throughout the study
    Scans approved or rejected
	SC	SC

Evaluate study scans for:
    Complete and error-free electronic transfer
    Adherence to protocol
    Consistency with previous scans
    Image quality
	SC, RE, Tech	SC, Tech

Repeat acquisition of rejected images	SC	PI, SC, Tech
Monitor and account for scanner hardware and software upgrades (prospectively or retrospectively)	SC, Tech	Tech

Analyze scans according to prespecified procedures with consideration of:
    Consistent operator for a given patient (semiautomated software)
    Consistent parameters used for a given patient (automated software)
	SC, Tech	—

Review and visually verify analysis results	SC, RE	—
After study		
Perform final quality assurance on analysis results	PI, RE	—
Archive raw MRI data	SC, Tech	SC, Tech
Archive MRI analysis results	SC, Tech	—

Abbreviations: PI, study or site principal investigator; RE, radiologist/imaging engineer/physicist in charge of the central MR imaging analysis center; SC, study coordinator; Tech, MR imaging technologist or other technical personnel.

used at the sites, which may come from a variety of manufacturers, use different software, and have different field strengths. A test scan usually is required from each study site before enrolling study subjects to ensure appropriate scan acquisition and data transfer procedures. Use of the same scanner or at least the same model and software at a particular site is important; scanner changes during a trial can have significant effects on the data acquired, for which even complex corrective postprocessing approaches may inadequately compensate.[16,98,99] Scanner upgrades and replacement usually are not under control of the study investigators, however. **Table 2** lists additional quality control measures and the responsible parties at the study site or the central MR imaging analysis center.

Data flow between the individual sites and the analysis center should be as rapid and seamless as possible. Accurate tracking of data and prompt assessment of transmitted studies allow efficient feedback to study sites. Analysis of imaging data on an ongoing basis is preferable to batch analysis at the end of a trial so that technical errors can be corrected before they are repeated. This approach also facilitates the provision of preliminary MR imaging data to the study team and data safety monitoring board.

Volumetric measurements can be performed by several techniques,[28] including manual tracing methods, semiautomated methods in which a user places a seed point at the edge of the structure of interest,[20,100,101] or automated methods based on signal intensities and spatial information.[102–104] Automated methods (as depicted in **Fig. 3**) are generally preferable in that (once established) they are less time- and labor-intensive, are unbiased, and have higher reproducibility.[105] Any method that does not use human oversight for error checking runs the risk for misclassifying tissue types, however.[17]

When individual lesions or regional atrophy is tracked over time, image registration is necessary. Consistent slice angle and level can be reproduced by repositioning of the subject in the scanner at each imaging session. This method is somewhat imprecise, however, and labor-intensive. Image registration through postprocessing is more accurate, places less demand on MR imaging personnel and subjects, and also can compensate for changes in magnetic field homogeneity. The latter issue is particularly relevant to newer echo-planar sequences, such as those used in DTI.

SUMMARY

MR imaging is an integral part of MS clinical trials. It provides the primary efficacy outcome of preliminary proof-of-concept studies and important corroborating data as secondary and exploratory outcomes in pivotal trials. At all stages of drug development, MR imaging provides important information on the kinetics and magnitude of treatment effect and insight into potential mechanisms of action. Attention to issues in scan acquisition, quantitative image processing, and statistical analysis is critical to generate high-quality data. Although it is unlikely that one single outcome measure can capture all aspects of the MS disease process, there is potential for MR imaging outcomes to evaluate inflammatory and degenerative components within clinical trials.

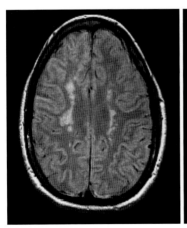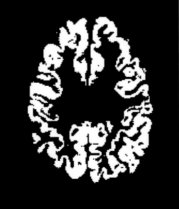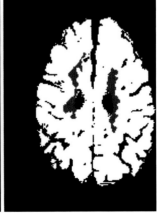

Fig. 3. Example of image analysis results using automated segmentation for a single slice. Left to right are the proton density–weighted image, GM mask, and brain lesion mask.

REFERENCES

1. Lublin FD, Reingold SC. Placebo-controlled clinical trials in multiple sclerosis: ethical considerations. National Multiple Sclerosis Society (USA) Task Force on Placebo-Controlled Clinical Trials in MS. Ann Neurol 2001;49(5):677–81.

2. Cohen JA, Rudick RA. Aspects of multiple sclerosis that relate to trial design and clinical management. In: Cohen JA, Rudick RA, editors. Multiple sclerosis therapeutics. 3rd edition. London: Informa Healthcare; 2007. p. 3–22.

3. Sormani MP, Rovaris M, Bagnato F, et al. Sample size estimations for MRI-monitored trials of MS comparing new vs standard treatments. Neurology 2001;57(10):1883–5.

4. Paty DW, Li DK, Oger JJ, et al. Magnetic resonance imaging in the evaluation of clinical trials in multiple sclerosis. Ann Neurol 1994;36(Suppl):S95–6.

5. Martinelli Boneschi F, Rovaris M, Comi G, et al. The use of magnetic resonance imaging in multiple sclerosis: lessons learned from clinical trials. Multiple Sclerosis 2004;10(4):341–7.

6. Prentice RL. Surrogate endpoints in clinical trials: definition and operational criteria. Stat Med 1989; 8(4):431–40.

7. Smith ME, Stone LA, Albert PS, et al. Clinical worsening in multiple sclerosis is associated with increased frequency and area of gadopentetate dimeglumine-enhancing magnetic resonance imaging lesions. Ann Neurol 1993;33(5):480–9.

8. Filippi M, Rovaris M, Capra R, et al. A multi-centre longitudinal study comparing the sensitivity of monthly MRI after standard and triple dose gadolinium-DTPA for monitoring disease activity in multiple sclerosis. Implications for phase II clinical trials. Brain 1998;121(Pt 10):2011–20.

9. Silver NC, Good CD, Sormani MP, et al. A modified protocol to improve the detection of enhancing brain and spinal cord lesions in multiple sclerosis. J Neurol 2001;248(3):215–24.

10. Molyneux PD, Filippi M, Barkhof F, et al. Correlations between monthly enhanced MRI lesion rate and changes in T2 lesion volume in multiple sclerosis. Ann Neurol 1998;43(3):332–9.

11. Stone LA, Albert PS, Smith ME, et al. Changes in the amount of diseased white matter over time in patients with relapsing-remitting multiple sclerosis. Neurology 1995;45(10):1808–14.

12. Simon JH, Miller DE. Measures of gadolinium enhancement, T1 black holes and T2-hyperintense lesions on magnetic resonance imaging. In: Cohen JA, Rudick RA, editors. Multiple sclerosis therapeutics. 3rd edition. London: Informa Healthcare; 2007. p. 113–42.

13. Li DK, Paty DW. Magnetic resonance imaging results of the PRISMS trial: a randomized, double-blind, placebo-controlled study of interferon-beta1a in relapsing-remitting multiple sclerosis. Prevention of relapses and disability by interferon-beta1a subcutaneously in multiple sclerosis. Ann Neurol 1999;46(2):197–206.

14. Rudick RA, Lee JC, Simon J, et al. Significance of T2 lesions in multiple sclerosis: a 13-year longitudinal study. Ann Neurol 2006;60(2):236–42.

15. Bakshi R, Ariyaratana S, Benedict RH, et al. Fluid-attenuated inversion recovery magnetic resonance imaging detects cortical and juxtacortical multiple sclerosis lesions. Arch Neurol 2001; 58(5):742–8.

16. Filippi M, Rocca MA, Gasperini C, et al. Interscanner variation in brain MR lesion load measurements in multiple sclerosis using conventional spin-echo, rapid relaxation-enhanced, and fast-FLAIR sequences. AJNR Am J Neuroradiol 1999;20(1): 133–7.

17. Sanfilipo MP, Benedict RH, Sharma J, et al. The relationship between whole brain volume and disability in multiple sclerosis: a comparison of normalized gray vs. white matter with misclassification correction. Neuroimage 2005;26(4):1068–77.

18. van Walderveen MA, Kamphorst W, Scheltens P, et al. Histopathologic correlate of hypointense lesions on T1-weighted spin-echo MRI in multiple sclerosis. Neurology 1998;50(5):1282–8.

19. Simon JH, Lull J, Jacobs LD, et al. A longitudinal study of T1 hypointense lesions in relapsing MS: MSCRG trial of interferon beta-1a. Multiple Sclerosis Collaborative Research Group. Neurology 2000;55(2):185–92.

20. Bermel RA, Sharma J, Tjoa CW, et al. A semiautomated measure of whole-brain atrophy in multiple sclerosis. J Neurol Sci 2003;208(1–2):57–65.

21. Paolillo A, Pozzilli C, Gasperini C, et al. Brain atrophy in relapsing-remitting multiple sclerosis: relationship with 'black holes,' disease duration and clinical disability. J Neurol Sci 2000;174(2):85–91.

22. Rudick RA, Fisher E, Lee JC, et al. Use of the brain parenchymal fraction to measure whole brain atrophy in relapsing-remitting MS. Multiple Sclerosis Collaborative Research Group. Neurology 1999; 53(8):1698–704.

23. Miller DH, Barkhof F, Frank JA, et al. Measurement of atrophy in multiple sclerosis: pathological basis, methodological aspects and clinical relevance. Brain 2002;125(Pt 8):1676–95.

24. Bermel RA, Bakshi R. The measurement and clinical relevance of brain atrophy in multiple sclerosis. Lancet Neurol 2006;5(2):158–70.

25. Paolillo A, Piattella MC, Pantano P, et al. The relationship between inflammation and atrophy in clinically isolated syndromes suggestive of multiple sclerosis: a monthly MRI study after triple-dose gadolinium-DTPA. J Neurol 2004;251(4):432–9.

26. Brex PA, Jenkins R, Fox NC, et al. Detection of ventricular enlargement in patients at the earliest clinical stage of MS. Neurology 2000;54(8): 1689–91.

27. Fisher E, Rudick RA, Cutter G, et al. Relationship between brain atrophy and disability: an 8-year follow-up study of multiple sclerosis patients. Mult Scler 2000;6(6):373–7.

28. Pelletier D, Garrison K, Henry R. Measurement of whole-brain atrophy in multiple sclerosis. [Review] [53 refs]. J Neuroimaging 2004;14(3 Suppl). 11S–9S.

29. Simon JH. Linear and regional measures of brain atrophy in multiple sclerosis. In: Zivadinov R, Bakshi R, editors. Hauppauge (NY): Nova Science; 2004. p. 15–27.

30. Ge Y, Grossman RI, Udupa JK, et al. Brain atrophy in relapsing-remitting multiple sclerosis and secondary progressive multiple sclerosis: longitudinal quantitative analysis. Radiology 2000;214(3):665–70.

31. Smith SM, Zhang Y, Jenkinson M, et al. Accurate, robust, and automated longitudinal and cross-sectional brain change analysis. Neuroimage 2002;17(1):479–89.

32. Collins DL, Montagnat J, Zijdenbos AP, et al. Automated estimation of brain volume in multiple sclerosis with BICCR. Lect Notes Comput Sci 2001;2082:141–7.

33. Fox NC, Jenkins R, Leary SM, et al. Progressive cerebral atrophy in MS: a serial study using registered, volumetric MRI. Neurology 2000;54(4): 807–12.

34. Smith SM, De Stefano N, Jenkinson M, et al. Normalized accurate measurement of longitudinal brain change. J Comput Assist Tomogr 2001; 25(3):466–75.

35. Chard DT, Parker GJ, Griffin CM, et al. The reproducibility and sensitivity of brain tissue volume measurements derived from an SPM-based segmentation methodology. J Magn Reson Imaging 2002;15(3):259–67.

36. Anderson VM, Bartlett JW, Fox NC, et al. Detecting treatment effects on brain atrophy in relapsing remitting multiple sclerosis: sample size estimates. J Neurol 2007;254(11):1588–94.

37. Zivadinov R, Grop A, Sharma J, et al. Reproducibility and accuracy of quantitative magnetic resonance imaging techniques of whole-brain atrophy measurement in multiple sclerosis. J Neuroimaging 2005;15(1):27–36.

38. Jones CK, Riddehough A, Li DKB, et al. MRI cerebral atrophy in relapsing-remitting MS: results from the PRISMS trial. Neurology 2001;56(Suppl 3):A379 [abstract].

39. Filippi M, Rovaris M, Inglese M, et al. Interferon beta-1a for brain tissue loss in patients at presentation with syndromes suggestive of multiple sclerosis: a randomised, double-blind, placebo-controlled trial. Lancet 2004;364(9444):1489–96.

40. Fox RJ, Fisher E, Tkach J, et al. Brain atrophy and magnetization transfer ratio following methylprednisolone in multiple sclerosis: short-term changes and long-term implications. Mult Scler 2005;11(2):140–5.

41. Kappos L, Moeri D, Radue EW, et al. Predictive value of gadolinium-enhanced magnetic resonance imaging for relapse rate and changes in disability or impairment in multiple sclerosis: a meta-analysis. Gadolinium MRI Meta-analysis Group. Lancet 1999;353(9157):964–9.

42. Sormani MP, Bruzzi P, Beckmann K, et al. MRI metrics as surrogate endpoints for EDSS progression in SPMS patients treated with IFN beta-1b. Neurology 2003;60(9):1462–6.

43. Paolillo A, Coles AJ, Molyneux PD, et al. Quantitative MRI in patients with secondary progressive MS treated with monoclonal antibody Campath 1H. Neurology 1999;53(4):751–7.

44. Rice GP, Filippi M, Comi G. Cladribine and progressive: clinical and MRI outcomes of a multicenter controlled trial. Cladribine MRI Study Group. Neurology 2000;54(5):1145–55.

45. Filippi M, McGowan JC, Tortorella C. Measures of magnetization transfer in multiple sclerosis. In: Cohen JA, Rudick RA, editors. Multiple sclerosis therapeutics. 3rd edition. London: Informa Healthcare; 2007. p. 143–71.

46. van Waesberghe JH, Kamphorst W, De Groot CJ, et al. Axonal loss in multiple sclerosis lesions: magnetic resonance imaging insights into substrates of disability. Ann Neurol 1999;46(5):747–54.

47. Phillips MD, Grossman RI, Miki Y, et al. Comparison of T2 lesion volume and magnetization transfer ratio histogram analysis and of atrophy and measures of lesion burden in patients with multiple sclerosis. AJNR Am J Neuroradiol 1998;19(6):1055–60.

48. Cercignani M, Iannucci G, Rocca MA, et al. Pathologic damage in MS assessed by diffusion-weighted and magnetization transfer MRI. Neurology 2000;54(5):1139–44.

49. Filippi M, Iannucci G, Tortorella C, et al. Comparison of MS clinical phenotypes using conventional and magnetization transfer MRI. Neurology 1999; 52(3):588–94.

50. Kalkers NF, Hintzen RQ, van Waesberghe JH, et al. Magnetization transfer histogram parameters reflect all dimensions of MS pathology, including atrophy. J Neurol Sci 2001;184(2):155–62.

51. Inglese M, van Waesberghe JH, Rovaris M, et al. The effect of interferon beta-1b on quantities derived from MT MRI in secondary progressive MS. Neurology 2003;60(5):853–60.

52. van Waesberghe JH, van Walderveen MA, Castelijns JA, et al. Patterns of lesion development

in multiple sclerosis: longitudinal observations with T1-weighted spin-echo and magnetization transfer MR. AJNR Am J Neuroradiol 1998;19(4):675–83.

53. Richert ND, Ostuni JL, Bash CN, et al. Interferon beta-1b and intravenous methylprednisolone promote lesion recovery in multiple sclerosis. Mult Scler 2001;7(1):49–58.

54. Kita M, Goodkin DE, Bacchetti P, et al. Magnetization transfer ratio in new MS lesions before and during therapy with IFNbeta-1a. Neurology 2000;54(9):1741–5.

55. Horsfield MA, Barker GJ, Barkhof F, et al. Guidelines for using quantitative magnetization transfer magnetic resonance imaging for monitoring treatment of multiple sclerosis. J Magn Reson Imaging 2003;17(4):389–97.

56. Rocca MA, Cercignani M, Iannucci G, et al. Weekly diffusion-weighted imaging of normal-appearing white matter in MS. Neurology 2000;55(6):882–4.

57. Werring DJ, Brassat D, Droogan AG, et al. The pathogenesis of lesions and normal-appearing white matter changes in multiple sclerosis: a serial diffusion MRI study. Brain 2000;123(Pt 8):1667–76.

58. Cassol E, Ranjeva JP, Ibarrola D, et al. Diffusion tensor imaging in multiple sclerosis: a tool for monitoring changes in normal-appearing white matter. Mult Scler 2004;10(2):188–96.

59. Fox RJ, Sakaie K, Lee JC, et al. A validation study of multi-centre diffusion tensor imaging. Mult Scler 2007;13(Suppl 7):S76.

60. Bjartmar C, Battistuta J, Terada N, et al. N-acetylaspartate is an axon-specific marker of mature white matter in vivo: a biochemical and immunohistochemical study on the rat optic nerve. Ann Neurol 2002;51(1):51–8.

61. Matthews PM, Pioro E, Narayanan S, et al. Assessment of lesion pathology in multiple sclerosis using quantitative MRI morphometry and magnetic resonance spectroscopy. Brain 1996;119(Pt 3):715–22.

62. Fu L, Matthews PM, De Stefano N, et al. Imaging axonal damage of normal-appearing white matter in multiple sclerosis. Brain 1998;121(Pt 1):103–13.

63. Khan O, Shen Y, Caon C, et al. Axonal metabolic recovery and potential neuroprotective effect of glatiramer acetate in relapsing-remitting multiple sclerosis. Mult Scler 2005;11(6):646–51.

64. Sarchielli P, Presciutti O, Tarducci R, et al. 1H-MRS in patients with multiple sclerosis undergoing treatment with interferon beta-1a: results of a preliminary study. J Neurol Neurosurg Psychiatry 1998;64(2):204–12.

65. Parry A, Corkill R, Blamire AM, et al. Beta-interferon treatment does not always slow the progression of axonal injury in multiple sclerosis. J Neurol 2003;250(2):171–8.

66. Inglese M, Ge Y, Filippi M, et al. Indirect evidence for early widespread gray matter involvement in relapsing-remitting multiple sclerosis. Neuroimage 2004;21(4):1825–9.

67. Rovaris M, Gambini A, Gallo A, et al. Axonal injury in early multiple sclerosis is irreversible and independent of the short-term disease evolution. Neurology 2005;65(10):1626–30.

68. De Stefano N, Filippi M, Miller D, et al. Guidelines for using proton MR spectroscopy in multicenter clinical MS studies. Neurology 2007;69(20):1942–52.

69. Simon JH. Brain and spinal cord atrophy in multiple sclerosis. Neuroimaging Clin N Am 2000;10(4):753–70.

70. Stevenson VL, Leary SM, Losseff NA, et al. Spinal cord atrophy and disability in MS: a longitudinal study. Neurology 1998;51(1):234–8.

71. Sailer M, Fischl B, Salat D, et al. Focal thinning of the cerebral cortex in multiple sclerosis. Brain 2003;126(Pt 8):1734–44 [see comment].

72. De Stefano N, Matthews PM, Filippi M, et al. Evidence of early cortical atrophy in MS: relevance to white matter changes and disability. Neurology 2003;60(7):1157–62.

73. Tiberio M, Chard DT, Altmann DR, et al. Gray and white matter volume changes in early RRMS: a 2-year longitudinal study. Neurology 2005;64(6):1001–7.

74. Sastre-Garriga J, Ingle GT, Chard DT, et al. Grey and white matter atrophy in early clinical stages of primary progressive multiple sclerosis. Neuroimage 2004;22(1):353–9.

75. Sanfilipo MP, Benedict RH, Weinstock-Guttman B, et al. Gray and white matter brain atrophy and neuropsychological impairment in multiple sclerosis. Neurology 2006;66(5):685–92.

76. Benedict RH, Zivadinov R, Carone DA, et al. Regional lobar atrophy predicts memory impairment in multiple sclerosis. AJNR Am J Neuroradiol 2005;26(7):1824–31.

77. Filippi M, Rocca MA, Colombo B, et al. Functional magnetic resonance imaging correlates of fatigue in multiple sclerosis. Neuroimage 2002;15(3):559–67.

78. Polman CH, Reingold SC, Edan G, et al. Diagnostic criteria for multiple sclerosis: 2005 revisions to the "McDonald Criteria." Ann Neurol 2005;58(6):840–6.

79. Martinez-Yelamos S, Martinez-Yelamos A, Martin Ozaeta G, et al. Regression to the mean in multiple sclerosis. Mult Scler 2006;12(6):826–9.

80. Katz D, Taubenberger JK, Cannella B, et al. Correlation between magnetic resonance imaging findings and lesion development in chronic, active multiple sclerosis. Ann Neurol 1993;34(5):661–9.

81. Panitch HS, Hirsch RL, Schindler J, et al. Treatment of multiple sclerosis with gamma interferon: exacerbations associated with activation of the immune system. Neurology 1987;37(7):1097–102.

82. The Lenercept Multiple Sclerosis Study Group and The University of British Columbia MS/MRI Analysis Group. TNF neutralization in MS: results of a randomized, placebo-controlled multicenter study. Neurology 1999;53(3):457–65.

83. Bielekova B, Goodwin B, Richert N, et al. Encephalitogenic potential of the myelin basic protein peptide (amino acids 83-99) in multiple sclerosis: results of a phase II clinical trial with an altered peptide ligand. Nat Med 2000;6(10):1167–75.

84. Chen JT, Collins DL, Atkins HL, et al. Brain atrophy after immunoablation and stem cell transplantation in multiple sclerosis. Neurology 2006;66(12):1935–7.

85. Langer-Gould A, Atlas SW, Green AJ, et al. Progressive multifocal leukoencephalopathy in a patient treated with natalizumab. N Engl J Med 2005;353(4):375–81.

86. Kappos L, Antel J, Comi G, et al. Oral fingolimod (FTY720) for relapsing multiple sclerosis. N Engl J Med 2006;355(11):1124–40.

87. Tubridy N, Behan PO, Capildeo R, et al. The effect of anti-alpha4 integrin antibody on brain lesion activity in MS. The UK Antegren Study Group. Neurology 1999;53(3):466–72.

88. Bielekova B, Richert N, Howard T, et al. Humanized anti-CD25 (daclizumab) inhibits disease activity in multiple sclerosis patients failing to respond to interferon beta. Proc Natl Acad Sci U S A 2004;101(23):8705–8.

89. O'Connor P, Miller D, Riester K, et al. Relapse rates and enhancing lesions in a phase II trial of natalizumab in multiple sclerosis. Mult Scler 2005;11(5):568–72.

90. Polman CH, O'Connor PW, Havrdova E, et al. A randomized, placebo-controlled trial of natalizumab for relapsing multiple sclerosis. N Engl J Med 2006;354(9):899–910.

91. Rudick RA, Stuart WH, Calabresi PA, et al. Natalizumab plus interferon beta-1a for relapsing multiple sclerosis. N Engl J Med 2006;354(9):911–23.

92. Sormani MP, Molyneux PD, Gasperini C, et al. Statistical power of MRI monitored trials in multiple sclerosis: new data and comparison with previous results. J Neurol Neurosurg Psychiatry 1999;66(4):465–9.

93. Filippi M, Yousry T, Campi A, et al. Comparison of triple dose versus standard dose gadolinium-DTPA for detection of MRI enhancing lesions in patients with MS. Neurology 1996;46(2):379–84.

94. Gasperini C, Pozzilli C, Bastianello S, et al. The influence of clinical relapses and steroid therapy on the development of Gd-enhancing lesions: a longitudinal MRI study in relapsing-remitting multiple sclerosis patients. Acta Neurol Scand 1997;95(4):201–7.

95. Goodin DS. Magnetic resonance imaging as a surrogate outcome measure of disability in multiple sclerosis: have we been overly harsh in our assessment? Ann Neurol 2006;59(4):597–605.

96. Filippi M, Rocca MA, Comi G. The use of quantitative magnetic-resonance-based techniques to monitor the evolution of multiple sclerosis. Lancet Neurol 2003;2(6):337–46.

97. Molyneux PD, Miller DH, Filippi M, et al. The use of magnetic resonance imaging in multiple sclerosis treatment trials: power calculations for annual lesion load measurement. J Neurol 2000;247(1):34–40.

98. Han X, Jovicich J, Salat D, et al. Reliability of MRI-derived measurements of human cerebral cortical thickness: the effects of field strength, scanner upgrade and manufacturer. Neuroimage 2006;32(1):180–94.

99. Gasperini C, Rovaris M, Sormani MP, et al. Intra-observer, inter-observer and inter-scanner variations in brain MRI volume measurements in multiple sclerosis. Mult Scler 2001;7(1):27–31.

100. Molyneux PD, Wang L, Lai M, et al. Quantitative techniques for lesion load measurement in multiple sclerosis: an assessment of the global threshold technique after non uniformity and histogram matching corrections. Eur J Neurol 1998;5(1):55–60.

101. Raff U, Rojas GM, Hutchinson M, et al. Quantitation of T2 lesion load in patients with multiple sclerosis: a novel semiautomated segmentation technique. Acad Radiol 2000;7(4):237–47.

102. Alfano B, Brunetti A, Larobina M, et al. Automated segmentation and measurement of global white matter lesion volume in patients with multiple sclerosis. J Magn Reson Imaging 2000;12(6):799–807.

103. Anbeek P, Vincken KL, van Osch MJ, et al. Automatic segmentation of different-sized white matter lesions by voxel probability estimation. Med Image Anal 2004;8(3):205–15.

104. Wu Y, Warfield SK, Tan IL, et al. Automated segmentation of multiple sclerosis lesion subtypes with multichannel MRI. Neuroimage 2006;32(3):1205–15.

105. Achiron A, Gicquel S, Miron S, et al. Brain MRI lesion load quantification in multiple sclerosis: a comparison between automated multispectral and semi-automated thresholding computer-assisted techniques. Magn Reson Imaging 2002;20(10):713–20.

Variants of Multiple Sclerosis

Jack H. Simon, MD, PhD[a,b,*], B.K. Kleinschmidt-DeMasters, MD[c]

KEYWORDS

- Devic's Neuromyelitis optica
- Balo's concentric sclerosis • Marburg MS
- Schilder's disease

The so-called variants of multiple sclerosis (MS) although relatively rare are clinically important as they cause considerable diagnostic uncertainty and, sometimes, misdiagnosis. As new more aggressive and more targeted treatments for MS and its variants are developed, accurate diagnosis becomes more critical. The variants of MS are also instructive as they force imagers, clinicians, and basic scientists to consider the factors that result in variant imaging for these unusual clinical/immunologic presentations. One variant, Devic's Neuromyelitis optica (NMO), has been central to discovery of an entirely new pathophysiology involving water channels, which was revealed in recent years.

Controversies and history that are central features in many discussions of the MS variants have been previously addressed.[1] For this article, the authors' approach is to discuss the currently clinically most important MS variants, ie, those that are most likely to be seen or considered in clinical practice, including NMO, Balo's concentric sclerosis (BCS), Marburg MS, and Schilder's disease. Acute disseminated encephalomyelitis (ADEM) is briefly discussed as its clinical presentation, imaging, and pathologic features frequently elicit a discussion of the MS variants **Table 1**.

DEVIC'S NEUROMYELITIS OPTICA

NMO has been classified as an inflammatory, demyelinating disease with features that overlap with MS. However, with recent discoveries that related initially to serum markers (immunoglobulins) and subsequently to the specific targets of these immunoglobulins (aquaporins), NMO is now accepted as distinct from MS. The NMO serum biomarker, an autoantibody called NMO-IgG, first aroused interest as it showed promise as a more specific measure for NMO,[2] potentially distinguishing NMO from MS, but it also distinguished MS from ADEM and possibly Asian forms of MS with stronger spinal-optic presentations. NMO-IgG was subsequently found to specifically target aquaporin-4 (AQP4), the most abundant water channel in the central nervous system (CNS).[3] The current hypothesis is that action at the AQP4-rich sites in the CNS may be an underlying pathophysiologic mechanism for NMO,[4–7] in contrast to the mostly unknown pathophysiologic mechanisms in MS and the other MS variants.

Clinical

NMO is characterized clinically by acute visual loss, often bilateral, and/or acute transverse myelitis, but with the visual and spinal cord signs and symptoms often presenting nearly simultaneously. The visual symptoms of NMO usually precede the spinal symptoms, but the reverse is not uncommon. Severe visual symptoms with blindness may become total and permanent within a few days and bilateral optic neuritis is most common. This is in contrast to MS where bilateral optic neuritis is relatively uncommon and the initial visual compromise is usually limited and reversible. In patients who present with visual system

[a] Imaging, Portland VA Medical Center, Mail Stop P2IMAG, 3710 SW Veterans Hospital Road, Portland, OR 97207, USA

[b] Departments of Radiology and Neurology, Oregon Health and Sciences University, Portland, OR, USA

[c] Departments of Pathology, Neurology and Neurosurgery, University of Colorado Health Sciences Center, Denver, CO, USA

* Corresponding author.

E-mail address: jack.simon3@va.gov (J.H. Simon).

Neuroimag Clin N Am 18 (2008) 703–716
doi:10.1016/j.nic.2008.06.003
1052-5149/08/$ – see front matter. Published by Elsevier Inc.

Table 1
Classical features of the MS variants compared with acute disseminated encephalomyelitis and relapsing MS

	Relapsing MS	Acute Disseminated Encephalomyelitis	Devic's Neuromyelitis Optica	Balo's Concentric Sclerosis	Schilder's Disease	Marburg MS
Age	Childhood to adult	Childhood to adult	Childhood to adult	Childhood to adult	Predominantly children	Typically in young adult
Typical clinical course	Early events often subclinical Early deficits mostly reversible Most relapsing early, later progressive	Acute onset Encephalopathy, headaches, vomiting, drowsiness, fever and lethargy Mostly monophasic, some polyphasic Preceding illness, vaccination	Acute onset Nearly synchronous myelopathy and optic neuropathy (either first) Fixed & severe deficits with each attack Monophasic or relapsing	Symptoms suggesting mass may occur Typical lesions (one or few) at presentation, may suggest mass Rarely can occur during course of typical relapsing MS Historically acute, severe but highly variable. By MRI more common and more benign	Acute onset Headache, vomiting seizures, visual problems No prodrome Variable course	Acute onset, poorly responsive Death not uncommon in weeks-months Typically monophasic
MR imaging brain	Brain with multifocal lesions, periventricular moreso than peripheral white, but both Lesions suggest dissemination in time Chronic T1 hypointensities (black holes)	Multifocal, large lesions, may involve brain stem Basal ganglia and thalamus may contain symmetric lesions Often (but not strictly) synchronous enhancement (lesions of similar age initially)	Brain white matter normal, or non-specific. More rarely, an unusual periependymal pattern	Lamellar lesions in isolation or accompanying typical MS-like lesions	Typical large (2-3 cm), bihemispheric centrum ovale white matter lesions	Multifocal diffuse white matter lesions in brain or brainstem, highly destructive, impressively progressive over time

						MS-like
MR imaging spinal cord	Vertical oriented but length ≤2 vertebra Partial transverse involvement Acute mild at most swelling T1- hypointensity extreme rare, acute or chronic stages	May have long vertical pathology greater than for MS May have prominent swelling	May have long vertical pathology greater than for MS Prominent swelling common Near full transverse involvement T1-hypointensity in acute and chronic stages is common			
Pathology	Multifocal demyelination, variable injury, not restricted to perivenous regions. Lesions of differing ages; most old lesions well demarcated from surrounding white matter, with sharp borders	Perivenous inflammation, demyelination	Demyelination and necrosis with severe axonal injury and cavitation; damage predominantly or exclusively in optic nerve and spinal cord, often affected long segments of cord	Concentric zones of normal myelin alternating with demyelination	Severe myelin loss; large, well demarcated, bilateral white matter plaques involving cerebral hemispheric white matter	Severe acute myelin loss with numerous Luxol fast blue-positive macrophages; widely distributed, becoming confluent.

difficulties, transverse myelitis characteristically develops within a few weeks, with severe paraplegia, sensory loss with a distinct level, and sphincter disturbances. Fixed weakness from onset, rather than improvement over time after the initial event is the typical course, again in contrast to MS where weakness is frequently reversible in the early stages and where the spinal cord involvement, both clinically and by imaging, is usually partial transverse (asymmetric and/or limited) myelitis. The interval separating the visual and spinal syndromes may be days or weeks, but in most cases is within 3 months.[8–13] The clinical course following the presentation of NMO is variable but is most often monophasic, that is, without recurrent attacks (but with fixed deficits), or, less frequently, multiphasic with the patient experiencing multiple severe relapses with step-wise neurologic deterioration.[8,11,12] NMO may also follow an acute progressive and potentially fatal course with respiratory failure and death after cervical myelitis. Rarely, there can be complete clinical recovery without relapse. Prognosis is poor compared with classic MS, with most patients left with severe visual loss or inability to ambulate without assistance within five years of onset.

Neuropathology

NMO is characterized pathologically by considerably more tissue destruction and greater loss of axons than is seen in typical MS, with necrotizing demyelination in the spinal cord and optic nerves. The tissue involvement often extends over numerous spinal cord segments and the cord may be swollen. Over time there may be considerable shrinkage of the cord and cavitation due to tissue destruction.[9] NMO may show a greater B cell component, more prominent eosinophilic and neutrophilic infiltrates, complement activation, and vascular fibrosis, all rare in typical MS, along with more MS-like features including T cell infiltrates and the presence of macrophages.[10]

Imaging

Spinal cord

By magnetic resonance (MR) imaging, NMO lesions of the spinal cord tend to be vertically extensive, often exceeding three vertebral segments (**Fig. 1**), and a lesion on axial imaging will often extend across much or all of spinal cord area. Both the gray and white matter as well as the central cord may be abnormal, and the spinal cord may be swollen.[11,14] This characteristic appearance is in contrast to typical MS[15,16] where spinal cord involvement, although also vertically oriented, is usually two segments or fewer in length,

and on axial images, lesion is asymmetrically distributed across the spinal cord cross section. Although the spinal cord can be swollen in MS in the acute stages of a focal lesion, relative to NMO, the swelling is most often mild, if perceived at all by visual criteria.

Another difference between MS and NMO is the limited hypointensity of spinal cord lesion on T1-weighted imaging even in acute MS lesions,[17] compared with the often striking T1-hypointense changes that are seen in NMO. Chronic T1-hypointensity in the spinal cord (T1-black holes) are also notably absent in MS, but they occur in NMO, probably related to more severe and more extensive injury, including necrosis by histopathology. In NMO, there may be longitudinally extensive and central enhancement of the spinal cord as compared with MS where enhancement may be difficult to detect, is more spotty and ill defined, and more fleeting.

Spinal cord atrophy does occur frequently in MS, but most often by visual criteria, it is apparent as localized and segmental. In NMO, over time, spinal cord atrophy may be readily apparent, and may occur over long segments.

Anterior visual system

Imaging findings in the optic nerves and optic chiasm, including T2-hyperintensity, swelling or enhancement, may be less helpful in distinguishing NMO from typical MS. When present, lesions follow similar patterns to the spinal cord in extent and intensity, beyond what is often observed in MS.

Brain

Despite the striking extent and distribution of clinically or imaging–apparent lesion in the anterior visual pathways and spinal cord, patients with "pure" NMO show remarkably limited neurologic signs or symptoms or demyelination in other regions of the CNS. Most series suggest that the majority of cases will be characterized by a normal or near normal brain MRI at presentation (see **Fig. 1**), and, when positive, with only limited nonspecific white matter abnormalities.[11,14,18] However, other series suggest that these nonspecific patterns are not so rare.[5] The nonspecific T2-hyperintensities that are described in NMO may not abut the ventricular surfaces, and they are not accompanied by acute or chronic T1-hypointense lesions that are more typical in MS. On follow-up, cases of NMO are less likely to accumulate new T2-hyperintensites, in contrast to typical MS where new lesions are frequent.[14]

Support for a different lesion distribution in MS and NMO comes from studies of the normal appearing white matter (NAWM), where magnetization transfer ratios tend to be normal for NMO,

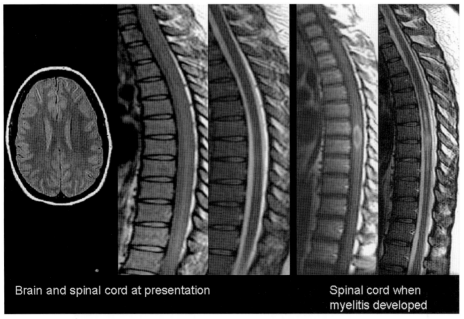

Fig. 1. Devic's neuromyelitis optica (NMO). Initially the patient presented with optic neuritis. The spinal cord was normal as shown in second (proton density) and third (T2-weighted) panels, and the brain was characteristically normal (proton density image, left panel). Weeks later, when transverse myelitis developed, the cord showed a cavitary enhancing lesion (fourth panel), and a long hyperintense lesion on on T2-weighted series. In addition to the length, often three segments or greater, the spinal cord lesions in NMO extend across the cross section of cord (not shown).

in contrast to MS where the NAWM is more typically abnormal.[14,19]

Another NMO lesion by imaging?

Cases of NMO have been observed that meet NMO diagnostic criteria clinically, yet have relatively specific patterns of brain involvement beyond the optic nerve.[5] In these cases, T2-hyperintense lesions were observed in the hypothalamus, bilateral periventricular surfaces surrounding the third ventricle, in the region of area postrema, and more symmetrically than expected for MS around the base of the fourth ventricle (**Fig. 2**). This distribution was noted to overlap with regions of high AQP4 expression in the periependymal regions, potentially linking disturbances of water homeostasis and the imaging findings. The lesions in brainstem have been noted to be relatively assymptomatic and reversible.

A current hypothesis encompasses two basic pathologies in NMO,[7] both of which are associated with loss of AQP4 immunoreactivity, the most prevalent pathology involving the spinal cord and optic nerves, with AQP4 loss in the context of vasculocentric immune complex deposition, active demyelination and vascular hyperplasia with hyalinization. The less frequent pathology in the spinal cord and medulla extending into the area postrema appears to be highly inflammatory. In the latter,

AQP4 loss was associated with vasculocentric IgG and IgM deposits, complement activation, and tissue rarefaction, but there was no evidence of demyelination.

Current Diagnosis

Despite remarkable improvements in laboratory criteria and stronger imaging criteria, no single criterion is specific for NMO, including the current serum autoantibody test, which is based on NMO-IgG seropositive status. Cerebrospinal fluid (CSF) oligoclonal bands, less likely in NMO than MS, are not specific or sensitive. NMO-IgG is moderately sensitive, and increasingly accepted as moderately or strongly specific, but it does not provide a definitive diagnostic test in itself. Consequently, diagnostic criteria based on multiple factors have been proposed,[13] requiring optic neuritis and acute myelitis (clinical considerations), and two of three supportive criteria which can include MR imaging contiguous spinal cord involvement extending over three vertical segments, a brain MR imaging study not meeting MS diagnostic criteria, or NMO-IgG seropositive status.

BALO'S CONCENTRIC SCLEROSIS

BCS shows a peculiar pattern of pathology (most often in the cerebral hemispheric white matter)

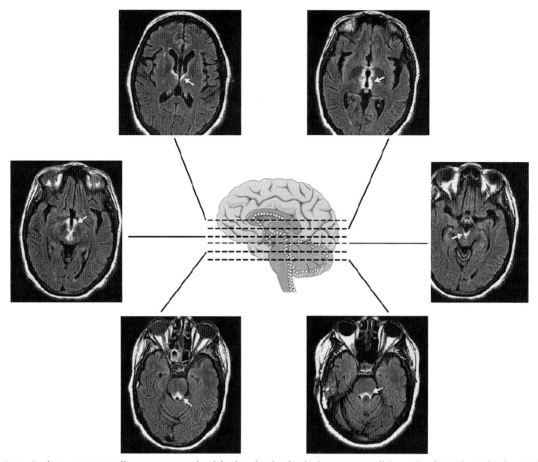

Fig. 2. Lesions corresponding to aquaporin rich sites in the brain in neuromyelitis optica (NMO). Multiple axial fluid attenuated inversion recovery (FLAIR) slices from a patient in the series reported by Pittock et al. show hyperintense lesions at ther base of the fourth ventricle, in the hypothalamus, and periependymal regions that correspond anatomically to high aquaporin 4 protein expression. Aquaporin 4 is the predominant water channel in the brain, highly concentrated in astrocytic foot processes at the blood-brain barrier. The brain in NMO is typically normal or shows only nonspecific white matter lesions. However, a minority of cases show this unusual pattern in addition to anterior visual and/or spinal cord lesions. (*From* Pittock SJ, Weinshenker BG, Lucchinetti CF, et al. Neuromyelitis optica brain lesions localized at sites of high aquaporin 4 expression. Arch Neurol 2006;63(7):966; with permission.)

consisting of a concentric configuration of alternating bands of white matter of different pathology, with relatively preserved myelination alternating with regions of demyelination (**Fig. 3**).[20] The BCS pathologic patterns can be found throughout the neuroaxis including the spinal cord, optic chiasm, brainstem, cerebellum, and supratentorial brain.

Clinical

The original description and early literature concerning BCS emphasized an aggressive form of demyelination with poor outcome.[21] Disease typically was described as progressing over weeks to months, with severe disability or death as the typical outcome; clinical symptoms include headache, aphasia, cognitive or behavioral dysfunction, and/or seizures.

Because these cases were diagnosed at autopsy, there was a strong case selection bias toward worst-case outcomes. Using MR imaging, BCS lesions have been found that co-exist with typical MS-like lesions[22] and in patients with a typical MS course, although some patients are severely affected. Reports of BCS–like cases by imaging often have favorable clinical and imaging outcomes.

BCS lesions have been found rarely to develop after a typical relapsing-remitting course of MS, and Balo-like bands have been described along the periphery of acute MS plaques.[23]

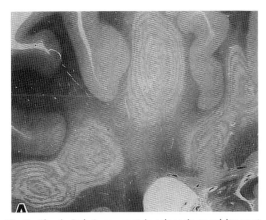

Fig. 3. Classic Balo's concentric sclerosis as white matter lesions (single or in this case multiple) with concentric rings containing partially myelinated alternating with demyelinated bands of tissue. Section stained with Luxol fast blue. (*From* Yao DL, Webster HD, Hudson LD, et al. Concentric sclerosis (Balo): morphometric and in situ hybridization study of lesions in six patients. Ann Neurol 1994;35(1): 18–30; with permission.)

Co-existence of BCS lesions with typical MS-like (nonconcentric) lesions is now well recognized in the neuropathology literature.

The clinical course of the more "benign" BCS has been described as monophasic with resolution of pathology and clinical findings over time, and as MS-like with a multiphasic but self-limited course, and responsive to therapy. A detailed review of the literature is presented in Mowry and colleagues.[24]

Neuropathology

Although the early pathology literature suggested that the abnormal bands (intermingled with normal bands) were the result of partial remyelination, more recent evidence suggests that the abnormal bands are more often areas of incomplete demyelination alternating with preserved myelin.[20] The mechanisms responsible for this peculiar pathology remains a mystery, but the visually fascinating BCS patterns, although rare, have attracted much attention. It is thought that the process that gives rise to the concentric layers may arise through inflammatory demyelination. In some individuals, a zone of protective preconditioning of oligodendrocytes is located in the surrounding layer of immediately adjacent white matter. This zone is therefore preserved from demyelination as the inflammatory process spreads outward. However, inflammation reaches the next, more peripheral region, which contains susceptible oligodendrocytes, and this zone is susceptible to injury.[20,25]

Imaging

BCS lesions are readily identified on proton density or T2-weighted images, but the concentric pattern may also be apparent on T1-weighted images. The rings in BCS may show contrast enhancement; the enhancing regions are thought to correspond to zones of demyelination. Synchronously enhancing, sequentially enhancing, and transiently enhancing rings have been reported.

BCS may present as classic large tumors in isolation associated with a fulminant clinical course, or as cases in which less impressive BCS–like lesions co-exist with typical MS lesions (**Fig. 4**).[26–29] There is also increasing recognition of borderline BCS–like lesions with only a few lamellae or rings, but the relationship of these to more classic Balo's patterns is uncertain (**Fig. 5**).

By proton MR spectroscopy, the principal metabolite ratios are similar to those observed in very large MS lesions,[24,30] including: an increase in the choline to creatine ratio; a decrease in the N-acetylaspartate to creatine ratio; and increased lactate. On follow-up, there may be a return toward normal ratios and values. Restricted diffusion along the surfaces of some BCS lesions may occur. These findings may normalize or become regions with increased diffusivity.[24]

ACUTE MS (MARBURG TYPE)

Rarely, an acute, idiopathic, inflammatory, demyelinating disease may be very rapidly progressive with frequent and severe relapses. These cases with a particularly malignant course may fall within the term Marburg MS.

Clinical

One of Marburg's original cases presented with sleepiness, headache, nausea, vomitting, and left hemiparesis. The post mortem study showed widespread acute and subacute demyelinating lesions.[31] Other cases may be more typical of MS with an aggressive course. This relatively rare process may be unresponsive to conventional therapy, resulting in death often within one year, or severe residual deficits, and may then be classified as acute MS of the Marburg Type. Death may also occur early, within weeks to months, either from severe widespread cerebral lesions or more likely from acute involvement of the lower brainstem or upper cervical cord.[32]

Neuropathology

Marburg's by neuropathology falls within the MS spectrum, with multiple severe focal demyelinating lesions of variable age and injury.[9,33] In contrast to

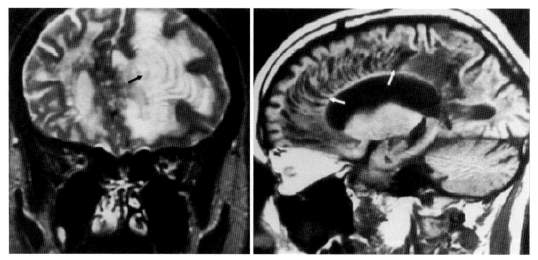

Fig. 4. Balo's concentric sclerosis (BCS). The classic lesion by MRI, confirmed by autopsy. The literature contains descriptions of BCS lesions that are far less developed than in this set of images, some co-existing with typical MS-like lesions. (*From* Poser, Brinar. The nature of multiple sclerosis. Clin Neurol Neurosurg 2004;106:166; with permission.)

the pathology of ADEM (see below), lesions tend to be widely distributed and not primarily perivenous. The focal lesions may show various developmental ages as the disease progresses, with more destructive change compared with typical MS. In the Marburg type of acute MS, abundant Luxol fast blue-positive macrophages (reflecting recent rather than remote degradation) are seen throughout the hypercellular demyelinating lesions.

Imaging

The classic MR imaging appearance at first clinical presentation may include multiple, some large, often confluent lesions that may involve the brainstem but which more commonly affecting the cerebral hemispheric white matter. Lesions may show enhancement and perilesional edema is often present. This appearance is not pathognomonic (**Fig. 6**). Aggressive changes over time accompanied by

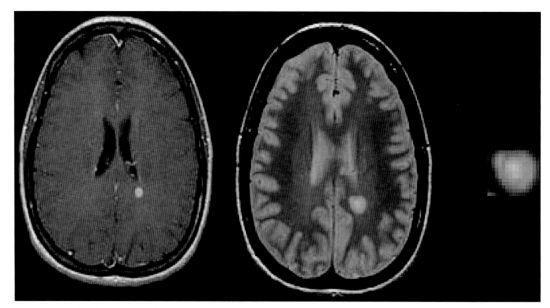

Fig. 5. MS, with a lesion resembling a minimal Balo's concentric sclerosis (BCS) pattern. Left panel shows a ring-enhancing lesion. Proton density-weighted image, middle panel, shows a central area of hyperintensity with a T2-hypointense rim, surrounded by a T2-hyperintense area, the latter likely edema. This appearance is not rare in typical MS, but can be mistaken for BCS.

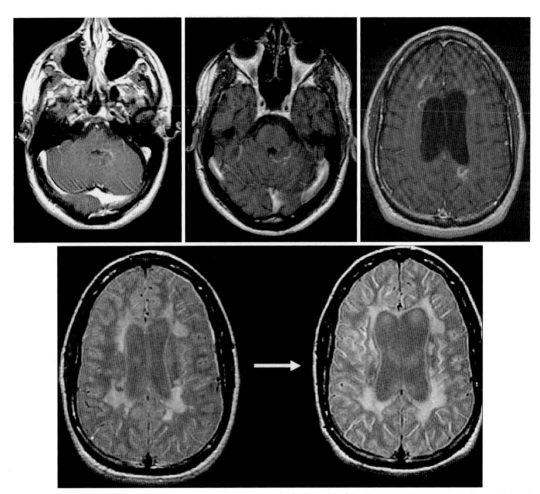

Fig. 6. Aggressive MS over two years, in a pattern that is indistinguishable from Marburg MS. Patient with relatively early disease onset at age 15 and death 7 years later, related to MS. Disease was initially relapsing–remitting but converted relatively quickly to secondary progressive MS (progression without relapses). Top row shows multiple contrast enhancing lesions with relatively rare edge enhancement patterns. Bottom left proton density-weighted image image shows the initial moderate lesion burden, which increased rapidly to include confluent lesions over only two years, with considerable brain volume loss.

clinical deterioration may be required to differentiate Marburg's type MS from severe MS. In contrast to ADEM, in which lesions may tend initially to be similar (but not strictly so) in age based on their contrast enhancement pattern, in Marburg's the more likely appearance will include a mixture of acute and nonacute lesions.

SCHILDER'S DISEASE

Schilder's disease, also known as diffuse myelinoclastic sclerosis, is a rare demyelinating disorder with an interesting but still confusing history. Schilder's original three cases, under the umbrella of an entity known as encephalitis periaxialis diffusa, described in 1912, 1913, and 1924, were subsequently found to be three different disorders. The

1912 case was myelinoclastic diffuse sclerosis; the 1913 case was a leukodystrophy; the 1924 case was subacute sclerosing panencephalitis.[1]

Classic Schilder's disease is a form of acute MS that occurs almost entirely in childhood. One practical definition proposed by Poser[34] includes the following components: (1) a subacute or chronic myelinoclastic disorder with one or two roughly symmetric plaques at least 2 × 3 cm (large) in two of three dimensions; (2) involvement of the centrum semiovale; (3) these being the only lesions based on clinical, paraclinical or imaging findings; (4) adrenoleukodystropy must be excluded.

Small MS-like lesions have been described in some cases accompanying the large areas of demyelination. There is controversy regarding applying a firm line to include or exclude these cases as Schilder's disease,[1,31] however, cases with large lesions are often described as Schilder's disease. Cases with multiple additional macroscopic abnormalities may be more characteristic of MS or disseminated encephomyelitis in the appropriate setting.[1]

Clinical

Disease duration and clinical course are variable. Lesions may respond to treatment, and may recur.

Neuropathology

By neuropathology, a defining feature of Schilder's disease is sharply demarcated, giant coalescent plaques of demyelination, usually involving the majority of bilateral cerebral hemispheric white matter. Histologically, the features of Schilder's disease are nearly identical to MS. Using the eponymic designation more broadly to include cases of all ages that show massive bilateral cerebral white matter disease affected the centrum semiovale, "Schilder's disease" is not distinguishable from severe MS.[9,35]

Imaging

Imaging reveals large, bihemispheric lesions (**Fig. 7**).[36–42] The lesions occurring in two hemispheres may be bridged by abnormal signal in the corpus callosum.

Multiple small lesions in addition to the dominant lesions may favor MS or Marburg type MS. Patients with ADEM may have a typical preceding vaccination or infection, and a more typical lesion distribution (see below) without bihemisheric dominant, nearly symmetric, lesions.

Acute Disseminated Encephalomyelitis

ADEM is a monophasic immune-mediated demyelinating disease predominantly affecting children, associated with a preceding viral or bacterial infection, or vaccination.[43] ADEM has also been described in adults.[44] It has been estimated that 29% of children diagnosed with ADEM will have a final diagnosis of MS,[45] this fraction being even higher in adults.[44] As prognosis and optimal therapy vary, the distinction becomes increasingly important. ADEM may mimic MS at the time of the initial presentation but also over months and sometimes several years following presentation. Although oligoclonal bands favor MS over ADEM, the findings are not specific for either.

ADEM, while not usually considered a variant of MS, is discussed briefly here in the context of MS variants because it is often included in the differential diagnosis of the MS variants, for example, in Schilder's disease (both with large cerebral lesions, acute, severe CNS signs, symptoms), NMO (acute myelopathy and extensive, swollen spinal cord lesions in both), and Marburg's type MS (in their severe clinical presentations and multifocal demyelinating lesions).

Clinical

ADEM in children commonly presents with nonspecific symptoms, including headaches, vomiting, drowsiness, fever and lethargy, which

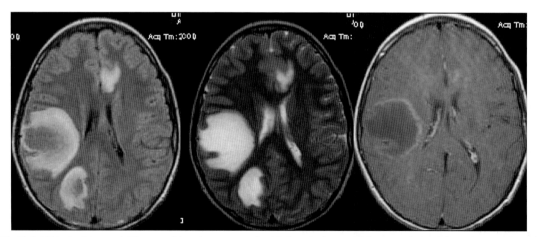

Fig. 7. Schilder's disease. A 10-year old male presented with headache, vomiting, ataxia and foot drop. Left and middle panels (proton density and T2-weighted images, respectively) show multiple large hemispheric lesions, with an enhancing rim (*right panel*). By neuropathology findings were consistent with Schilder's disease. Acute disseminated encephalomyelitis is included in the differential for such lesions. The most classic form of Schilder's disease would include only the centrum semiovale lesions. (*Courtesy of* John Strain, MD, The Childrens Hospital, Denver, CO.)

are relatively uncommon in MS, as well as hemiparesis, ataxia, and cranial nerve findings.[46,47]

Recently, the definition of pediatric ADEM has been refined,[48] emphasizing encephalalopathy (eg, mental status and/or behavioral changes) to help distinguish ADEM from a clinically isolated syndrome, the latter the first indication of MS in most cases. Repeated episodes (dissemination in time and space) reclassifies the disease as MS, although there remain subtleties and controversy regarding phasic (single protracted episodes), and multiphasic ADEM (relapse within months or years). The prognosis for children with ADEM tends to be favorable.

Neuropathology

ADEM classically is characterized by pronounced perivascular inflammation, with relatively minor demyelination restricted to the region of inflammation. In contrast, the dominant feature in MS is more extensive and widespread inflammation and demyelination.

Imaging

On MR imaging, typically large, multifocal assymmetrically distributed lesions are observed in the supra- and infratentorial white matter (**Fig. 8**).[49] ADEM lesions may have poorly defined margins by imaging.[46,49] Although the early MR imaging literature emphasized synchronous contrast enhancement in ADEM, this finding is not strictly required, as there are now series documenting cases with no enhancement, and others showing a mixture of enhancing and nonenhancing lesions.[49,50] Cortical gray matter, thalamic, and basal ganglia lesions are more common in ADEM

than in MS, and often show some symmetry, while the white matter involvement in ADEM tends to be asymmetric as in MS. In ADEM, spinal cord lesions may be large and swollen, more so than in MS,[46,50] and similar to the spinal cord in acute lesions of NMO. Most important, follow-up MR scans may be very useful in the diagnostic work-up, because lesions in ADEM frequently may completely or partially resolve, with minimal residual qualitative or quantitative evidence for injury,[51] with no or minimal new lesions being formed.

OTHER VARIANTS OF MS

Based on immunopathologic studies from biopsy and autopsy material, there is a growing body of evidence that MS may be best characterized as a heterogeneous pathology. However, the pathology-based forms of MS are relatively homogeneous within individuals.[52] The underlying pathology in MS in Pattern I is T cell/macrophage associated. Pattern II includes antibody/complement components. Pattern III is characterized by oligodendrogliopathy. Pattern IV is relatively rare, and is characterized by oligodendrocyte degeneration in the periplaque white matter.[52] This classification is being tested in an international collaborative research study with worldwide collection of specimens.

There is some overlap of this disease pattern classification with the pathology described for the MS variants. For example, the demyelinating component of NMO may have some overlap with Pattern II, based on its neuropathology including antibody/complement components.[53] BCS has been associated with pattern III pathology.[24,53]

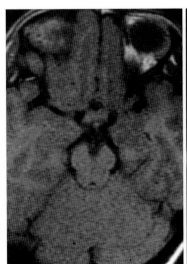 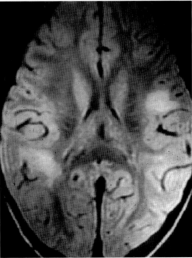

Fig. 8. Acute disseminated encephalomyelitis. In this child, the optic chiasm is swollen as shown in the left panel. Right panel shows classic large asymmetric white matter lesions without sharp borders. ADEM often includes additional symmetric lesions involving the deep gray matter.

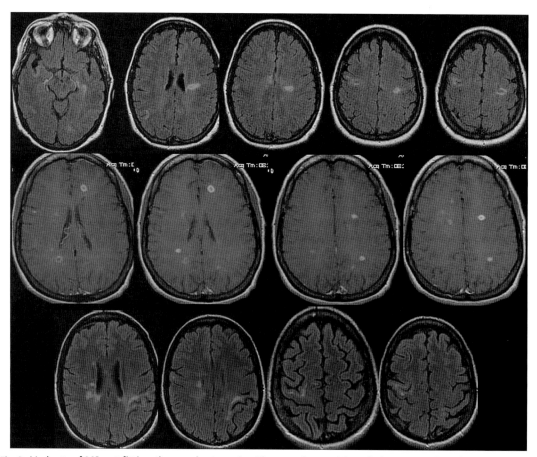

Fig. 9. Variants of MS not fitting the usual categories. Three patients with well-documented MS have unusual lesion patterns that are all different yet relatively homogeneous within each individual. In the top panel, a patient with mostly gray matter lesions at multiple locations. The patient in the middle panel forms almost exclusively ring enhancing lesions corresponding to typical white matter T2-hyperintensities (not shown). In the lower panel, a patient shows a pattern with multiple unusually long juxtacortical lesions.

By imaging criteria, well-documented cases of MS may also show considerable variation in characteristics, including those based on degree of tissue injury (eg, chronic T1 hypointensity) and atrophy. These variations, which can be striking, are well-accepted as variations within the typical range of the MS pathology. Idiopathic inflammatory, demyelinating lesions of the brain, although usually MS-like in appearance, rarely may be atypical appearing,[54] as large ring-like, megacystic, Balo-like and diffusely infiltrating. The authors have observed other variations that may be more subtle, with single dominant patterns within individuals that fall within the expected imaging variations for MS (**Fig. 9**).

SUMMARY

The classic multiple sclerosis variants including Devic's neuromyelitis optica (NMO), Balo's concentric Sclerosis, Schilder's disease, and Marburg MS are both interesting and instructive from a disease pathophysiology perspective. Although rare, the variants are important as they often arise in the differential diagnosis for severe, acute demyelinating disease, including MS and ADEM. In the case of NMO, an originally unsuspected and entirely new pathophysiology based on water channels has been described, only after the recent original description of the more specific diagnostic test for NMO based on serum immunoglobulin.

REFERENCES

1. Poser CM, Brinar W. The nature of multiple sclerosis. Clin Neurol Neurosurg 2004;106:159–71.
2. Lennon VA, Wingerchuk DM, Kryzer TJ, et al. A serum autoantibody marker of neuromyelitis

optica: distinction from multiple sclerosis. Lancet 2004;364(9451):2106–12.

3. Lennon VA, Kryzer TJ, Pittock SJ, et al. IgG marker of optic-spinal multiple sclerosis binds to the aquaporin-4 water channel. J Exp Med 2005; 202(4):473–7.

4. Hinson SR, Pittock SJ, Lucchinetti CF, et al. Pathogenic potential of IgG binding to water channel extracellular domain in neuromyelitis optica. Neurology 2007;69(24):2221–31.

5. Pittock SJ, Lennon VA, Krecke K, et al. Brain abnormalities in neuromyelitis optica. Arch Neurol 2006;63(3):390–6.

6. Pittock SJ, Weinshenker BG, Lucchinetti CF, et al. Neuromyelitis optica brain lesions localized at sites of high aquaporin 4 expression. Arch Neurol 2006; 63(7):964–8.

7. Roemer SF, Parisi JE, Lennon VA, et al. Pattern-specific loss of aquaporin-4 immunoreactivity distinguishes neuromyelitis optica from multiple sclerosis. Brain 2007;130(Pt 5):1194–205.

8. Wingerchuk DM, Lennon VA, Lucchinetti CF, et al. The spectrum of neuromyelitis optica. Lancet Neurol 2007;6(9):805–15.

9. Kleinschmidt-Demasters BK, JH Simon. Dysmyelinating and demyelinating disorders. Ch 5. In RA Prayson, editor. Neuropathology. Philadelphia: Elsevier; 2005. p. 181–222.

10. Lucchinetti CF, Mandler RN, McGavern D, et al. A role for humoral mechanisms in the pathogenesis of Devic's neuromyelitis optica. Brain 2002;125(Pt 7): 1450–61.

11. O'Riordan JI, Gallagher HL, Thompson AJ, et al. Clinical, CSF, and MRI findings in Devic's neuromyelitis optica. J Neurol Neurosurg Psychiatry 1996; 60(4):382–7.

12. Wingerchuk DM, Weinshenker BG. Neuromyelitis optica: clinical predictors of a relapsing course and survival. Neurology 2003;60(5):848–53.

13. Wingerchuk DM, Lennon VA, Pittock SJ, et al. Revised diagnostic criteria for neuromyelitis optica. Neurology 2006;66(10):1485–9.

14. Filippi M, Rocca MA, Moiola L, et al. MRI and magnetization transfer imaging changes in the brain and cervical cord of patients with Devic's neuromyelitis optica. Neurology 1999;53(8):1705–10.

15. Lycklama G, Thompson A, Filippi M, et al. Spinal-cord MRI in multiple sclerosis. Lancet Neurol 2003; 2(9):555–62.

16. Simon JH. Update on Multiple Sclerosis. Radiol Clin North Am 2006;44(1):79–100.

17. Gass A, Filippi M, Rodegher ME, et al. Characteristics of chronic MS lesions in the cerebrum, brainstem, spinal cord, and optic nerve on T1-weighted MRI. Neurology 1998;50(2):548–50.

18. Ghezzi A, Bergamaschi R, Martinelli V, et al. Clinical characteristics, course and prognosis of relapsing

Devic's Neuromyelitis Optica. J Neurol 2004; 251(1):47–52.

19. Rocca MA, Agosta F, Mezzapesa DM, et al. Magnetization transfer and diffusion tensor MRI show gray matter damage in neuromyelitis optica. Neurology 2004;62(3):476–8.

20. Stadelmann C, Ludwin S, Tabira T, et al. Tissue preconditioning may explain concentric lesions in Balo's type of multiple sclerosis. Brain 2005;128(Pt 5): 979–87.

21. Pearce JM. Balo's encephalitis periaxialis concentrica. Eur Neurol 2007;57(1):59–61.

22. Wang C, Zhang KN, Huang G, et al. Balo's disease showing benign clinical course and co-existence with multiple sclerosis-like lesions in Chinese. Multiple Sclerosis 2008;14:418–24.

23. Moore GR, Berry K, Oger JJ, et al. Balo's concentric sclerosis: surviving normal myelin in a patient with a relapsing-remitting clinical course. Mult Scler 2001;7(6):375–82.

24. Mowry Ellen M, Woo John H, Ances Beau M. Technology insight: can neuroimaging provide insights into the role of ischemia in Baló's concentric sclerosis? Nat Clin Pract Neurol 2007;3: 341–8.

25. Love S. Establishing preconditions for Balo's concentric sclerosis. Brain 2005;128(Pt 5):960–2.

26. Yao DL, Webster HD, Hudson LD, et al. Concentric sclerosis (Balo): morphometric and in situ hybridization study of lesions in six patients. Ann Neurol 1994; 35(1):18–30.

27. Iannucci G, Mascalchi M, Salvi F, et al. Vanishing Balo-like lesions in multiple sclerosis. J Neurol Neurosurg Psychiatry 2000;69(3):399–400.

28. Ng SH, Ko SF, Cheung YC, et al. MRI features of Balo's concentric sclerosis. Br J Radiol 1999; 72(856):400–3.

29. Karaarslan E, Altintas A, Senol U, et al. Balo's concentric sclerosis: clinical and radiologic features of five cases. AJNR Am J Neuroradiol 2001;22(7): 1362–7.

30. Khiat A, Lesage J, Boulanger Y. Quantitative MRS study of Balo's concentric sclerosis lesions. Magn Reson Imaging 2007;25(7):1112–5.

31. Wegner C. Pathological differences in acute inflammatory demyelinating diseases of the central nervous system. Int MS J 2005;12(1):13–9, 12.

32. Mendez MF, Pogacar S. Malignant monophasic multiple sclerosis or "Marburg's disease". Neurology 1988;38(7):1153–5.

33. Bitsch A, Wegener C, da Costa C. Lesion development in Marburg's type of acute multiple sclerosis: from inflammation to demyelination. Mult Scler 1999;vol. 5(No. 3):138–46.

34. Poser CM. Myelinoclastic diffuse sclerosis. In: Koetsier JC, editor. Handbook of clinical neurology. New York: Elsevier; 1985. p. 419–28.

35. Gallucci M, Caulo M, Cerone G, et al. Acquired inflammatory white matter disease. Childs Nerv Syst 2001;17(4–5):202–10.
36. Afifi AK, Bell WE, Menezes AH, et al. Myelinoclastic diffuse sclerosis (Schilder's disease): report of a case and review of the literature. J Child Neurol 1994;9(4):398–403.
37. Barth PG, Derix MM, de Krom MC, et al. Schilder's diffuse sclerosis: case study with three years' follow-up and neuro-imaging. Neuropediatrics 1989;20(4):230–3.
38. Garrido C, Levy-Gomes A, Teixeira J, et al. [Schilder's disease: two new cases and a review of the literature]. Rev Neurol 2004;39(8):734–8 [in Spanish].
39. Kurul S, Cakmakçi H, Dirik E, et al. Schilder's disease: case study with serial neuroimaging. J Child Neurol 2003;18(1):58–61, 36.
40. Fitzgerald MJ, Coleman LT. Recurrent myelinoclastic diffuse sclerosis: a case report of a child with Schilder's variant of multiple sclerosis. Pediatr Radiol 2000;30(12):861–5.
41. Hainfellner JA, Schmidbauer M, Schmutzhard E, et al. Devic's neuromyelitis optica and Schilder's myelinoclastic diffuse sclerosis. J Neurol Neurosurg Psychiatry 1992;55(12):1194–6 [No abstract available].
42. Mehler MF, Rabinowich L. Inflammatory myelinoclastic diffuse sclerosis (Schilder's disease):neuroradiologic findings. AJNR Am J Neuroradiol 1989;10(1):176–80.
43. Menge T, Hemmer B, Nessler S, et al. Acute disseminated encephalomyelitis: an update. Arch Neurol 2005;62(11):1673–80.
44. Schwarz S, Mohr A, Knauth M, et al. Acute disseminated encephalomyelitis. A follow-up study of 40 adult patients. Neurology 2001;56:1313–8.
45. Belman AL, Chitnis T, Renoux C. Challenges in the classification of pediatric multiple sclerosis and future directions. Neurology 2007;68(16 Suppl 2):S70–4.
46. Dale RC, de Sousa C, Chong WK, et al. Acute disseminated encephalomyelitis, multiphasic disseminated encephalomyelitis and multiple sclerosis in children. Brain 2000;123(Pt 12):2407–22.
47. Hynson JL, Kornberg AJ, Coleman LT, et al. Clinical and neuroradiologic features of acute disseminated encephalomyelitis in children. Neurology 2001;56(10):1257–60.
48. Banwell B, Shroff M, Ness JM, et al. MRI features of pediatric multiple sclerosis. Neurology 2007;68(16 Suppl 2)):S46–53.
49. Tenembaum S, Chitnis T, Ness J, et al. Acute disseminated encephalomyelitis. Neurology 2007;68(16 Suppl 2):S23–36.
50. Baum PA, Barkovich AJ, Koch TK, et al. Deep gray matter involvement in children with acute disseminated encephalomyelitis. AJNR Am J Neuroradiol 1994;15(7):1275–83.
51. Inglese M, Salvi F, Iannucci G, et al. Magnetization transfer and diffusion tensor MR imaging of acute disseminated encephalomyelitis. AJNR Am J Neuroradiol 2002;23(2):267–72.
52. Lucchinetti CF, Bruck W, Lassmann H. Evidence for pathogenic heterogeneity in multiple sclerosis. Ann Neurol 2004;56(2):308.
53. Stadelmann C, Bruck W. Lessons from the neuropathology of atypical forms of multiple sclerosis. Neurol Sci 2004;(25 Suppl 4):S319–22.
54. Seewann A, Enzinger C, Filippi M, et al. MRI characteristics of atypical idiopathic inflammatory demyelinating lesions of the brain: a review of reported findings. J Neurol 2008;255(1):1–10.

Index

Note: Page numbers of article titles are in **boldface** type.

Neuroimag Clin N Am 18 (2008) 717–719
doi:10.1016/S1052-5149(08)00104-4

United States Postal Service

Statement of Ownership, Management, and Circulation
(All Periodicals Publications Except Requestor Publications)

1. Publication Title	2. Publication Number	3. Filing Date
Neuroimaging Clinics of North America	0 1 0 - 5 4 8	9/15/08

4. Issue Frequency	5. Number of Issues Published Annually	6. Annual Subscription Price
Feb, May, Aug, Nov	4	$240.00

7. Complete Mailing Address of Known Office of Publication (Not printer) (Street, city, county, state, and ZIP+4)

Elsevier Inc.
360 Park Avenue South
New York, NY 10010-1710

Contact Person
Stephen Bushing

Telephone (Include area code)
215-239-3688

8. Complete Mailing Address of Headquarters or General Business Office of Publisher (Not printer)

Elsevier Inc., 360 Park Avenue South, New York, NY 10010-1710

9. Full Names and Complete Mailing Addresses of Publisher, Editor, and Managing Editor (Do not leave blank)

Publisher (Name and complete mailing address)

John Schrefer, Elsevier, Inc., 1600 John F. Kennedy Blvd. Suite 1800, Philadelphia, PA 19103-2899

Editor (Name and complete mailing address)

Lisa Richman, Elsevier, Inc., 1600 John F. Kennedy Blvd. Suite 1800, Philadelphia, PA 19103-2899

Managing Editor (Name and complete mailing address)

Catherine Bewick, Elsevier, Inc., 1600 John F. Kennedy Blvd. Suite 1800, Philadelphia, PA 19103-2899

10. Owner (Do not leave blank. If the publication is owned by a corporation, give the name and address of the corporation immediately followed by the names and addresses of all stockholders owning or holding 1 percent or more of the total amount of stock. If not owned by a corporation, give the names and addresses of the individual owners. If owned by a partnership or other unincorporated firm, give its name and address as well as those of each individual owner. If the publication is published by a nonprofit organization, give its name and address.)

Full Name	Complete Mailing Address
Wholly owned subsidiary of	4520 East-West Highway
Reed/Elsevier, US holdings	Bethesda, MD 20814

11. Known Bondholders, Mortgagees, and Other Security Holders Owning or Holding 1 Percent or More of Total Amount of Bonds, Mortgages, or Other Securities. If none, check box ☐ None

Full Name	Complete Mailing Address
N/A	

2. Tax Status (For completion by nonprofit organizations authorized to mail at nonprofit rates) (Check one)
The purpose, function, and nonprofit status of this organization and the exempt status for federal income tax purposes:
☐ Has Not Changed During Preceding 12 Months
☐ Has Changed During Preceding 12 Months (Publisher must submit explanation of change with this statement)

PS Form 3526, September 2006 (Page 1 of 3 (Instructions Page 3)) PSN 7530-01-000-9931 PRIVACY NOTICE: See our Privacy policy in www.usps.com

---

13. Publication Title	14. Issue Date for Circulation Data Below
Neuroimaging Clinics of North America	August 2008

15. Extent and Nature of Circulation		Average No. Copies Each Issue During Preceding 12 Months	No. Copies of Single Issue Published Nearest to Filing Date
a. Total Number of Copies (Net press run)		2500	2500
b. Paid Circulation (By Mail and Outside the Mail)	(1) Mailed Outside-County Paid Subscriptions Stated on PS Form 3541. (Include paid distribution above nominal rate, advertiser's proof copies, and exchange copies)	1374	1320
	(2) Mailed In-County Paid Subscriptions Stated on PS Form 3541 (Include paid distribution above nominal rate, advertiser's proof copies, and exchange copies)		
	(3) Paid Distribution Outside the Mails Including Sales Through Dealers and Carriers, Street Vendors, Counter Sales, and Other Paid Distribution Outside USPS®	481	458
	(4) Paid Distribution by Other Classes Mailed Through the USPS (e.g. First-Class Mail®)		
c. Total Paid Distribution (Sum of 15b (1), (2), (3), and (4)) ▲		1855	1778
d. Free or Nominal Rate Distribution (By Mail and Outside the Mail)	(1) Free or Nominal Rate Outside-County Copies Included on PS Form 3541	77	72
	(2) Free or Nominal Rate In-County Copies Included on PS Form 3541		
	(3) Free or Nominal Rate Copies Mailed at Other Classes Mailed Through the USPS (e.g. First-Class Mail).		
	(4) Free or Nominal Rate Distribution Outside the Mail (Carriers or other means)		
e. Total Free or Nominal Rate Distribution (Sum of 15d (1), (2), (3) and (4)) ▲		77	72
f. Total Distribution (Sum of 15c and 15e) ▲		1932	1850
g. Copies not Distributed (See instructions to publishers #4 (page #3)) ▲		568	650
h. Total (Sum of 15f and g) ▲		2500	2500
i. Percent Paid (15c divided by 15f times 100) ▲		96.01%	96.11%

16. Publication of Statement of Ownership

☐ If the publication is a general publication, publication of this statement is required. Will be printed in the November 2008 issue of this publication.   ☐ Publication not required

17. Signature and Title of Editor, Publisher, Business Manager, or Owner

Jean Fancici — Executive Director of Subscription Services

Date
September 15, 2008

I certify that all information furnished on this form is true and complete. I understand that anyone who furnishes false or misleading information on this form or who omits material or information requested on the form may be subject to criminal sanctions (including fines and imprisonment) and/or civil sanctions (including civil penalties).

PS Form 3526, September 2006 (Page 2 of 3)

Moving?

Make sure your subscription moves with you!

To notify us of your new address, find your **Clinics Account Number** (located on your mailing label above your name), and contact customer service at:

E-mail: elspcs@elsevier.com

800-654-2452 (subscribers in the U.S. & Canada)
314-453-7041 (subscribers outside of the U.S. & Canada)

Fax number: 314-523-5170

Elsevier Periodicals Customer Service
11830 Westline Industrial Drive
St. Louis, MO 63146

*To ensure uninterrupted delivery of your subscription, please notify us at least 4 weeks in advance of move.

ELSEVIER